Imaging of Head and Neck Spaces for Diagnosis and Treatment

Editors

SANGAM G. KANEKAR, KYLE MANNION

OTOLARYNGOLOGIC CLINICS OF NORTH AMERICA

www.oto.theclinics.com

December 2012 • Volume 45 • Number 6

ELSEVIER

1600 John F. Kennedy Boulevard • Suite 1800 • Philadelphia, Pennsylvania 19103-2899

http://www.theclinics.com

OTOLARYNGOLOGIC CLINICS OF NORTH AMERICA Volume 45, Number 6
December 2012 ISSN 0030-6665, ISBN-13: 978-1-4557-5870-8

Editor: Joanne Husovski
Development Editor: Donald Mumford

Otolaryngologic Clinics of North America (ISSN 0030-6665) is published bimonthly by Elsevier, Inc., 360 Park Avenue South, New York, NY 10010-1710. Months of issue are February, April, June, August, October, and December. Business and Editorial Offices: 1600 John F. Kennedy Blvd., Suite 1800, Philadelphia, PA 19103-2899. Customer Service Office: 6277 Sea Harbor Drive, Orlando, FL 32887-4800. Periodicals postage paid at New York, NY and additional mailing offices. Subscription prices is $335.00 per year (US individuals), $628.00 per year (US institutions), $161.00 per year (US student/resident), $442.00 per year (Canadian individuals), $789.00 per year (Canadian institutions), $496.00 per year (international individuals), $789.00 per year (international institutions), $248.00 per year (international & Canadian student/resident). Foreign air speed delivery is included in all *Clinics'* subscription prices. All prices are subject to change without notice. **POSTMASTER:** Send address changes to *Otolaryngologic Clinics of North America*, Elsevier Health Sciences Division, Subscription Customer Service, 3251 Riverport Lane, Maryland Heights, MO 63043. **Telephone: 1-800-654-2452 (U.S. and Canada); 314-447-8871 (outside U.S. and Canada). Fax: 314-447-8029. E-mail: journalscustomerservice-usa@elsevier.com (for print support); journalsonlinesupport-usa@elsevier.com (for online support).**

Reprints. For copies of 100 or more of articles in this publication, please contact the Commercial Reprints Department, Elsevier Inc., 360 Park Avenue South, New York, NY 10010-1710. Tel.: 212-633-3812; Fax: 212-462-1935; E-mail: reprints@elsevier.com.

Otolaryngologic Clinics of North America is also published in Spanish by McGraw-Hill Interamericana Editores S.A., P.O. Box 5-237, 06500 Mexico D.F., Mexico.

Otolaryngologic Clinics of North America is covered in *MEDLINE/PubMed (Index Medicus), Current Contents/Clinical Medicine, Excerpta Medica, BIOSIS, Science Citation Index,* and *ISI/BIOMED.*

Printed and bound by CPI Group (UK) Ltd, Croydon, CR0 4YY

Transferred to digital print 2012

Contributors

GUEST EDITORS

SANGAM G. KANEKAR, MD
Division of Neuroradiology, Associate Professor, Department of Radiology; Associate Professor, Departments of Neurology and Otolaryngology,The Milton S. Hershey Medical Center, The Pennsylvania State University, Hershey, Pennsylvania

KYLE MANNION, MD, FACS
Assistant Professor, Department of Otolaryngology/Head and Neck Surgery, Vanderbilt University Medical Center, Nashville, Tennessee

AUTHORS

AMIT K. AGARWAL, MD
Assistant Professor of Radiology, Division of Neuroradiology, Department of Radiology, Hershey Medical Center, Penn State University, Hershey, Pennsylvania

JOSEPH M. AULINO, MD
Neuroradiology Section, Department of Radiology and Radiological Sciences, Vanderbilt University Medical Center, Nashville, Tennessee

THOMAS C. BRYSON, MD
Department of Radiology, University of Michigan Hospital and Health Systems, Ann Arbor, Michigan

J. LEVI CHAZEN, MD
Department of Radiology, New York-Presbyterian Hospital, Weill Cornell Medical College, New York, New York

ASIM F. CHOUDHRI, MD
Department of Radiology; Department of Neurosurgery, University of Tennessee Health Science Center; Department of Radiology, Le Bonheur Neuroscience Institute, Le Bonheur Children's Hospital, Memphis, Tennessee

J. MATTHEW DEBNAM, MD
Associate Professor, Radiology, Section of Neuroradiology, MD Anderson Cancer Center, The University of Texas, Houston, Texas

DHEERAJ GANDHI, MD
Professor of Radiology, Neurology, and Neurosurgery, Department of Radiology, University of Maryland Medical Center, Baltimore, Maryland

JOSEPH GEMMETE, MD
Associate Professor of Radiology, Department of Radiology, University of Michigan Health System, Ann Arbor, Michigan

DAVID GOLDENBERG, MD, FACS
Division of Otolaryngology-Head and Neck Surgery, The Milton S. Hershey Medical Center, The Pennsylvania State University, Hershey, Pennsylvania

NANDITA GUHA-THAKURTA, MD
Professor, Radiology, Section of Neuroradiology, MD Anderson Cancer Center, The University of Texas, Houston, Texas

AJAY GUPTA, MD
Assistant Professor of Radiology, New York-Presbyterian Hospital, Weill Cornell Medical College, New York, New York

BENJAMIN Y. HUANG, MD, MPH
Assistant Professor of Radiology, Department of Radiology, University of North Carolina School of Medicine, Chapel Hill, North Carolina

GAURAV JINDAL, MD
Assistant Professor of Interventional Neuroradiology, Department of Radiology, University of Maryland Medical Center, Baltimore, Maryland

SANGAM G. KANEKAR, MD
Division of Neuroradiology, Associate Professor, Department of Radiology; Associate Professor, Departments of Neurology and Otolaryngology, The Milton S. Hershey Medical Center, The Pennsylvania State University, Hershey, Pennsylvania

CLINTON KUWADA, MD
Head & Neck/Microvascular Reconstructive Surgery Fellow, Department of Otolaryngology/Head & Neck Surgery, Vanderbilt University Medical Center, Nashville, Tennessee

PHILIP LOBERT, MD
Department of Radiology, University of Michigan Health Systems, Ann Arbor, Michigan

KYLE MANNION, MD, FACS
Assistant Professor, Department of Otolaryngology/Head & Neck Surgery, Vanderbilt University Medical Center, Nashville, Tennessee

DANIEL E. MELTZER, MD
Assistant Clinical Professor of Radiology, Department of Radiology, Albert Einstein College of Medicine, St. Luke's-Roosevelt Hospital Center, New York, New York

ROBERT E. MORALES, MD
Department of Radiology, Division of Neuroradiology, University of Maryland, Baltimore, Maryland

SURESH K. MUKHERJI, MD, FACR
Professor, Neuroradiology, Head and Neck Radiology, Department of Radiology, University of Michigan Hospital and Health Systems, Ann Arbor, Michigan

HEMANT A. PARMAR, MD
Associate Professor, Neuroradiology, Department of Radiology, University of Michigan, Ann Arbor, Michigan

C. DOUGLAS PHILLIPS, MD, FACR
Professor of Radiology and Director of Head and Neck Imaging, Department of Radiology, New York-Presbyterian Hospital, Weill Cornell Medical College, New York, New York

MARTHA SHOWALTER, MD
Department of Radiology, Penn State University and Hershey Medical Center,
Pennsylvania

GAURANG V. SHAH, MD
Associate Professor, Radiology, Department of Radiology, University of Michigan
Hospital and Health Systems, Ann Arbor, Michigan

DEBORAH R. SHATZKES, MD
Associate Professor of Clinical Radiology, Columbia College of Physicians and Surgeons,
Department of Radiology, Lenox Hill Hospital, New York, New York

MICHAEL SOLLE, MD, PhD
Adjunct Professor of Radiology, Department of Radiology, University of North Carolina
School of Medicine, Chapel Hill, North Carolina; Staff Radiologist, VHA National
Teleradiology Program, Durham, North Carolina

ASHOK SRINIVASAN, MBBS, MD
Associate Professor of Radiology, Division of Neuroradiology, Department of Radiology,
University of Michigan Health Systems, Ann Arbor, Michigan

DANIEL WARSHAFSKY, MD
Division of Otolaryngology-Head and Neck Surgery, The Milton S. Hershey Medical
Center, The Pennsylvania State University, Hershey, Pennsylvania

MARK C. WEISSLER, MD, FACS
Joseph P. Riddle Distinguished Professor of Otolaryngology/Head and Neck Surgery;
Chief, Division of Head and Neck Oncology, Department of Otolaryngology/Head and
Neck Surgery, University of North Carolina School of Medicine, Chapel Hill, North Carolina

THOMAS ZACHARIA, MD
Department of Radiology, Penn State University and Hershey Medical Center, Hershey,
Pennsylvania

Contents

appearance of tumors and lesions on computed tomography or magnetic resonance imaging is presented, and their differential diagnosis is discussed. The image of each carotid disease is presented, and the discussion concludes with treatment recommendations and considerations.

Cross-sectional imaging plays an important role in the evaluation of the retropharyngeal space (RPS) and the prevertebral space (PVS). Because of their deep location within the neck, lesions arising within these spaces are difficult, if not impossible, to evaluate on clinical examination. This article details the cross-sectional anatomy and imaging appearances of primary and secondary diseases involving the RPS and PVS, including metastasis and spread from adjacent spaces. The role of image-guided biopsy is also discussed.

The mylohyoid muscle divides the lower part of the oral cavity into 2 spaces: the sublingual space, which is located superior to the muscle, and the submandibular space, inferior to the muscle but superior to the hyoid bone. Although the submandibular and sublingual spaces are small, a wide range of pathologic processes may involve these spaces. They include cystic lesions, inflammatory conditions with various causes, rare vascular lesions, and benign and malignant neoplasms. This article outlines the radiologic anatomy of the region, describes the various pathologic processes that may affect it, and discusses the use of imaging in their evaluation.

Imaging with CT, MRI, or fluorodeoxyglucose F 18–positron emission tomography is often an important complement to laryngoscopy for diagnosis and management of laryngeal pathology. At most centers, CT is the most popular modality for general laryngeal imaging given its widespread availability, ease of acquisition, and familiarity to clinicians, whereas MRI and positron emission tomography are used as problem-solving tools. Frequent indications for laryngeal imaging include cancer staging, suspected submucosal abnormalities, vocal cord paralysis, laryngeal trauma, and laryngotracheal stenosis. This article reviews the primary imaging modalities used for evaluation of, normal cross-sectional anatomy of, and radiologic features of common diseases of the larynx.

This article discusses the rationale for imaging cervical lymph nodes and reviews nodal anatomy and common drainage patterns, imaging features of pathologic lymph nodes, and the advantages of various imaging modalities available for evaluation and diagnosis of the lymph nodes.

OTOLARYNGOLOGIC CLINICS
OF NORTH AMERICA

Preface

Otolaryngology and Radiology: Partners in Diagnosing and Managing Head and Neck Disease

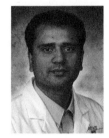 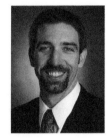

Sangam G. Kanekar, MD   Kyle Mannion, MD, FACS
Guest Editors

Diagnostic imaging plays a major role in both diagnosis and treatment planning for inflammatory, infectious, vascular, and neoplastic processes in the head and neck. Cross-sectional imaging has become the integral part in the evaluation of patients with head and neck disorders. As technology has evolved, the imaging modalities available, as well as the way they are employed, have evolved as well.

This *Otolaryngologic Clinics of North America* issue strives to describe the current state of imaging in the head and neck, covering both imaging techniques and specific pathologies. We chose to divide this issue based on the fascial spaces of the neck. This necessitates some overlap between articles as many of the pathologies discussed can occur in more than one fascial space or may extend from one space to another. These fascial planes provide important barriers and anatomic knowledge of the tissues involved is integral to treatment planning. Beyond anatomic overviews of head and neck spaces, evaluation of lymph nodes and applications of the various interventional procedures for neck lesions are discussed. Our hope is that experienced practicing head and neck surgeons and otolaryngology residents can all benefit from this concise yet comprehensive, image-rich review of imaging of neck spaces.

The newer imaging modalities discussed in these articles hint at a future that will improve on or replace techniques currently existing for otolaryngologists. This makes close cooperation and knowledge sharing between otolaryngologists and radiologists key to continued optimal care of our shared patients.

We thank all the authors for their excellent contributions that make this issue an outstanding and comprehensive review on "Imaging of the head and neck for diagnosis and treatment." We wish to thank the departments of radiology, otolaryngology,

Otolaryngol Clin N Am 45 (2012) xi–xii
http://dx.doi.org/10.1016/j.otc.2012.09.002
0030-6665/12/$ – see front matter © 2012 Elsevier Inc. All rights reserved.

oto.theclinics.com

and oncology at both Penn State Milton S. Hershey Medical Center and Vanderbilt University. We also wish to thank *Otolaryngologic Clinics of North America* manager, Joanne Husovski, and the staff at Elsevier for their assistance. Finally, we thank our families for their overwhelming support.

Sangam G. Kanekar, MD
Department of Radiology and Neurology
Penn State University and Hershey Medical Center
500 University Drive
Hershey, PA 17033, USA

Kyle Mannion, MD, FACS
Department of Otolaryngology/Head and Neck Surgery
Vanderbilt University Medical Center
1215 21st Avenue South
Nashville, TN 37232, USA

E-mail addresses:
skanekar@hmc.psu.edu (S.G. Kanekar)
Kyle.mannion@vanderbilt.edu (K. Mannion)

Imaging Anatomy of Deep Neck Spaces

Daniel Warshafsky, MD[a], David Goldenberg, MD[a],
Sangam G. Kanekar, MD[b,c,d],*

KEYWORDS

- Deep neck spaces • Head and neck • Neck space • Neck fascia • Anatomy

KEY POINTS

- There are many opinions about what defines the neck spaces and how to best organize them into useful clinical tools.
- A solid understanding of the anatomy and relationship of the various neck spaces is valuable in diagnosing and treating diseases of the neck.
- The neck has 2 layers of fascia, the superficial and deep layers.
- The superficial cervical fascia is a thin layer that consists mainly of loose areolar connective tissue and adipose tissue that extends from the head to the thorax and the shoulders to the axilla.
- The deep cervical fascia, or fascia colli, is subdivided into 3 layers:
  1. Superficial layer of deep cervical fascia
  2. Middle layer of deep cervical fascia
  3. Deep layer of deep cervical fascia

FASCIA OF THE NECK

The anatomy of the neck is complex and, as a result, not very well understood. There are many opinions about what defines the neck spaces and how to best organize them into useful clinical tools. This article presents a comprehensive analysis of the neck fascia and neck spaces that are formed by the interplay of the different fascial layers.

[a] Division of Otolaryngology-Head and Neck Surgery, The Milton S. Hershey Medical Center, The Pennsylvania State University, 500, University Drive, Hershey, PA 17033, USA; [b] Division of Neuroradiology, Department of Radiology, The Milton S. Hershey Medical Center, The Pennsylvania State University, 500, University Drive, Hershey, PA 17033, USA; [c] Department of Neurology, The Milton S. Hershey Medical Center, The Pennsylvania State University, 500, University Drive, Hershey, PA 17033, USA; [d] Department of Otolaryngology, The Milton S. Hershey Medical Center, The Pennsylvania State University, 500, University Drive, Hershey, PA 17033, USA
* Corresponding author. Department of Radiology, Neurology and Otolaryngology, The Milton S. Hershey Medical Center, The Pennsylvania State University, 500, University Drive, Hershey, PA 17033.
E-mail address: skanekar@hmc.psu.edu

Otolaryngol Clin N Am 45 (2012) 1203–1221
http://dx.doi.org/10.1016/j.otc.2012.08.001
0030-6665/12/$ – see front matter © 2012 Elsevier Inc. All rights reserved.

Abbreviations: Deep Neck Spaces	
ACS	Anterior cervical space
AMS	Aerodigestive mucosal space
CS	Carotid space
DS	Danger space
DDCF	Deep layer of deep cervical fascia
IHN	Infrahyoid neck
MDCF	Middle layer of deep cervical fascia
MS	Masticator space
PCS	Posterior cervical space
PMS	Pharyngeal mucosal space
PPS	Parapharyngeal space
PS	Parotid space
PTS	Peritonsillar space
PVS	Perivertebral space
RPS	Retropharyngeal space
SCF	Superficial cervical fascia
SDCF	Superficial layer of deep cervical fascia
SHN	Suprahyoid neck
SLS	Sublingual space
SMS	Submandibular space
SQCCA	Squamous cell carcinoma
VS	Visceral space

A solid understanding of the anatomy and relationship of the various neck spaces is valuable in diagnosing and treating diseases of the neck (**Table 1**).

The neck has 2 layers of fascia, the superficial and deep layers. The superficial cervical fascia is a thin layer that consists mainly of loose areolar connective tissue and adipose tissue that extends from the head to the thorax and the shoulders to the axilla.[1] It lies between the dermis of the skin and the deep cervical fascia and contains the platysma, muscles of facial expression, cutaneous nerves, blood vessels, and lymphatics.[2]

The deep cervical fascia, or fascia colli, is subdivided into 3 layers (**Fig.1**)[1]: (1) superficial layer of deep cervical fascia, (2) middle layer of deep cervical fascia, and (3) deep layer of deep cervical fascia.

The superficial layer of deep cervical fascia lies between the superficial cervical fascia and the muscles of the neck. It attaches anteriorly to the hyoid bone and superiorly to the lower border of the mandible, the mastoid process, the superior nuchal line, and the external occipital protuberance, to invest all the superficial neck structures.[3] It splits to encircle the sternocleidomastoid and trapezius muscles to blend posteriorly with the ligamentum nuchae and splits again between the angle of the mandible and the mastoid process to enclose the parotid gland.[4] Inferiorly, it attaches to the spine and acromion of the scapula, the clavicle, and the manubrium.[2]

The middle layer of deep cervical fascia extends from the skull base superiorly to the mediastinum inferiorly and anteriorly from the hyoid bone to the thoracic inlet. It is divided into the muscular division and visceral divisions. The muscular division surrounds the strap muscles, the sternohyoid, sternothyroid, omohyoid, and thyrohyoid[3] and forms a pulley through which the intermediate tendon of the digastrics muscles passes to suspend the hyoid bone.[4] Over the sternocleidomastoid, it fuses with the superficial layer of deep cervical fascia. The visceral division, which is also called the *buccopharyngeal* in the suprahyoid neck, encloses the visceral structures of the neck: the pharynx, larynx, esophagus, trachea, thyroid, and parathyroid glands; periesophageal lymph nodes; and the recurrent laryngeal nerve.[4] This layer attaches posteriorly to the prevertebral fascia and blends with the investing fascia at the lateral borders of the infrahyoid muscles.[1]

Table 1
Leading diagnoses by space and type

Space	Congenital	Inflammatory	Benign Neoplasm	Malignant Neoplasm	Other
Masticator	Fibrous dysplasia	Odontogenic abscess	Schwannoma	AMS SQCCA, sarcoma	
Parapharyngeal space	Branchial cleft cyst	Pharyngitis spread	Pleomorphic adenoma	AMS SQCCA, adenoid cystic carcinoma	
Parotid	Branchial cleft cyst	Sialadenitis, HIV cysts	Pleomorphic adenoma	Mucoepidermoid carcinoma	Cranial nerve VII schwannoma
Carotid space	Branchial cleft cyst	Thrombophlebitis	Schwannoma, paraganglioma	Lymphadenopathy	Carotid dissection, pseudoaneurysm
Retropharyngeal space	Medial carotid deviation	Adenitis, abscess	Lipoma, hemangioma	AMS SQCCA, Nodes	
Perivertebral space	Lymphangioma	Discitis, osteomyelitis	Schwannoma, chordoma	Metastases to bones, lymph nodes	Sarcomas

Data from Yousem D. Suprahyoid spaces of the head and neck. Semin Roentgenol 2000;35(1):63–71.

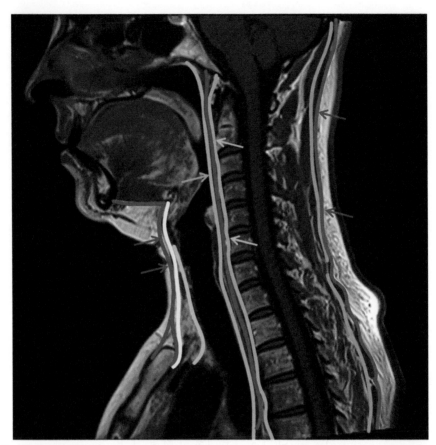

Fig. 1. Sagittal T1-weighted image with line the fascias of the neck. Three layers of the deep cervical fascia encompassing the anatomic structures of the neck are the superficial layer (investing fascia, *red arrow*), middle layer (buccopharyngeal fascia, *blue arrow*), and the deep layer (prevertebral fascia, *green arrow*).

The deep layer of deep cervical fascia surrounds the deep muscles of the neck and the cervical vertebrae. Extending from the skull base into the mediastinum, the deep cervical fascia has 2 distinct divisions: the alar and prevertebral layers.[1,4] The alar layer forms the posterior and lateral walls of the retropharyngeal space and bridges the transverse processes of the vertebrae. The prevertebral layer encloses the paraspinal muscles: the longus colli and longus capitis muscles; the anterior, middle, and posterior scalene muscles; and the levator scapulae.[2,3] The prevertebral fascia also surrounds the brachial plexus trunks, phrenic nerve, cervical plexus, vertebral artery, and vertebral vein, with the cervical sympathetic trunk fixed into the anterior part of the fascia.[1-3]

NECK SPACES

The suprahyoid neck spaces comprise the area from the base of the skull to the hyoid bone excluding the orbits, paranasal sinuses, and the oral cavity. In the suprahyoid region, the spaces of the neck include the sublingual space, submandibular space, peritonsillar space (PTS), parapharyngeal space, pharyngeal mucosal space, masticator space, parotid space, carotid space (**Fig. 2**), retropharyngeal space, danger space (DS), and perivertebral space.

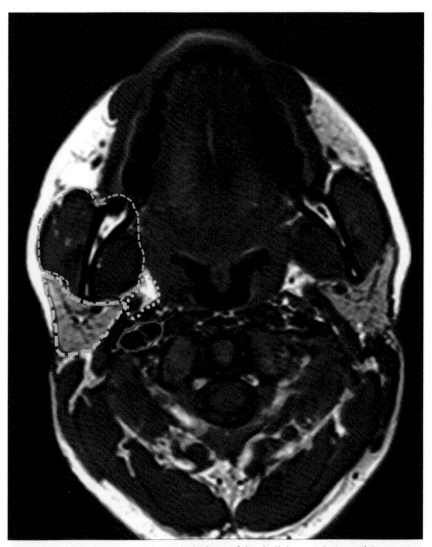

Fig. 2. Axial T1-weighted image through the base of the skull shows relations of the masticator space (*blue*), parotid space (*yellow*), parapharyngeal space (*green*), and carotid space (*red*).

In the infrahyoid neck, the visceral space is present, whereas the masticator space, parapharyngeal space, and parotid space are no longer present. The carotid space, retropharyngeal space, DS, and the perivertebral space span the suprahyoid and infrahyoid compartments.[1–4]

THE SUPRAHYOID NECK
Sublingual Space

Overview
The sublingual space is a potential space that lies entirely within the oral cavity and, as such, has no fascial margins. It is a paired space, but the 2 sides communicate anteriorly through an isthmus under the frenulum of the tongue.[5]

Extent

The sublingual space is a small space within the oral tongue that is bordered anteriorly by the mandible, inferolaterally by the mylohyoid muscle, and medially by the genioglossus and geniohyoid muscles[1,5] (**Fig. 3**).

Anatomic relationships

At the posterior margin of the mylohyoid, the sublingual space communicates directly with the parapharyngeal space and the submandibular space.[5]

Contents

The sublingual space encompasses part of hypoglossus muscle, lingual nerve, CN IX and XI, Wharton's duct, lingual artery and vein, sublingual gland, and deep portion of the submandibular gland and duct.[1-3]

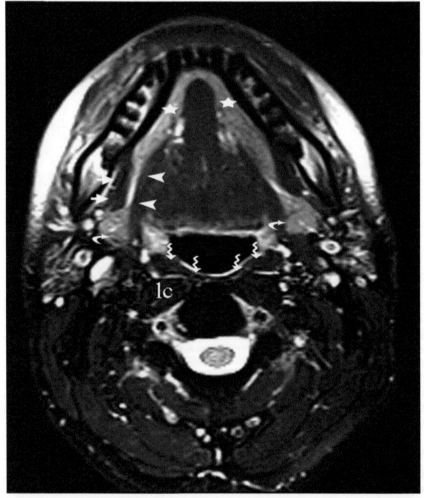

Fig. 3. Axial T2-weighted image shows sublingual space (*white stars*), mylohyoid muscle (*straight arrows*), genioglossus muscle (*arrowhead*), submandibular gland in submandibular space (*curved arrows*), retropharyngeal space (*zig-zag arrows*), and longus coli muscle (lc).

Submandibular Space

Overview
The submandibular space is located deep to the platysma and is enclosed by the superficial layer of deep cervical fascia.[5]

Extent
The submandibular space extends from the hyoid bone to the floor of the mouth (mylohyoid muscle) and is bordered anterolaterally by the mandible and inferiorly by the superficial layer of deep cervical fascia.[4,5]

Anatomic relationships
The posterior portion of the submandibular space has no fascial boundary, so the submandibular space communicates freely with the posterior of the sublingual space and the inferior of the parapharyngeal space (**Fig. 3**). [1]

Contents
The submandibular space contains the anterior belly of digastrics, submandibular and submental lymph nodes, submandibular gland, facial artery and vein, and the inferior loop CN XII.[5]

Peritonsillar Space

Overview
The PTS is an area of loose connective tissue between the palatine tonsil and the superior constrictor muscle.[3]

Extent
The PTS is bounded anteriorly and posteriorly by the anterior and posterior tonsillar pillars, respectively, and inferiorly by the posterior tongue. Its medial border is the capsule of the palatine tonsil, and its lateral border is the superior pharyngeal constrictor.[3]

Anatomic relationships
The peritonsillar space borders the parapharyngeal space medially.[3]

Contents
The contents of the peritonsillar space are the superior constrictor muscles and connective tissue.[3]

Parapharyngeal Space

Overview
The parapharyngeal space is a unique neck space that is central to all the other suprahyoid neck spaces.[6] It contains few contents and consists mostly of fat. Additionally, it is the most mobile of neck spaces because of its incomplete covering by the deep cervical fascia. The parapharyngeal space is the key space in the suprahyoid neck for how it reacts to masses in adjacent spaces, which allows for better evaluation and targeting of these masses, and as a pathway between the other suprahyoid neck spaces.[7]

Extent
The parapharyngeal space is an inverted pyramid–shaped space in the center of the head and neck that extends from the petrous apex at the base of the skull to the greater cornu of the hyoid. It includes the jugular foramen, hypoglossal foramen, and the foramen lacerum.[8] It is bounded medially by the buccopharyngeal fascia,

laterally by the superficial layer of deep cervical fascia, posteriorly by the preverte-bral fascia, and anteriorly by the pterygomandibular raphe and the medial pterygoid muscle.[7] The parapharyngeal space is divided further into 2 compartments by the fascia that joins the styloid process to the tensor veli palatini: the prestyloid compartment and the poststyloid compartment.[2,8] However, some investigators consider the poststyloid portion of the parapharyngeal space to be part of the carotid space.[7]

Anatomic relationships

The parapharyngeal space is a central connection between the other deep neck spaces. Inferiorly, it is continuous with the submandibular space, because there is no fascia separating the parapharyngeal space from the submandibular space, so infection or malignancy can travel freely between these regions.[5,8,9] It is found antero-lateral to the retropharyngeal space, posteromedial to the masticator space and peri-tonsillar space, medial to the parotid space, and lateral to the visceral space.[6] The carotid space passes directly through the posterior of the parapharyngeal space to the mediastinum.[3,8]

Contents

The prestyloid compartment contains mostly fat and the styloglossus and stylo-pharyngeus muscles, the deep lobe of the parotid gland, the internal maxillary artery, and the inferior alveolar, lingual, and auriculotemporal nerves[7] (**Fig. 4**). The poststyloid compartment contains the carotid artery; internal jugular vein; sympa-thetic chain and cranial nerves IX, X, XI, and XII; and, rarely, ectopic salivary glands.[3,8]

Parapharyngeal infections usually arise from the tonsils or through dental manipula-tion. Symptoms typical of parapharyngeal infections or masses may include trismus, pain, dysphagia, neck stiffness, and a "hot potato" voice.[3]

Pharyngeal Mucosal Space

Overview

The pharyngeal mucosal space is all of the tissues on the airway side of the middle layer of deep cervical fascia, essentially the mucosal surface of the nasopharynx, oropharynx, and hypopharynx.[2] On the airway side of the pharyngeal mucosal space, there is no fascial boundary, and it is connected to the parapharyngeal space and ret-ropharyngeal space.[10]

Extent

The pharyngeal mucosal space extends from the skull base to the cricoid cartilage. It is bordered superiorly by the aponeurosis of the superior constrictor muscle where it merges with the middle layer of deep cervical fascia.[2]

Anatomic relationships

The pharyngeal mucosal space lays anteromedially to the parapharyngeal space and directly anterior to the retropharyngeal space.[10]

Contents

The pharyngeal mucosal space contains mucosa, lymphoid tissue of Waldeyer's ring, adenoids, tonsils, minor salivary glands, the torus tubarius, pharyngobasilar fascia, and the cartilage of the Eustachian tubes (**Fig. 5**). The muscles of the pharyngeal mucosal space are the superior and middle constrictor muscles, the levator palatini, the palatoglossus, the palatopharyngeus, and the salpingopharyngeus.[3]

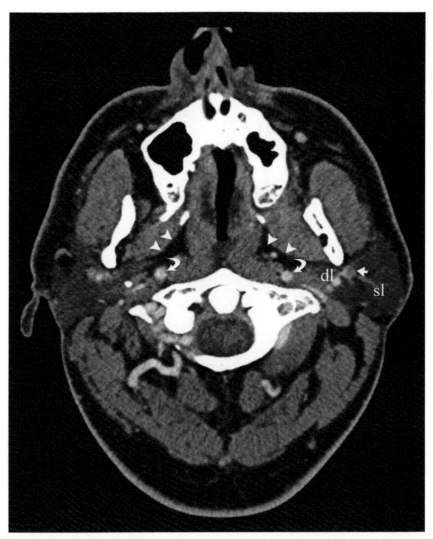

Fig. 4. Axial contrast-enhanced computed tomogoraphy scan through the neck shows relationship of the carotid artery in the carotid sheath (*curved arrows*) to the prestyloid parapharyngeal space (*arrowheads*). The superficial (sl) and deep lobe (dl) of the parotid gland are divided by retromandibular vein (*arrow*) seen within the gland posterior to the mandible.

Masticator Space

Overview

The masticator space is enveloped by 2 layers of the superficial fascia. The superficial fascia splits at the inferior border of the mandible into medial and lateral components.[3] The medial fascia goes over the pterygoid muscles and masseter muscle to the skull base, including the foramen ovale and foramen spinosum, whereas the lateral fascia runs over the temporalis muscle to insert at the zygomatic arch.[2,6]

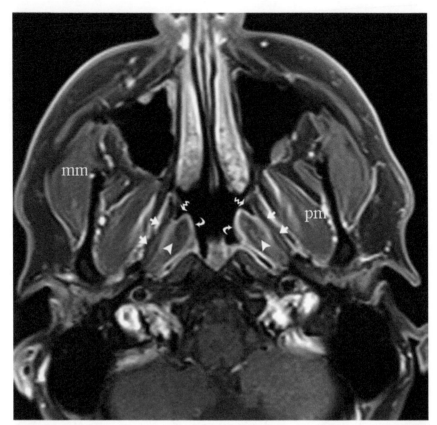

Fig. 5. Axial gadolinium-enhanced T1-weighted image through the base of the skull shows pharyngeal mucosal space. Shown are the torus tubarius (*curved arrows*), tensor veli palatine muscle (*straight arrows*) levator veli palatine muscle (*arrowheads*), and Eustachian tube opening (*zig zag arrows*). mm, masseter muscle; pm, lateral pterygoid muscle.

Extent

The masticator space is a large space that goes from the high parietal calvarium to the mandibular angle and is divided into medial and lateral compartments by the ramus of the mandible.[11]

Anatomic relationships

The masticator space is separated from the adjacent neck spaces by the superficial cervical fascia.[7] This space is not present superiorly, where the masticator space directly connects with the external temporal fossa, considered by some to be an extension of the masticator space. The masticator space lays posterior to the buccal space, anterior to the parotid space, anterolateral to the parapharyngeal space, superior to the submandibular and sublingual spaces, and inferior to the skull base.[11] The masticator space is an important route of communication with other deep neck spaces. The medial compartment connects to the infratemporal fossa through the foramen ovale and the pterygopalatine fossa through the pterygopalatine foramen,[11] which then communicate with the middle space and Meckel's cave through the foramen rotundum, with the orbit through the inferior orbital fissure, and with the palate through the palatine foramen.[11] The masticator space can serve as a conduit for perineural intracranial spread of malignancy, along the trigeminal nerve, through the foramen ovale into Meckel's cave.[1]

Contents

The masticator space contains most of the buccal fat pad and the 4 muscles of mastication: the masseter, temporalis, medial pterygoid, and lateral pterygoid (**Fig. 6**). Bony structures of the masticator space include the ramus and posterior body of the mandible, coronoid process, condylar process, and the temporomandibular joint.[1] Additionally, through it run the mandibular (V3) branches of the trigeminal nerve: the masticator branch, which innervates the muscles of mastication; the mylohyoid branch, which innervates the anterior belly of the digastrics and mylohyoid muscles; the inferior alveolar branch, which provides sensory innervation to the mandible and chin; the lingual nerve, which provides sensory innervation to the anterior two-thirds of the tongue and the floor of the mouth; and the auriculotemporal nerve, which provides sensory innervations to the area of the external

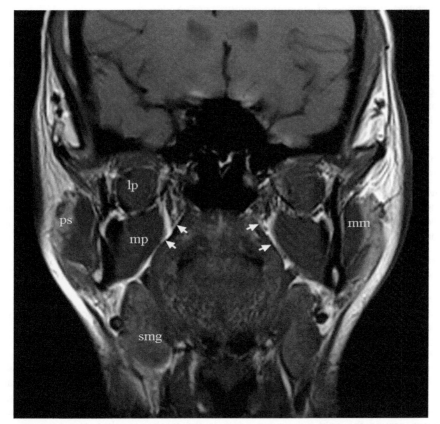

Fig. 6. Coronal T1-weighted image image shows relationship of parotid space (ps), masticator space with muscles of mastication and parapharyngeal space (*arrows*). lp, lateral pterygoid muscle; mm, masseter muscle; mp, medial pterygoid muscle; smg, submandibular gland.

auditory canal and temporomandibular joint.[3,11] The vascular components of the masticator space are the internal maxillary artery and the pterygoid venous plexus.[2] Additionally, the parotid duct runs along the anterior of the masseter muscle before opening into the oral cavity, and along its route there can be accessory parotid tissue.[5]

Parotid Space

Overview
The parotid space is formed by the superficial layer of deep cervical fascia as it splits to surround the parotid gland.[12]

Extent
The parotid space extends from the external auditory canal to the angle of the mandible.[12]

Anatomic relationships
The parotid space is found posterior to the masticator space and lateral to the carotid space and parapharyngeal space. The parotid space is not enclosed by fascia at the superiomedial aspect of the gland, which allows for direct communication with the prestyloid component of the parapharyngeal space.[1,12]

Contents
The parotid space comprises the parotid gland, with the superficial lobe taking up two-thirds of the parotid space, and the proximal portion of the parotid duct, which emerges from the parotid gland to run over the masseter muscle[12] (**Fig. 7**; see **Fig. 4**). In addition, the parotid space contains the extracranial portion of the facial nerve, branches of the trigeminal nerve, external carotid artery retromandibular vein, posterior facial vein, and intraparotid lymph nodes.[3]

THE INFRAHYOID NECK
Visceral Space

Overview
The visceral space (VS) is a cylindrical, central, infrahyoid space enclosed by the middle layer of deep cervical fascia. It is the largest space in the infrahyoid neck and the only space that is found entirely in the infrahyoid neck.[13]

Extent
The visceral space extends from the hyoid bone down into the mediastinum.[14]

Anatomic relationships
Lateral to the visceral space are the paired anterior cervical spaces, posterolateral are the paired carotid spaces, and directly posterior is the retropharyngeal space.[13,14]

Contents
The infrahyoid neck comprises the viscera of the larynx, trachea, hypopharynx, esophagus, and thyroid and parathyroid glands.[14] Also contained within the visceral space is the recurrent laryngeal nerve, which, on the left, recurs at the level of the aortic arch where it passes through the aortopulmonic window and, on the right, recurs around the right subclavian artery in the tracheoesophageal groove up to the larynx.[15] The level VI groups of lymph nodes, the paratracheal, prelaryngeal, and pretracheal nodes, are all found within the visceral space as well as in the infrahyoid strap muscles.[13]

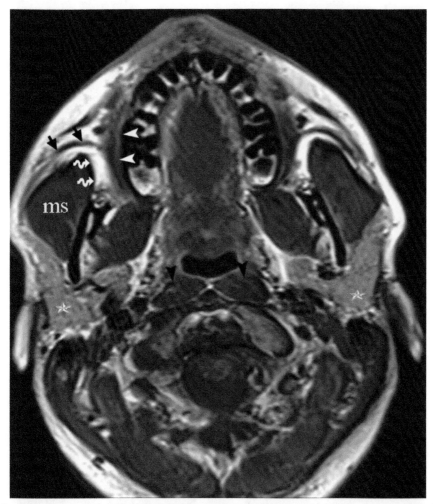

Fig. 7. Axial T1-weighted image shows parotid gland (*white star*), with parotid duct (*black arrows*) running over the masseter muscle (ms) and piercing the buccinators muscle (*white arrowheads*). Buccal space (*curved arrows*) is seen anterior to the masticator space.

Entire Neck Spaces

Retropharyngeal space
Overview The retropharyngeal space is a fat-filled space formed between the middle layer of deep cervical fascia anteriorly and the alar layer of fascia posteriorly and laterally[2,3,16] (**Fig. 8**).

Extent The retropharyngeal space extends from the skull base to the level of the T4 vertebral body posteriorly or approximately the level of the tracheal bifurcation in the mediastinum anteriorly.[15] It is bordered posteriorly by alar fascia of deep layer and anteriorly by the buccopharyngeal fascia of middle layer that lines the esophagus and pharynx.[16]

Anatomic Relationships In the suprahyoid neck, the retropharyngeal space is found posterior to the visceral space, anterior to the danger space and perivertebral space,

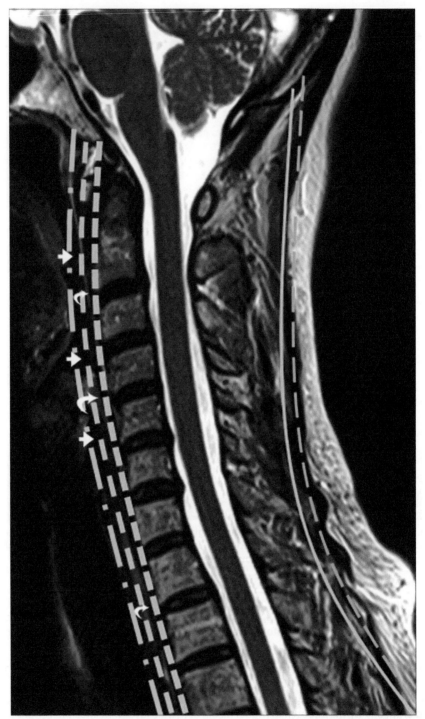

Fig. 8. Sagittal T1-weighted image with line diagram shows retropharyngeal space (*straight arrows*) between the middle layer (buccopharyngeal fascia) and the deep layer (prevertebral fascia) of the deep cervical fascia and dangerous space (*curved arrows*) between the 2 leaves of deep layer of deep cervical fascia.

and medial to the carotid space[16] (**Fig. 9**). In the infrahyoid neck, the retropharyngeal space is posterior to the hypopharynx and cervical esophagus, medial to the carotid space, and anterior to the danger space, into which it empties inferiorly at T3.[2,15,16]

Contents The main component of the retropharyngeal space is fat. In the suprahyoid neck it contains the deep cervical lymph nodes, also known as the *nodes of Rouviere*, that typically atrophy in childhood, beginning around age 4.[16,17] These lymph nodes travel on the lateral sides of the retropharyngeal space and can become infected in childhood, leading to retropharyngeal abscesses.[17] In adults, retropharyngeal abscesses are caused by penetrating injuries or infectious spread from other neck spaces.

Danger space

Overview Named the danger space because of the potential for rapid spread of infection to the posterior mediastinum through its loose areolar tissue, the danger space is a potential space between the alar and prevertebral layers of the deep layer of deep cervical fascia[15,17] (see **Fig. 8**).

Extent The danger space extends from the skull base to the diaphragm. It is bordered anteriorly by the alar fascia, posteriorly by the prevertebral fascia, and laterally by the transverse processes.[1]

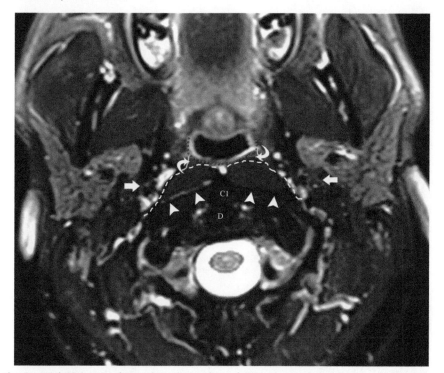

Fig. 9. Axial T2 image shows the relationship of retropharyngeal and prevertebral space. Curved arrow is the retropharyngeal space between the middle layer of deep cervical fascia (*red dotted line*) and deep layer of deep cervical fascia (*yellow dotted line*) and laterally bounded by alar fascia (*blue line*). *Arrowheads* outline the anterior margin of C1 vertebral body. Posterior to the deep layer of deep cervical fascia is prevertebral space. Carotid space (*arrows*) is antero-lateral to the prevertebral space. C1, axis vertebra; D, dens.

Anatomic Relationships The danger space is located posterior to the retropharyngeal space and anterior to the prevertebral space.[1,17]

Contents The danger space contains fat.[1]

Perivertebral space
Overview The perivertebral space is a large midline space enclosed entirely by the deep layer of deep cervical fascia.[1,16]

Extent The perivertebral space is formed by the prevertebral fascia anteriorly and the vertebral bodies posteriorly.[16] It extends from the divus of the skull base to the coccyx and is divided in to 2 main divisions, the prevertebral and paraspinal spaces, by the lateral fascial attachments to the vertebral transverse processes[1,15] (**Fig. 10**).

Anatomic Relationships The prevertebral space lies directly behind the danger space.[15] It is bounded anterolaterally by the carotid space and laterally by the anterior aspect of the posterior cervical spine.[15] The paraspinal space lies deep to the

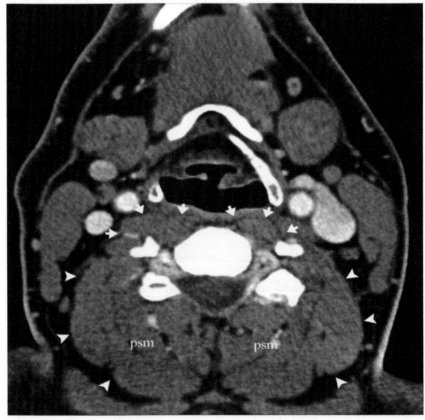

Fig. 10. Axial contrast-enhanced CT scan shows perivertebral space. Space anterior to the vertebral body is a prevertebral component (*arrows*) and the posterior component is called paraspinal component (*arrowheads*), which has posterior paraspinal muscles (psm).

posterior cervical space and posterior to the transverse processes of the cervical spine.[16]

Contents Within the prevertebral portion of the perivertebral space are the prevertebral muscles; the longus colli and longus capitis; the anterior, middle, and posterior scalene muscles; the roots of the brachial plexus; the phrenic nerve; the vertebral artery; and vein and the vertebral bodies.[1] The paraspinal space contains the paraspinal muscles, posterior vertebral column, and proximal brachial plexus.[15,16] The C5-T1 roots of the brachial plexus travel in a complex route through the prevertebral space. Theses roots exit the cervical neural foramina and pass between the anterior and middle scalene muscles before going through an opening in the deep layer of deep cervical space. From there they enter the posterior cervical space while heading toward the axilla.[16]

Carotid space

Overview The carotid space is the area enclosed by the carotid sheath, a structure formed from all 3 layers of the fascia.[9] The fascia is incomplete in the area above the angle of the mandible, so its contents lie within the greater area of the parapharyngeal space.[7] This area of the carotid space is sometimes referred to as the *retrostyloid portion* of the parapharyngeal space.[6]

Extent The carotid space begins at the aortic arch and extends to the inferior margin of the jugular foramen-carotid canal. It is divided into 4 major segments: nasopharyngeal, oropharyngeal, cervical, and mediastinal.[1,2]

Anatomic Relationships The carotid space abuts the retropharyngeal space medially, visceral space anteromedially, parapharyngeal space and anterior cervical space anteriorly, parotid space laterally, posterior cervical space posterolaterally, and the prevertebral space posteromedially.[9]

Contents The suprahyoid neck carotid space contains the internal carotid artery; internal jugular vein; CN IX, X, XI, XII; and the sympathetic plexus and lymph nodes[1,2,9] (**Fig. 11**). The infrahyoid neck carotid space contains the common carotid artery, internal jugular vein, and only CN X. The internal jugular nodal chain is associated with but not in the infrahyoid neck carotid space.[1,9]

 A vitally important fact about the carotid space is its role as the so-called Lincoln Highway of the neck. The carotid space is a route of travel of infection or malignancy from the neck into the mediastinum, such as descending necrotizing mediastinitis, or from the mediastinum into the neck.[18]

Cervical Spaces

Overview

The anterior cervical space and the posterior cervical space are 2 well-defined spaces that are not enclosed by their own fascia. They extend from the skull base to the clavicles and are composed primarily of fat.[1,19]

Anterior cervical space The anterior cervical space is a small space in the anterolateral neck. It is not enclosed by fascia and contains only fat. The anterior cervical space lies lateral to the visceral space and anterior to the carotid space.[19]

Posterior cervical space The posterior cervical space lies posterolateral to the carotid space and lateral to the paraspinal space. It contains mostly fat as well as the spinal accessory nerve and spinal accessory chain of deep cervical lymph nodes.[19]

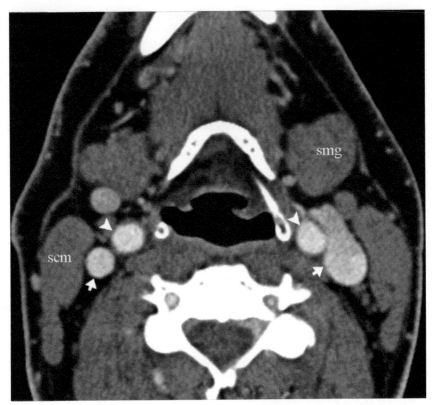

Fig. 11. Axial contrast-enhanced CT scan shows carotid space with carotid artery (*arrowheads*) and internal jugular vein (*arrows*). smg, submandibular gland.

REFERENCES

1. Williams DW III. An Imager's guide to normal neck anatomy. Semin Ultrasound CT MR 1997;18(3):157–81.
2. Brown W, Gleeson M. Scott-Brown's otolaryngology, head and neck surgery. 7th edition. London: Hodder Arnold; 2008.
3. Cummings C, Flint P. Cummings otolaryngology - head and neck surgery. 5th edition, revision. Philadelphia: Mosby Elsevier; 2010. p. 201–8.
4. Moore K, Dalley A, Agur A. Clinically oriented anatomy. 6th edition. Philadelphia: Wolters Kluwer; 2010.
5. Gervasio A, D'Orta G, Mujahed I, et al. Sonographic anatomy of the neck: the suprahyoid region. J Ultrasound 2011;14(3):130–5.
6. Chong V, Mukherji S, Goh C. The suprahyoid neck: normal and pathological anatomy. J Laryngol Otol 1999;113:501–8.
7. Yousem D. Suprahyoid spaces of the head and neck. Semin Roentgenol 2000; 35(1):63–71.
8. Babbel R, Harnsberger H. The parapharyngeal space: the key to unlocking the suprahyoid neck. Semin Ultrasound CT MR 1990;11(6):444–59.
9. Fruin M, Smoker W, Harnsberger H. The carotid space in the suprahyoid neck. Semin Ultrasound CT MR 1990;11(6):504–19.

10. Parker G, Harnsberger H, Jacobs J. The Pharyngeal mucosal space. Semin Ultrasound CT MR 1990;11(6):460–75.
11. Faye N, Lafitte F, Williams M, et al. The Masticator space: from anatomy to pathology. J Neuroradiol 2009;36:121–30.
12. Pollei S, Harnsberger H. The Radiologic evaluation of the parotid space. Semin Ultrasound CT MR 1990;11(6):486–503.
13. Babbel R, Smoker W, Harnsberger H. The visceral space: the unique infrahyoid space. Semin Ultrasound CT MR 1991;12(3):204–23.
14. Smoker W. Normal anatomy of the infrahyoid neck. Semin Ultrasound CT MR 1991;12(3):192–203.
15. Gervasio A, Mujahed I, Biasio A, et al. Ultrasound anatomy of the neck: the infra-hyoid region. J Ultrasound 2010;13:85–9.
16. Davis W, Smoker W, Harnsberger H. The normal and diseased retropharyngeal and prevertebral spaces. Semin Ultrasound CT MR 1990;11(6):520–33.
17. Reynolds S, Chow A. Severe soft tissue infections of the head and neck: a primer for critical care physicians. Lung 2009;187(5):271–9.
18. Kono T, Kohno A, Kuwashima S, et al. CT findings of descending necrotizing me-diastinitis via the carotid space ('Lincoln Highway'). Pediatr Radiol 2001;31(2):84–6.
19. Parker G, Harnsberger H, Smoker W. The anterior and posterior cervical spaces. Semin Ultrasound CT MR 1991;12(3):257–73.

Imaging Evaluation of the Parapharyngeal Space

Ajay Gupta, MD, J. Levi Chazen, MD, C. Douglas Phillips, MD*

KEYWORDS

- Parapharyngeal space - Head and neck imaging - Computed tomography
- Magnetic resonance imaging

KEY POINTS

- The division of the parapharyngeal space into the prestyloid and retrostyloid spaces, as divided by the tensor–vascular–styloid fascia, is significant to the surgical approach of head and neck surgeons, because this fascial plane acts as a landmark to the great vessels and cranial nerves located just deep to this plane in the carotid sheath.
- Given the significantly varied imaging differential diagnoses of the parapharyngeal and carotid spaces, it is advantageous in imaging to approach these spaces as separate imaging entities to increase the precision of diagnoses.

NORMAL IMAGING ANATOMY OF THE PARAPHARYNGEAL SPACE

The parapharyngeal space is a largely fat-filled spaced in the suprahyoid neck that has been variably described by anatomists, head and neck surgeons, and radiologists.[1–6] The bilateral parapharyngeal spaces are regions in neck that have historically been subdivided by surgeons into prestyloid and retrostyloid compartments.[4] The more anterior prestyloid compartment lies deep to the masticator space and lateral to the pharyngeal mucosa, with the deep lobe of the parotid extending into its lateral aspect. The posterior retrostyloid compartment corresponds with the carotid sheath and its components, and has more recently been termed the carotid space. The craniocaudal extent of the parapharyngeal space runs from the skull base to the angle of the mandible.

The division of the parapharyngeal space into the prestyloid and retrostyloid spaces, as divided by the tensor–vascular–styloid fascia, is significant to the surgical approach of head and neck surgeons, because this fascial plane acts as a landmark to the great vessels and cranial nerves located just deep to this plane in the carotid sheath. However, from an imaging perspective, we along with other authors[6] favor separating the parapharyngeal space from the carotid space given the significantly

Department of Radiology, New York-Presbyterian Hospital, Weill Cornell Medical College, 525 East 68th Street, New York, NY 10065, USA
* Corresponding author.
E-mail address: dphillips@med.cornell.edu

Otolaryngol Clin N Am 45 (2012) 1223–1232
http://dx.doi.org/10.1016/j.otc.2012.08.002
0030-6665/12/$ – see front matter © 2012 Elsevier Inc. All rights reserved.

oto.theclinics.com

varied imaging differential diagnoses of these 2 regions. We approach these spaces as separate imaging entities. This point is worth emphasizing because, to a large degree, the existing literature on the "parapharyngeal space" includes more general and broad definition of this space, which includes portions of the deep lobe of the parotid gland (an obvious component of the parotid space) and carotid space. In the era of cross-sectional imaging, we are able to reliably separate these spaces and will do for the purpose of this review to increase the precision of image-specific differential diagnoses.

Defined as such, we consider the parapharyngeal space as bilateral, crescent-shaped, fat-filled regions extending from the skull base to the hyoid bone (**Fig. 1**). The parapharyngeal space contacts the skull base in a triangular region along the inferior surface of the petrous temporal bone; there are no significant bony foramina. Inferiorly, the parapharyngeal space fat is contiguous with the fat of the posterior margin of the submandibular space. The incomplete fascial planes surrounding the parapharyngeal space are complex and include the middle layer of the deep cervical fascia separating the parapharyngeal space from the medially located pharyngeal mucosal space, the medial slip of the superficial layer of the deep cervical fascia separating the parapharyngeal space from the masticator and parotid spaces, and the combined fascia of the carotid sheath and the deep layer of the deep cervical fascia separating the parapharyngeal space from the carotid and retropharyngeal spaces posteriorly.[6]

The parapharyngeal space is of particular interest to head and neck radiologists given its high degree of conspicuity. Fat is easily delineated from other soft tissues on both magnetic resonance imaging (MRI) and computed tomography (CT), and the parapharyngeal space is accordingly relatively easily identified, even with significant displacement and distortion by mass effect arising from lesions in the bordering spaces of the neck. Although the frequency of lesions primary to the parapharyngeal

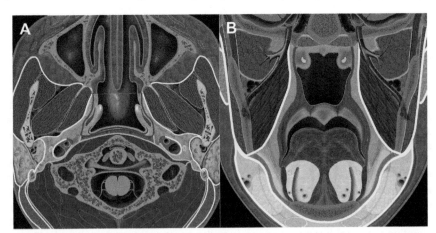

Fig. 1. Axial (*A*) and coronal (*B*) illustrations of the suprahyoid neck. Note the large craniocaudal extent of the PPS (*orange*) to the skull base and close proximity to the PMS, MS, PS, and CS. All 3 layers of the cervical fascia contribute to the parapharyngeal space—deep (*cyan*), middle (*magenta*), and superficial (*yellow*). CS (*red*), carotid space; MS (*purple*), masticator space; PCS (*magenta*), posterior cervical space; PMS (*blue*), pharyngeal mucosal space; PPS (*orange*), parapharyngeal space; PS (*green*), parotid space; PVS (*gray*), paravertebral space; SLS (*light green*), sublingual space; SMS (*light blue*), submandibular space. (*From* Harnsberger HR. Anatomy: Parapharyngeal Space. Salt Lake City: Amirsys 2011. Available at: https://my.statdx.com/STATdxMain.jsp?rc=false#anatomyContent;parapharyngeal_space_neuro.   Accessed Dec 15, 2011; Used with permission from Amirsys, Inc.)

space is relatively rare (and discussed in depth below), the importance of the parapharyngeal space as an imaging sign revealing the site of origin of adjacent neck pathology cannot be overstated. The parapharyngeal space is surrounded by multiple adjacent spaces in the suprahyoid neck, including the pharyngeal mucosa space, masticator space, parotid space, carotid space, and the lateral margin of the retropharyngeal space. Lesions arising from these spaces tend to displace the parapharyngeal fat in predictable patterns—a point that can be of critical importance in localizing the space of origin of a neck lesion. For instance, a carotid space mass pushes the parapharyngeal space fat anteriorly (**Fig. 2**). A lesion in the masticator space pushes the parapharyngeal space fat posteriorly (**Fig. 3**). Similarly, lesions in the pharyngeal mucosal space and lateral retropharyngeal deviate the parapharyngeal fat laterally and anterolaterally, respectively.

Furthermore, clinical evaluation of the parapharyngeal space is limited, further improving the utility of cross-sectional imaging. Typically, only large masses within the parapharyngeal space are palpable by bimanual examination given its location lateral to the pharyngeal mucosa and deep to the masticator space and mandibular ramus. These lesions can grow to a relatively large size before clinical detection. For this reason, imaging can add significantly to the diagnosis and treatment plan of a patient with a suspected parapharyngeal space lesion.

IMAGING STRATEGIES FOR PARAPHARYNGEAL SPACE LESIONS

The choice of imaging modality to evaluate this region is limited to CT or MRI given absence of a reliable sonographic window to this relatively inaccessible space. Contrast-enhanced CT is often more easily accessible, requires less patient cooperation, and can be done in patients with contraindications to MRI such as implanted

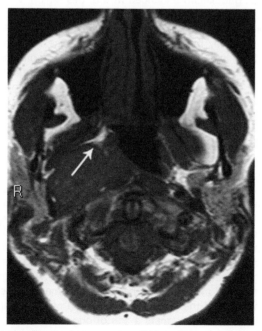

Fig. 2. Axial T1-weighted image demonstrates a T1 hypointense lesion arising from the right carotid space displacing the parapharyngeal space fat stripe anteromedially (*arrow*).

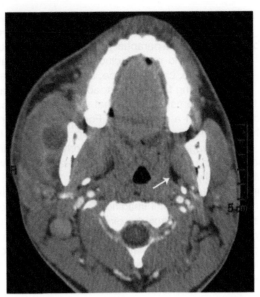

Fig. 3. Axial CT image showing a heterogeneous mixed-density lesion arising in the right masticator space with distortion and medial displacement of the right parapharyngeal space fat. Note the normal left-sided parapharyngeal space fat (*arrow*).

pacing devices or cochlear implants. However, beside the radiation exposure and potential toxicities of iodinated contrast, contrast-enhanced CT generally provides less information than gadolinium-enhanced MRI of this region, which in most cases is the preferred technique for evaluating primary lesions of the parapharyngeal space. Although gadolinium-enhanced MRI is not without its own potential toxicities,[7] lesions of this region are generally better characterized with the information provided by MRI in 3 planes. At our institution, suspected or known parapharyngeal masses are evaluated with the following sequences from the skull base to just below the hyoid bone: Axial T2- and T1-weighted, fat-saturated post-contrast images; coronal T1-, T2-fat-saturated, and T1-weighted fat-saturated post-contrast images; and sagittal T1-weighted fat-saturated post-contrast images. The use of fat-saturated pre-contrast T1-weighted imaging should be abandoned; the fat is a critical element of evaluating lesions in this region.

Before evaluating the imaging characteristics of a lesion primary to the parapharyngeal space, it is critical to confirm that the space of origin is in fact the parapharyngeal space and not secondary extension of an adjacent lesion from a bordering space. Demonstrating a margin of fat separating the lesion from the adjacent spaces of the neck is necessary to confidently place a lesion in the parapharyngeal space. Failure to visualize an intervening fat plane between a lesion and an adjacent space on any section implies that the lesion is not primary to the parapharyngeal space, or has invaded a contiguous space. A classic example of this imaging dilemma is a benign mixed tumor arising from the deep lobe of the parotid gland. Although on initial review of MRI (**Fig. 4**) this lesion may seem to be located primary in the parapharyngeal space, close examination of the posterolateral margin of the parapharyngeal mass shows no clear fat plane and suggests a site of origin within the deep lobe of the parotid gland. Although the imaging features are consistent with a benign mixed tumor arising from salivary gland tissue (pleomorphic adenoma), the space of origin is the

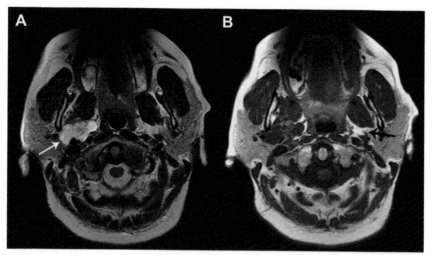

Fig. 4. Axial (*A*) T2- and axial (*B*) T1-weighted images demonstrate a T2-hyperintense, T1-hypointense multiobulated lesion arising from the deep lobe of the right parotid gland, characteristic of a parotid benign mixed tumor (*white arrow*). Note the normal left-sided T1-hyperintense fat stripe of the parapharyngeal fat (*black arrow*).

parotid gland with secondary deformation and mass effect on the parapharyngeal space.

LESIONS PRIMARY TO THE PARAPHARYNGEAL SPACE

A radiologic differential diagnosis for lesions in the parapharyngeal space depends largely on an understanding of the histology of the tissues present within the normal parapharyngeal space. Fortunately, the range of pathology and subsequent imaging differential diagnoses are limited by the fact that fat primarily occupies this space. Ectopic minor salivary gland rests are occasionally present, as is a portion of the pterygoid musculature venous plexus, which is centered in the adjacent masticator space. We discuss primary lesions within 2 main categories—neoplastic and congenital lesions—and present other miscellaneous, rarer lesions that have been reported in this space.

NEOPLASTIC LESIONS
Benign Lesions

Fewer than 0.5% of head and neck neoplasms originate in the parapharyngeal space.[8] Although no major salivary gland tissue is present in the normal parapharyngeal space, occasionally aberrant minor salivary gland rests are found in this space. These rests can give rise to the most common neoplasm of parapharyngeal space, a benign mixed tumor, or pleomorphic adenoma.[9–11] Typically, benign mixed tumors are well-circumscribed with noninfiltrative margins and are best characterized by MRI.[4,12–14] When small, these lesions tend to be spherical, but generally develop a lobulated appearance when larger than 2 cm. They are characteristically hypointense on T1-weighted images, markedly hyperintense on T2-weighted images, and can show patchy, heterogeneous enhancement (**Fig. 5**). The primary differential consideration is the more common deep lobe of the parotid benign mixed tumor, which has identical

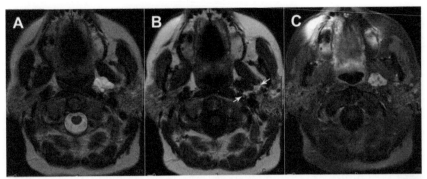

Fig. 5. Axial T2- (*A*), axial T1- (*B*) and axial T1-weighted post-contrast with fat saturation (*C*) images show a T2-hyperintense, T1-hypointense lesion arising in the left parapharyngeal space with avid contrast enhancement. Note the preserved fat plane from the along the margin of deep lobe the left parotid gland (*arrows*) demonstrating that this lesion is not primary to parotid space. These findings are characteristic of a benign mixed tumor primary to the parapharyngeal space.

imaging characteristics; T1 pre-contrast images remain the most accurate sequence to evaluate for the presence of fat surrounding the lesion. As noted, the appearance of benign mixed tumors is fairly characteristic on MRI and more nonspecific on contrast-enhanced CT, where a lesion of soft tissue attenuation can be seen on the background of hypodense fat. Rarely, calcifications or small areas of necrosis are also present in these lesions and detectable on CT or MRI.

Given the absence of muscle, bone, mucosa, lymph nodes, and nerves in the parapharyngeal space, the range of additional neoplastic lesions other than benign mixed tumors is relatively limited. Despite the abundance of fat in this space, lipomas of the parapharyngeal space are rare, with only a few scattered case reports noted in the literature.[15] Like lipomas elsewhere in the body, these are homogeneous, encapsulated tumors with fat attenuation on CT and fat signal characteristics on MRI (T1 hyperintense, T2 hyperintense, with complete suppression of signal on fat-suppressed images).

Malignant Parapharyngeal Space Tumors

Like salivary gland tissue elsewhere in the head and neck, malignant minor salivary gland tumors arising from the parapharyngeal space are possible, although exceedingly rare. Other malignant lesions such as a liposarcoma derived from the fatty elements in parapharyngeal space are also possible, but only rarely reported.[4] These and other malignant lesions primary to the parapharyngeal space demonstrate a more infiltrative and aggressive morphology, with a tendency to directly invade adjacent spaces of the neck. When this is the case, accurately characterizing the lesion as originating from the parapharyngeal space can be difficult.

CONGENITAL LESIONS

Developmental lesions can also rarely occur in the parapharyngeal space.[16,17] Second branchial cleft cysts most commonly occur at the anterior border of the sternocleidomastoid muscle at the level of the angle of the mandible (**Fig. 6**). However, they can occur anywhere along the course of the tonsillar fossa to the skin overlying the sternocleidomastoid muscle. Bailey type IV branchial cleft cysts can occur near the lateral pharyngeal wall, and relatively infrequently, in the parapharyngeal space itself. Like

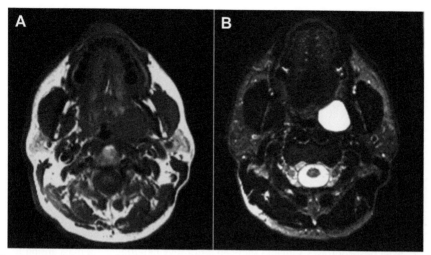

Fig. 6. Axial T1- (*A*) and axial T2-weighted with fat saturation (*B*) images demonstrate a unilocular T2-hyperintense lesion centered in the left parapharyngeal space, consistent with a second branchial cleft cyst.

other cystic lesions elsewhere in the neck, these are typically low density on CT with no evidence of enhancement. Similarly, these tend to be hypointense on T1-weighted images, fluid signal bright on T2-weighted images, and demonstrate no significant post-gadolinium enhancement. In the case of superinfected cyst, loss of normal simple fluid density and signal can be seen with associated wall thickening and irregular enhancement.

Other malformative, developmental lesions have also been described as occurring rarely in the parapharyngeal space, including lymphangiomas[18] and other rare vascular lesions such as hemangiomas.[19] Although normal arterial structures do not typically course through the parapharyngeal space, the posteromedial margin of a prominent pterygoid venous plexus can occasionally abut or extend into the fat of the parapharyngeal space; this should not be mistaken for pathology on contrast-enhanced imaging.

DIRECT EXTENSION OF ADJACENT NECK DISEASE INTO THE PARAPHARYNGEAL SPACE

As described, the direction in which the parapharyngeal space is pushed and deformed can be a critical imaging clue in the correct spatial localization of suprahyoid neck lesions. Most lesions adjacent to the parapharyngeal space tend to compress and push rather than frankly invade the parapharyngeal space. Recall the fascial planes separating this space from the adjacent masticator, parotid, carotid, pharyngeal mucosal, and lateral retropharyngeal spaces. Nonetheless, the most common lesion in the parapharyngeal space remains secondary lesions arising via direct transfascial extension. This typically occurs in the context of malignancy from an adjacent space (**Fig. 7**) or aggressive infection, such as can be seen from a peritonsillar abscess with secondary extension into the parapharyngeal fat (**Fig. 8**).

IMAGING IN PERCUTANEOUS BIOPSY OF PARAPHARYNGEAL SPACE LESIONS

Given the relative inaccessibility of the parapharyngeal space to direct palpation, percutaneous sonographic biopsy techniques that can be used elsewhere in the

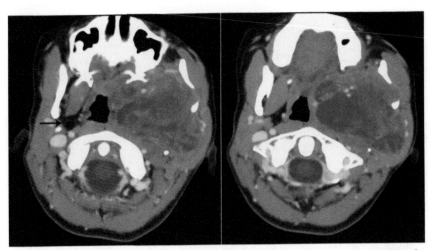

Fig. 7. Axial post-contrast CT images show an infiltrative heterogeneous mass arising from the left masticator space invading and obliterating the left parapharyngeal fat. Note the normal right-sided parapharyngeal fat (*arrow*).

head and neck cannot generally be applied to this region. However, given the benefits of preoperative lesion tissue sampling in planning operative approaches for parapharyngeal space masses, the performance of percutaneous biopsies can significantly add to patient care and possibly improve outcomes.[20] The use of CT guidance for percutaneous needle biopsy of deep neck lesions has been reported as well-tolerated, safe, and accurate in experienced hands.[21]

Our general approach for percutaneous CT biopsy uses a transfacial paramaxillary approach, employing the buccal space as a window. Briefly, a coaxial needle is introduced via the buccal space, which consists primarily of fat and is bound medially by

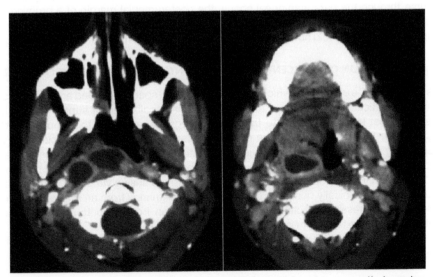

Fig. 8. Axial post-contrast CT images reveal peripherally enhancing, centrally hypodense, multiloculated retropharyngeal abscesses extending into the right parapharyngeal space.

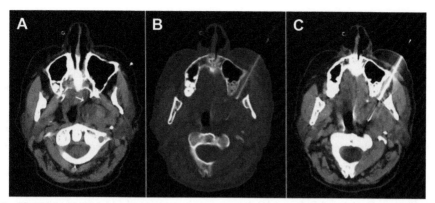

Fig. 9. Axial unenhanced CT images pre-biopsy (*A*), with needle advancement on bone windows (*B*) and with needle tip within the lesion (*C*) demonstrates a transfacial percutaneous approach to biopsy of a lesion invading the left parapharyngeal space. Note the left parapharyngeal space fat is displaced anteriorly (*arrow*).

the buccinator muscle and maxillary alveolar ridge and laterally by the zygomatic and risorius muscles. Anatomic structures within this space include the distal portion of Stenson's duct, the facial artery and vein, the buccal artery, and facial nerve branches. Risk of injury in minimized using a blunt tip stylet Hawkins-Akins needle. Care must be taken to identify the carotid vasculature on preprocedure contrast-enhancing imaging. Success rates are generally high with definitive pathologic diagnosis and low complication rates (**Fig. 9**).[22] Other approaches have been described in the literature including subzygomatic, submastoid, and retromandibular routes.[23,24]

SUMMARY

The parapharyngeal space, with its location deep in the neck surrounded by multiple adjacent spaces, is critical to evaluate in cross-sectional imaging studies. By accurately characterizing a lesion as originating in this space, a reasonable radiologic differential diagnosis of primary parapharyngeal space lesions can be made, especially keeping in mind the relatively few tissue types found in this region. However, the parapharyngeal space deserves close attention in all cases with suprahyoid neck masses, because the direction of mass effect on this parapharyngeal fat can help to localize lesions to specific spaces and thereby greatly assist in creating region-specific differential diagnoses.

REFERENCES

1. Hall C. The parapharyngeal space: an anatomical and clinical study. Ann Otol Rhinol Laryngol 1934;43:793–812.
2. Grodinsky M, Holyoke E. The fasciae and fascial spaces of the head, neck and adjacent regions. Am J Anatomy 1938;63:367–408.
3. Curtin HD. Separation of the masticator space from the parapharyngeal space. Radiology 1987;163(1):195–204.
4. Som PM, Curtin HD. Chapter 38-parapharyngeal and masticator space lesions. In: Som PM, Curtin HD, editors. Head and neck imaging. St. Louis (MO): Mosby; 2003. p. 1954–2003.

5. Som PM, Curtin HD. Chapter 34-fascia and spaces of the neck. In: Som PM, Curtin HD, editors. Head and neck imaging. St. Louis (MO): Mosby; 2003. p. 1805–27.

6. Harnsberger HR. Parapharyngeal space overview. In: Harnsberger HR, editor. Diagnostic imaging: head and neck. Altona (Canada): Amirsys; 2011. p. 2.

7. Gauden AJ, Phal PM, Drummond KJ. MRI safety: nephrogenic systemic fibrosis and other risks. J Clin Neurosci 2010;17(9):1097–104.

8. Hakeem AH, Hazarika B, Pradhan SA, et al. Primary pleomorphic adenoma of minor salivary gland in the parapharyngeal space. World J Surg Oncol 2009;7:85.

9. Mendelsohn AH, Bhuta S, Calcaterra TC, et al. Parapharyngeal space pleomorphic adenoma: a 30-year review. Laryngoscope 2009;119(11):2170–4.

10. Hughes KV 3rd, Olsen KD, McCaffrey TV. Parapharyngeal space neoplasms. Head Neck 1995;17(2):124–30.

11. Shahab R, Heliwell T, Jones AS. How we do it: a series of 114 primary pharyngeal space neoplasms. Clin Otolaryngol 2005;30(4):364–7.

12. Glastonbury C. Parapharyngeal space benign mixed tumor. In: Harnsberger HR, editor. Diagnostic imaging: head and neck. Altona (Canada): Amirsys; 2011. p. 2–4.

13. Miller FR, Wanamaker JR, Lavertu P, et al. Magnetic resonance imaging and the management of parapharyngeal space tumors. Head Neck 1996;18(1):67–77.

14. Som PM, Curtin HD. Lesions of the parapharyngeal space. Role of MR imaging. Otolaryngol Clin North Am 1995;28(3):515–42.

15. Ulku CH, Uyar Y. Parapharyngeal lipoma extending to skull base: a case report and review of the literature. Skull Base 2004;14(2):121–5.

16. Shin JH, Lee HK, Kim SY, et al. Parapharyngeal second branchial cyst manifesting as cranial nerve palsies: MR findings. AJNR Am J Neuroradiol 2001;22(3): 510–2.

17. Piccin O, Cavicchi O, Caliceti U. Branchial cyst of the parapharyngeal space: report of a case and surgical approach considerations. Oral Maxillofac Surg 2008;12(4):215–7.

18. Aygenc E, Fidan F, Ozdem C. Lymphatic malformation of the parapharyngeal space. Br J Oral Maxillofac Surg 2004;42(1):33–5.

19. Chrzanowski DS, Powers CN, Reiter ER. Parapharyngeal space hemangioma in a pediatric patient. Otolaryngol Head Neck Surg 2005;133(3):455–7.

20. Farrag TY, Lin FR, Koch WM, et al. The role of pre-operative CT-guided FNAB for parapharyngeal space tumors. Otolaryngol Head Neck Surg 2007;136(3):411–4.

21. Sherman PM, Yousem DM, Loevner LA. CT-guided aspirations in the head and neck: assessment of the first 216 cases. AJNR Am J Neuroradiol 2004;25(9): 1603–7.

22. Tu AS, Geyer CA, Mancall AC, et al. The buccal space: a doorway for percutaneous CT-guided biopsy of the parapharyngeal region. AJNR Am J Neuroradiol 1998;19:728–31.

23. Gupta S, Henningsen JA, Wallace MJ, et al. Percutaneous biopsy of head and neck lesions with CT guidance: various approaches and relevant anatomic and technical considerations. Radiographics 2007;27:371–90.

24. Harnsberger HR. Anatomy: parapharyngeal space. Amirsys; 2011. Available at: https://my.statdx.com/STATdxMain.jsp?rc=false#anatomyContent;parapharyngeal_space_neuro. Accessed December 15, 2011.

Masticator Space
Imaging Anatomy for Diagnosis

Daniel E. Meltzer, MD[a],*, Deborah R. Shatzkes, MD[b]

KEYWORDS

- Head and neck • Masticator space • Anatomy • Oral cavity • Schwannoma
- non-Hodgkin lymphoma • Odontogenic

KEY POINTS

- Differential diagnosis for disease of the masticator space depends largely on consideration of the structures that normally occupy the space, with the exception of infection, which tends to be from odontogenic causes.
- Noninfectious pathologic conditions may commonly involve neural structures, such as with schwannoma or perineural tumor spread.
- Neoplastic disease of the masticator space may arise from the musculoskeletal elements, such as sarcoma or non-Hodgkin lymphoma.
- Metastatic disease may affect the masticator space.
- Vascular disease is typified by vasoformative anomalies such as venous malformation, which has a propensity...such as lymphatic malformation or arteriovenous malformation.

INTRODUCTION

With the exception of infection, which tends to have odontogenic causes, the differential diagnosis for disease of the masticator space (MS) depends largely on consideration of the structures that normally occupy the space. Therefore, noninfectious pathologic conditions may commonly involve neural structures, with schwannoma or perineural tumor spread as representative examples. In addition to perineural tumor spread, neoplastic disease of the MS may arise from the musculoskeletal elements, such as sarcoma or non-Hodgkin lymphoma (NHL). Metastatic disease may also affect the MS. Vascular disease is typified by vasoformative anomalies such as venous malformations (VM), which have a propensity for the masticator muscles, and related entities such as lymphatic or arteriovenous malformations (AVM).

[a] Department of Radiology, Albert Einstein College of Medicine, St. Luke's-Roosevelt Hospital Center, 1000 Tenth Avenue, Suite 4B-14, New York, NY, USA; [b] Department of Radiology, Lenox Hill Hospital, North Shore - LIJ Health Systems, 100 E. 77th Street, New York, NY 10075, USA
* Corresponding author.
E-mail address: DMeltzer@chpnet.org

Otolaryngol Clin N Am 45 (2012) 1233–1251
http://dx.doi.org/10.1016/j.otc.2012.08.003
0030-6665/12/$ – see front matter © 2012 Elsevier Inc. All rights reserved.

Abbreviations: Masticator Space	
AVM	Arteriovenous malformation
LM	Lymphatic malformation
MPNST	Malignant peripheral nerve sheath tumor
MS	Masticator space
NF1	Neurofibromatosis type I
NHL	Non-Hodgkin lymphoma
NPCA	Nasopharyngeal carcinoma
ONJ	Osteonecrosis of the jaw
PNS	Perineural spread of tumor
PPS	Parapharyngeal space
VM	Venous malformation

PSEUDOLESIONS

There are several conditions that may simulate the presence of a mass lesion on cross-sectional imaging, and some of these may also represent diagnostic pitfalls on physical examination. The most common entities to be considered in this category are accessory parotid tissue, asymmetry of the pterygoid plexus, denervation of the muscles of mastication, and unilateral masseter hypertrophy.

At imaging, these entities are usually easily distinguishable from true pathologic entities owing to their characteristic appearances. Accessory parotid tissue appears identical to orthotopic parotid tissue and lies along the lateral aspect of the masseter. Similarly a hypertrophied masseter, as in the setting of bruxism, will otherwise resemble the normal contralateral muscle. Asymmetry of the pterygoid venous plexus is common, and easily recognized once the physician is aware of its existence.

In the acute setting, denervation may result in transient enlargement and enhancement of the affected muscles,[1] which may mimic an acute inflammatory or neoplastic process. The finding of an associated lesion affecting the mandibular or trigeminal nerves should allow correct diagnosis (**Fig. 1**).

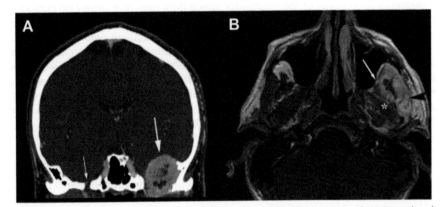

Fig. 1. Early denervation. A 36-year-old man with a left skull base mass that proved to be a giant cell tumor. (*A*) coronal soft tissue CT image shows an enhancing mass involving the left foramen ovale (*large arrow in A*). The contralateral normal foramen ovale is indicated for comparison (*small white arrow*). (*B*) Follow up at 3 months, post contrast T1-weighted MR image shows enhancement of the masseter (*black arrowhead*) and temporalis (*white arrow*) and, to a lesser extent, the pterygoids (*white asterisk*).

INFECTION

Odontogenic Infection

The teeth are considered to be a component of the oral cavity, rather than the MS. However, odontogenic infection is the most common pathologic condition to affect the MS. The classic presentation of a patient with an MS infection is facial swelling, pain, and trismus. The infection most commonly arises from the mandibular third molar (wisdom) tooth, followed in frequency by the more anterior molars and bicuspids.[2] The propensity of the third molar to become impacted may be related to its higher frequency of infection (as in the setting of pericoronitis). The lingual cortex of the mandible is thinner than the buccal cortex at this location, leading to more frequent involvement of the medial pterygoid muscle compared with the masseter muscle.[3]

The MS encompasses a portion of the posterior mandibular alveolar ridge. Infection may easily extend posteriorly along the alveolar ridge, tracking along the bone and/or periosteum and breaching the lingual cortex at the attachment of the medial pterygoid muscle. Alternatively, odontogenic infection may access the MS by tracking along the posterior alveolar ridge to the retromolar trigone, from which it may cross the fat space between the mandible and the medial pterygoid muscle.[3] This pathway of disease spread via the retromolar trigone has also been described in the setting of carcinoma of the mandibular gingiva.[4]

An infectious process in the MS may also traverse the parapharyngeal space (PPS) to involve the lateral oropharynx, potentially resulting in airway compromise (**Fig. 2**). Patients with PPS involvement may present with dyspnea or dysphagia, in addition to the more classic presenting symptoms previously described.[3]

OSTEOMYELITIS OF THE MANDIBLE

Osteomyelitis of the mandible is an infectious process that involves the cancellous and cortical portions of the bone. Osteomyelitis of the mandible has been described as both a precursor to and a result of soft tissue infection in the MS.[5] Historically, the disease process has been divided into acute (<1 month duration) or chronic (>1 month) forms. Chronic osteomyelitis may further be characterized as primary, with an insidious course that does not present with a typical acute phase, or secondary, which follows an acute episode.[6,7] The term subacute osteomyelitis refers to a transitional stage between acute and chronic.[8]

Mandibular osteomyelitis, either acute or chronic, may be a component of infection in the MS. Chronic mandibular osteomyelitis will typically manifest as abnormal sclerosis and cortical/periosteal thickening, which are best depicted on CT (**Fig. 3**). There may be associated myositis of the muscles of mastication. Classically, acute osteomyelitis will demonstrate CT findings of cortical thinning or erosion.[9] There may be progression to periosteal reaction, with thickening of the periosteum that may eventually sequester the diseased bone. Mandibular osteomyelitis may require subperiosteal drainage for effective treatment.[10]

INFECTION ARISING FROM NEIGHBORING SPACES

Infection of the spaces that border on the MS may secondarily involve the muscles of mastication. This is most commonly seen in the setting of parotitis. The inflammatory process in the parotid gland may be due to viral or bacterial infection. Parotitis may also be secondary to obstruction of the parotid duct by sialolithiasis, in which case there may be secondary inflammation of the masseter due to sialodochitis in the buccal space, immediately anterior to the muscle (**Fig. 4**). If there is accessory parotid

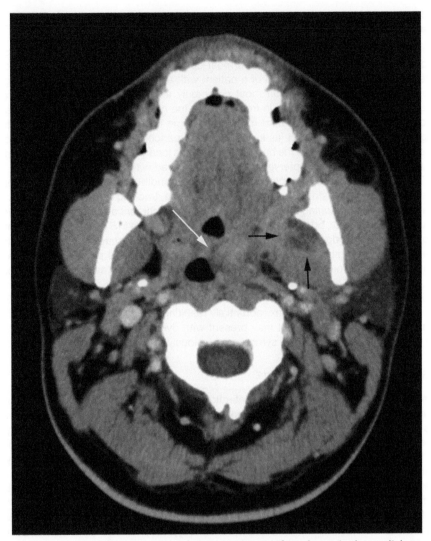

Fig. 2. Odontogenic infection. Axial soft tissue CT image of an abscess in the medial ptery-goid muscle (*black arrows*) of a 23-year-old man who had recent left wisdom tooth extrac-tion. There is edema extending medially across the anterior PPS resulting in mild abnormal thickening of the lateral oropharyngeal wall (*white arrow*).

tissue, the process may mimic an inflammatory process arising in the underlying masseter muscle.

Although the oropharynx is technically not a direct neighbor of the MS, it is common for infection of the lateral oropharyngeal wall (as in the setting of peritonsillar abscess) to cross the intervening PPS and involve the muscles of mastication (**Fig. 5**). The clinical finding of trismus is the classic sign of MS involvement. This lateral extension of the infec-tion may have implications for surgery, possibly requiring a percutaneous approach, instead of transoral. As with any infectious process, the severity of the infectious process

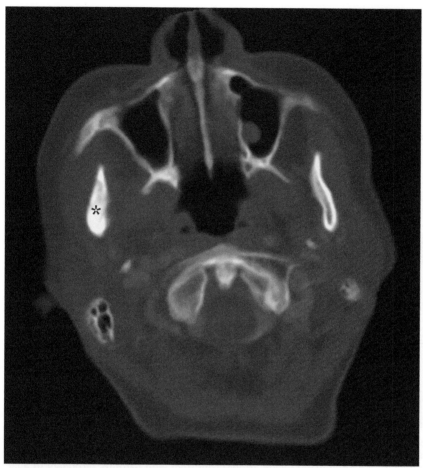

Fig. 3. Chronic osteomyelitis. Bone window CT image best depicts the abnormal sclerosis of the mandible (*asterisk*). The findings are consistent with chronic osteomyelitis.

at the time of imaging is variable. The progression is from edema to phlegmon and, finally, to mature abscess with liquefied content and a well-defined enhancing wall.

Otitis externa may occasionally involve the MS, with the classic symptom of trismus. The temporomandibular joint or parotid gland may become secondarily infected. The process may then spread anteriorly to the muscles of mastication, involving the intervening parotid tissue. This pattern of infection is more common in diabetic or immunocompromised patients.[10]

NEOPLASM

As elsewhere in the body, neoplasms arising in the MS may be categorized as benign or malignant, and the differential diagnosis will reflect the array of tissues normally found in this location. Benign lesions include nerve sheath tumors such as schwannoma or neurofibroma. Primary neoplasms of the muscles of mastication are rare; NHL may arise in the muscles, although it more commonly affects the mandible.

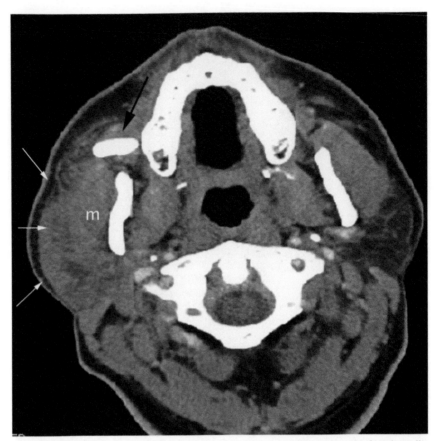

Fig. 4. Parotitis affecting the MS. A 50-year-old man presented with right facial swelling, evaluated with contrast-enhanced CT. Soft tissue axial CT image shows an enlarged and hyperenhancing parotid gland (*white arrows*) consistent with parotitis, secondary to a large sialolith (*black arrow*) in the parotid duct. The gland and the duct are visually indistinct from the masseter muscle (m), consistent with myositis, secondary to inflammation in the adjacent parotid and buccal spaces.

Benign or malignant osseous tumors of the mandible may arise within the MS. Soft tissue sarcomas may also arise in this space.

SCHWANNOMA OF THE TRIGEMINAL NERVE

Schwannoma is a benign nerve sheath tumor that may affect the cranial nerves as an isolated finding or in the setting of neurofibromatosis type II (NFII). When schwannoma affects the trigeminal nerve, the patient may present with facial paresthesia (less commonly pain) or difficulty chewing owing to related weakness of the ipsilateral muscles of mastication.[11] Trigeminal schwannoma, also known as neurinoma, accounts for approximately 0.2% of intracranial tumors.

The middle cranial fossa component of trigeminal schwannoma is considered interdural, maintaining the location between the layers of the lateral cavernous sinus wall that the ophthalmic and maxillary divisions normally occupy.[11] When present, the posterior fossa component also remains enveloped by dura, presumably stretching from the

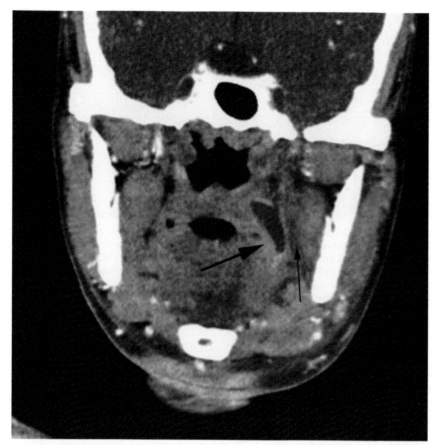

Fig. 5. Peritonsillar abscess affecting the MS. A 36-year-old woman presented with tragus, drooling, and trismus. Coronal contrast-enhanced CT image shows a peritonsillar abscess (*large arrow*). The infectious process is traversing the anterior aspect of the adjacent PPS to involve the left medial pterygoid muscle, where there is edema and possible phlegmon or early abscess formation (*small arrow*).

cavernous sinus or petrous apex, and may be considered subdural. This relationship to the dural layers may allow the surgeon, through a basal temporal surgical approach, to access the intracranial components without exposing the carotid artery or the venous space of the cavernous sinus.[11] For tumors with a large infratemporal component, a transmandibular or zygomatic infratemporal approach may be considered.[12]

Schwannoma typically has T2-signal hyperintensity and enhance briskly with intravenous contrast. As schwannomas enlarge, they may begin to show areas of cystic degeneration and more heterogeneous enhancement. The finding of trigeminal schwannoma should prompt careful search for other intracranial tumors that may signify underlying NFII (**Fig. 6**).

PLEXIFORM NEUROFIBROMA

Plexiform neurofibroma is a common manifestation of NF type I (NF1) and causes significant morbidity and cosmetic issues in patients with this disease. The term

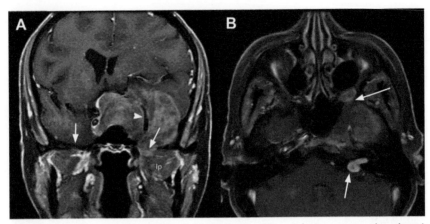

Fig. 6. (*A*) Coronal postcontrast T1-weighted imgage shows a heterogeneously enhancing mass with components in the left middle fossa and sellar region, consistent with schwannoma. The mass extends extracranially through foramen ovale into the MS, where is abuts the left lateral pterygoid (lp) muscle. The left foramen ovale (*long arrow*) is enlarged by the mass, compared to the normal contralateral foramen ovale (*small arrow*). The left internal carotid artery is enveloped by the tumor (*arrowhead*). (*B*) Axial postcontrast T1-weighted image shows that the mass also extends anteriorly through foramen rotundum into the pterygopalatine fossa (*long arrow*). There is an ipsilateral vestibular schwannoma in this patient with NFII (*short arrow*).

plexiform does not necessarily refer to involvement of a nerve plexus such as the lumbar or brachial plexus but, instead, to the network-like involvement of multiple fascicles of a nerve.[13] Plexiform neurofibroma may be revealed by imaging in about 50% of NF1 patients.[14] These tumors may undergo transformation into a malignant peripheral nerve sheath tumor (MPNST), a form of sarcoma. Patients with NF1 have 7% to 13% lifetime risk of MPNST, which most commonly arises from a plexiform neurofibroma or subcutaneous neurofibroma.[15] On T2-weighted MR imaging, the fascicles of plexiform neurofibroma have a classic target appearance when caught in cross-section, with relative hypointensity of the lesion's center (**Fig. 7**).

NHL

NHL of the MS may occur within the marrow cavity of the mandible but only rarely.[16] Extranodal location occurs in approximately 24% of cases of NHL, and only 0.6% of these arise in the mandible.[17] Most bone lymphomas are diffuse large B-cell type.[18] Patients may present with swelling, pain, numbness, tooth mobility, and cervical lymphadenopathy.[19] Tooth mobility and pain may also be seen in chronic infection, and chronic osteomyelitis is also an important diagnostic consideration.[17]

The CT imaging characteristics of osseous NHL are not particularly distinctive, and may mimic the appearance of other neoplasms such as metastatic disease or Ewing sarcoma, or may be confused with osteomyelitis. Lytic destruction is a common imaging finding, or a permeative pattern of lucency (moth-eaten appearance) may be seen in the cortex on CT.[19] On MRI, there may be loss of normal marrow signal, although this is also a nonspecific finding.

Involvement of skeletal muscle by NHL is also rare, particularly as the only involved organ, and accounts for approximately 1.4% to 5% of extranodal disease.[20] NHL

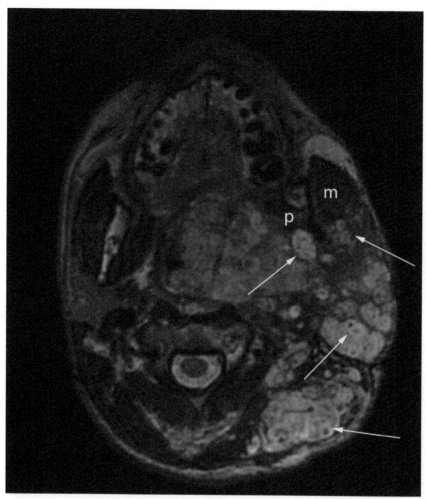

Fig. 7. Plexiform neurofibroma. Axial T2-weighted image of a 15-year-old boy with NFI. There are innumerable targetoid lesions (*arrows*) with central signal hypointensity, forming a left multispatial neck and face mass. The findings are consistent with a plexiform neurofibroma. There is encroachment on the posterior aspects of the left medial pterygoid (p) and masseter (m) muscles.

arising in the muscles of mastication is an even rarer occurrence, with a handful of cases reported in the literature. It is much more common for muscle involvement to occur as a manifestation of widespread disease.[21] Indeed, it may be difficult to tell if the MS disease started in the mandible or the masticator muscles. Lymphoma may also involve the mandibular nerve in the MS.

On CT, an infiltrative mass involving the masticator muscles may be seen, usually with enhancement, albeit heterogeneous. There may be associated osseous destruction. Lymphoma is classically described as having lower T2 signal intensity than other tumors on MRI (**Fig. 8**), as well as restricted diffusion, due to the high nuclear to cytoplasmic ratio of the lymphoma cells. However, this is a feature shared by other small round blue cell tumors, including sarcoma, one of the main differential considerations at imaging.

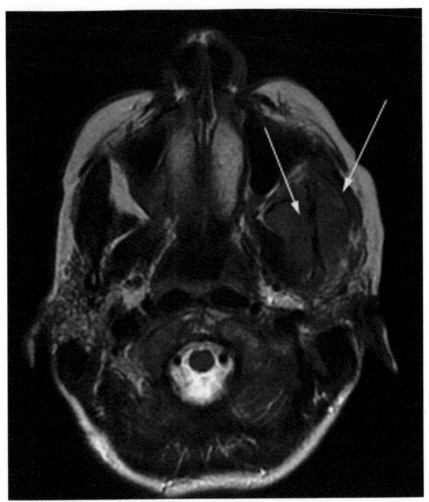

Fig. 8. NHL. A 45-year-old woman with HIV and NHL. T2-weighted MR image shows an infiltrative mass affecting the temporalis and masseter muscles (*arrows*). There is intermediate T2 signal of the involved muscles, typical of lymphoma.

METASTATIC DISEASE

Malignancies of the jaws are usually metastatic rather than primary, and occur more frequently in the mandible than in the maxilla.[22] Metastatic disease to the mandible is the first sign of underlying malignancy in a significant number of cases.[23] Metastatic lesions that affect the inferior alveolar nerve may present with ipsilateral chin paresthesia, also called numb chin syndrome.[24] Osseous erosion may be seen on CT imaging, and there may be loss of the expected fat in the inferior alveolar canal (**Fig. 9**).

SARCOMA OF THE MS

Sarcomas comprise less than 1% of malignancies of adults in the United States, with only a small portion of these arising in the head and neck.[25] Osteosarcoma, rhabdomyosarcoma, malignant fibrous histiocytoma, and angiosarcoma are the most

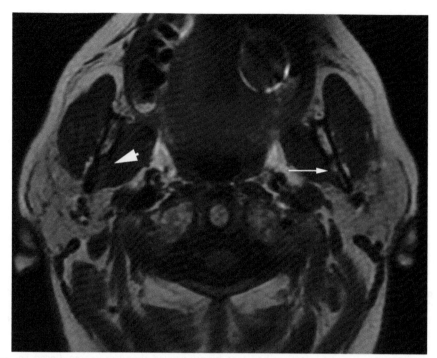

Fig. 9. Metastatic disease. A 71-year-old woman with a history of thyroid carcinoma presented with right chin numbness. The axial precontrast T1-weighted image shows loss of the expected hyperintense fat signal in the orifice of the right inferior alveolar canal (*white arrowhead*), compared with the contralateral side (*arrow*), consistent with the presence of neoplasm.

common sarcomas of the head and neck, but up to 20% of head and neck sarcomas remain unclassified.[25] Sarcomas of the head and neck may arise from either soft-tissue or osseous elements, with approximately 20% originating in bone or cartilage.[26] Certain subtypes have a higher occurrence in the mandible. Most notably, osteosarcoma, chondrosarcoma, and Ewing sarcoma have a propensity for involving osseous structures.[25] Malignancy of the mandible (primary and secondary) may be difficult to distinguish from infection because there may be periosteal reaction and soft tissue abnormality in both processes. The finding of permeative changes in the bone may help correctly identify a neoplastic process (**Fig. 10**).[27]

OSTEONECROSIS OF THE JAW

It is appropriate to mention osteonecrosis of the jaw (ONJ) in this section on malignancy. ONJ may have imaging findings that resemble mandibular neoplasm (primary or metastatic) or infection (**Fig. 11**). ONJ is most commonly a side effect of radiation therapy. However, in recent years it has been described in the setting of bisphosphonate therapy.[28] The most common imaging manifestation in bisphosphonate-related ONJ is progressive sclerosis.[29] Findings typically associated with osteomyelitis, such as periosteal bone formation and sequestrum-involucrum, have also been described. However, Phal and colleagues[29] found that these patients frequently have histologic findings suggesting a component of superimposed infection.

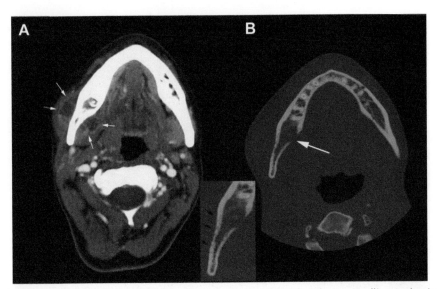

Fig. 10. Chondrosarcoma. A 23-year-old woman presented with right jaw swelling and pain. (*A*) Axial contrast-enhanced soft tissue CT image shows collections along the buccal and lingual cortical surfaces of the right posterior mandibular body, which appear to be subperiosteal in location (*small white arrows*). (*B*) Associated disease of the right posterior molar socket is visible on the bone algorithm image (*large white arrow*). The overall constellation of findings may suggest infection; however, biopsy proved chondrosarcoma. (*Inset*) There are permeative changes in the buccal cortex of the mandible (*small black arrows*), a finding that favors malignancy over infection.

MALIGNANCY FROM NEIGHBORING SPACES
Nasopharyngeal Carcinoma

Although the nasopharynx does not technically border the MS, the two spaces are separated below the skull base only by the thin anterior aspect of the PPS and its associated fascial boundaries. It is relatively common for nasopharyngeal carcinoma (NPCA) to spread laterally through the pharyngobasilar fascia into the PPS. From there, access to the MS may follow. It has been postulated that sclerosis of the pterygoid process may be a sign that this pattern of tumor spread has occurred and that involvement of the MS is present or imminent.[30] Involvement of the MS can have staging and therapeutic implications for patients with NPCA. Once in the MS, NPCA may also involve the mandibular nerve and extend intracranially through foramen ovale (**Fig. 12**).

PERINEURAL SPREAD OF TUMOR

With respect to terminology, perineural spread of tumor (PNS) must be distinguished from the words "perineural tumor" that may be seen in the histopathologic description of a tumor specimen. The latter term indicates physical proximity of tumor tissue to the nerve in question. In PNS, however, the nerve becomes a conduit for spread of tumor away from the primary lesion, leaving the adjacent tissues with a relatively normal appearance.[31] PNS may progress to skull base invasion and intracranial extension of tumor.

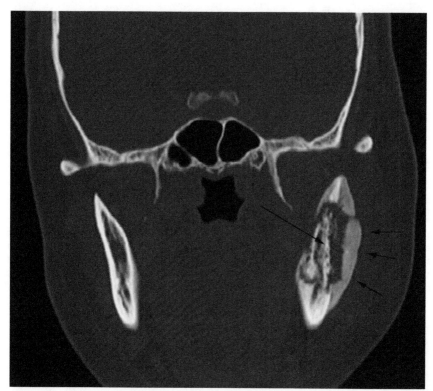

Fig. 11. ONJ. A 56-year-old woman with history of breast cancer and diffuse skeletal metastases. Coronal CT image shows a robust periosteal reaction (*short black arrows*) that resembles chronic osteomyelitis with sequestrum and involucrum. This abnormality proved to be a manifestation of bisphosphonate toxicity rather than metastatic disease. Metastatic disease may have a similar appearance. Although permeative change of the mandibular cortex usually favors malignancy, it is present in this case (*long arrow*).

PNS most commonly occurs centripetally, extending intracranially from the primary tumor. However, as tumor reaches connections to other nerve branches, spread may continue centrifugally, exiting the skull again. For example, there may be intracranial spread along the mandibular nerve to the trigeminal ganglion, and then extracranial extension along the maxillary nerve.[32–34] Because tumor cells extend along a nerve, there may be an imaging appearance of uninvolved segments, corresponding to microscopic tumor cell infiltration, particularly as the nerve passes through a skull base foramen, with more bulky tumor growth in the less confined space beyond the osseous channel.[35] The potential for these skip lesions implies that clear surgical margins may not guarantee the absence of PNS.[36]

Imaging findings in PNS include enhancement and/or enlargement of the involved nerve, foraminal enlargement or erosion, loss of normal fat at the extracranial openings of the neural foramina, and denervation atrophy of the involved muscles. Disease of the trigeminal nerve may also include asymmetric bulging of the cavernous sinus or loss of normal CSF density/signal in Meckel's cave.[37] MRI is the modality of choice to evaluate for PNS (**Fig. 13**).

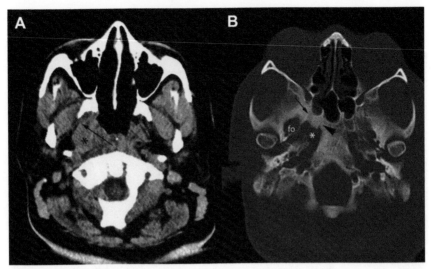

Fig. 12. NPCA. Axial CT images of a 43-year-old man with NPCA. (*A*) There is effacement of the right fossa of Rosenmüller by a nasopharyngeal mass (*asterisk*). There is extension of the mass across the anterior aspect of the PPS (*black arrow*). (*B*) Bone window image shows sclerosis of the ipsilateral pterygoid process (*arrowhead*). There is also abnormal expansion of foramen ovale (fo), the vidian canal (*small black arrow*) and of foramen lacerum (*asterisk*).

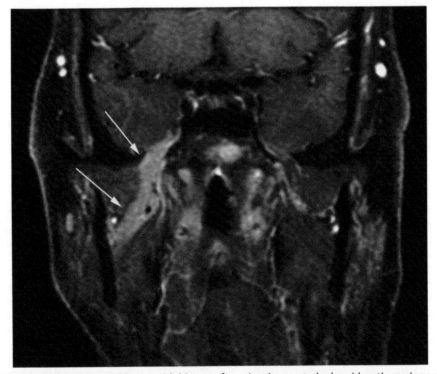

Fig. 13. PNS. A 46-year-old man with history of previously resected adenoid cystic carcinoma of the right submandibular gland. Postcontrast coronal fat-saturated T1-weighted image shows abnormal enhancement and expansion of the third division of the trigeminal nerve (*arrows*), extending from the inferior alveolar canal through foramen ovale into Meckel's cave.

VASCULAR LESIONS
VM

VM is a low-flow vascular lesion with vein-like walls. VM is present at birth and grows with the patient, commonly presenting in childhood.[38] VM is common in the head and neck with a predilection for certain muscles, including masseter and buccinator.[39] Spontaneous enlargement may accompany trauma, infection, and thrombosis.[40] Complete resection is usually not sought or achieved, owing to the infiltrative multi-spatial nature of the lesions, which puts vital structures at risk. Alleviation of symptoms and improved cosmesis are the typical aims of surgical and endovascular intervention.

VM frequently appears hypointense to skeletal muscle on CT. On MRI, it is typically T2 hyperintense and T1 hypointense. Though VM will typically enhance prominently on MRI, enhancement on CT is more variable. When present, phleboliths are highly specific for VM, visible on CT as rounded calcific densities. Phleboliths may be detected in MRI as roughly round foci of signal hypointensity (**Fig. 14**). Infiltrative involvement of the muscles of mastication is common and there may be involvement of the mandible or skull.

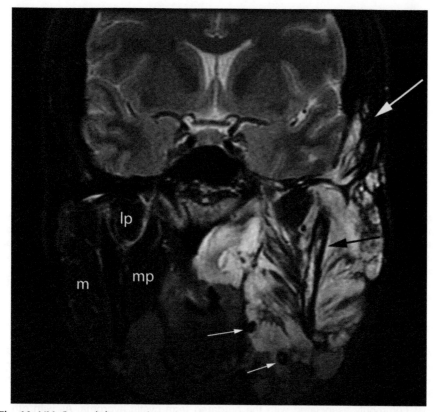

Fig. 14. VM. Coronal short tau inversion recovery MR image of a 15-year-old girl. The entire MS is involved, including the suprazygomatic portion of the temporalis muscle (*large white arrow*), with abnormal T2-signal intensity. There is also involvement of the mandible (*black arrow*). Phleboliths are visible in the submandibular region (*small white arrows*). The contra-lateral masseter (m), pterygoid (lp), and medial pterygoid (mp) muscles are labeled for reference.

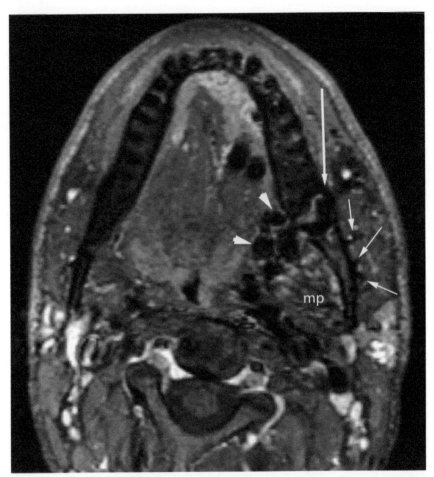

Fig. 15. AVM. A 38-year-old man. Axial postcontrast fat-saturated T1-weighted image shows abnormal vascular flow voids consistent with engorged veins adjacent to the left posterior mandibular body (*arrowheads*) and a large vein within the proximal left inferior alveolar canal (*long arrow*). There is enlargement and mild enhancement of the left medial ptery-goid muscle (mp), which may be a manifestation of impaired venous drainage. There is also mild enlargement of the left masseter, with additional flow voids visible along its medial aspect (*small arrows*).

LYMPHATIC MALFORMATION

Lymphatic malformation (LM) may have components that are microcystic or macro-cystic, and the two forms may coexist in the same lesion. Microcystic LM has very small cystic areas and propensity for an infiltrative multicompartmental distribution, whereas macrocystic LM has large fluid spaces and represents the appearance most commonly associated with the outdated term cystic hygroma. As with other complex vascular malformations of the face, the main goal of therapy for patients with LM is preservation of functional and aesthetic integrity.[41] Timing and extent of therapy will vary with the individual patient's symptoms and degree of impairment.

On MR imaging, microcystic LM may mimic solid tissue because of the enhance-ment of the walls and septations of the lesion's cystic units, with relatively little intervening fluid. Macrocystic LM may also have enhancement of its walls and internal septations, but has a more clearly fluid content. These larger components are prone to bleed internally, either spontaneously or in the setting of trauma or infection, in which instance they may enlarge precipitously. Imaging may show multiple hematocrit levels, especially in the macrocystic components.

AVM

AVM is a high flow vascular anomaly with connections between arteries and vein, without the normal arteriolar resistance vessels and capillaries.[42] A rare disease, cervicofacial AVM most commonly occurs in the cheek and ear, but it mainly involves the mandible or maxilla when intraosseous.[42] Fortunately, there is frequently reconstitution of bone following embolization. Cosmetic issues such as skin discoloration and distortion of facial features, and symptoms from bleeding and ulceration, are the main clinical features.[43]

Similar to other vasoformative anomalies in the face, AVM may be multicompartmental, affecting several contiguous fascial compartments. The imaging hallmarks are the presence of enlarged vascular structures and the absence of a well-defined mass. Typically, an area of edematous-appearing tissue is identified, with only mild T2 hyperintensity and little, if any, contrast enhancement. Occasionally, only the enlarged arteries and draining veins are identified without signal abnormality in the underlying tissue. A nidus is only rarely identified. In MRI, the abnormal vascular structures are best appreciated as curvilinear areas of T1-hypointense and T2-hypointense signal known as flow voids (**Fig. 15**).

SUMMARY

With the exception of infection, the differential diagnosis for disease of the MS depends largely on consideration of the normally occurring structures of that space. Therefore, noninfectious pathologic conditions may commonly involve neural structures, including schwannoma or perineural tumor spread. Also, neoplastic disease, such as sarcoma or NHL, may arise from the musculoskeletal elements. Metastatic disease may also affect the MS. Vascular disease includes vasoformative anomalies such as VM, which occurs in the muscles of mastication, and related entities such as lymphatic malformation or AVM.

REFERENCES

1. Russo CP, Smoker WR, Weissman JL. MR appearance of trigeminal and hypoglossal motor denervation. AJNR Am J Neuroradiol 1997;18:1375–83.
2. Flynn TR, Shanti RM, Levi MH, et al. Severe odontogenic infections, part 1: prospective report. J Oral Maxillofac Surg 2006;64:1093–103.
3. Ohshima A, Ariji Y, Goto M, et al. Anatomical considerations for the spread of odontogenic infection originating from the pericoronitis of impacted mandibular third molar: computed tomographic analyses. Oral Surg Oral Med Oral Pathol Oral Radiol Endod 2004;98:589–97.
4. Kimura Y, Sumi M, Sumi T, et al. Deep extension from carcinoma arising from the gingival: CT and MR imaging features. AJNR Am J Neuroradiol 2002;23:468–72.
5. Nyberg DA, Jeffrey RB, Brant-Zawadzki M, et al. Computed tomography of cervical infections. J Comput Assist Tomogr 1985;9:288–96.
6. Hudson JW. Osteomyelitis of the jaws: a 50-year perspective. J Oral Maxillofac Surg 1993;51:1294–301.

7. Schuknecht BF, Valavanis A. Osteomyelitis of the mandible. Neuroimaging Clin N Am 2003;13:605–18.

8. Schuknecht BF, Carls FR, Valavanis A, et al. Mandibular osteomyelitis: evaluation and staging in 18 patients, using magnetic resonance imaging, computed tomography and conventional radiographs. J Craniomaxillofac Surg 1977;25: 24–33.

9. Yoshiura K, Hijiya T, Ariji E, et al. Radiographic patterns of osteomyelitis in the mandible. Oral Surg Oral Med Oral Pathol 1994;78:116–24.

10. Chong VF, Fan YF. Pictorial review: radiology of the masticator space. Clin Radiol 1996;51:457–65.

11. Goel A, Shah A, Muzumdar D, et al. Trigeminal neurinomas with extracranial extension: analysis of 28 surgically treated cases. J Neurosurg 2010;113:1079–84.

12. Kouyialis AT, Stranjalis G, Papadogiorgakis N, et al. Giant dumbbell-shaped middle cranial fossa trigeminal schwannoma with extension to the infratemporal and posterior fossae. Acta Neurochir (Wien) 2007;149:959–64.

13. Korf BR. Plexiform neurofibromas. Am J Med Genet 1999;89:31–7.

14. Tonsgard JH, Kwak SM, Short MP, et al. CT imaging in adults with neurofibromatosis-1: frequent asymptomatic plexiform lesions. Neurology 1998;50:1755–60.

15. Evans DG, Baser ME, McGaughran J, et al. Malignant peripheral nerve sheath tumours in neurofibromatosis 1. J Med Genet 2002;39:311–4.

16. Longo F, De Maria G, Esposito P, et al. Primary non-Hodgkin's lymphoma of the mandible. Report of a case. Int J Oral Maxillofac Surg 2004;33:801–3.

17. Gusenbauer AW, Katsikeris NF, Brown A. Primary lymphoma of the mandible: report of a case. J Oral Maxillofac Surg 1990;43:409.

18. Weber AL, Rahemtulla A, Ferry JA. Hodgkin and non-Hodgkin lymphoma of the head and neck: clinical, pathologic and imaging evaluation. Neuroimaging Clin N Am 2003;13:371–92.

19. Piatelli A, Croce A, Tete S, et al. Primary non-Hodgkin's lymphoma of the mandible: a case report. J Oral Maxillofac Surg 1997;55:1162–6.

20. Connor SE, Chavda SV, West R. Recurrence of non-Hodgkin's lymphoma isolated to the right masticator and left psoas muscles. Eur Radiol 2000;10:841–3.

21. Glazer HS, Lee JK, Balfe DM, et al. Non-Hodgkin lymphoma: computed tomographic demonstration of unusual extranodal involvement. Radiology 1983; 149(1):211–7.

22. D'Silva NJ, Summerlin D, Cordell KG, et al. Metastatic tumors in the jaws A retrospective study of 114 cases. J Am Dent Assoc 2006;137(12):1667–72.

23. Hirschberg A, Leibovich P, Buchner A. Metastatic tumors to the jawbones: analysis of 390 cases. J Oral Pathol Med 1994;23(8):337–41.

24. Halachmi S, Madeb R, Madjar S, et al. Numb chin syndrome as the presenting symptom of metastatic prostate carcinoma. Urology 2000;55:286i–286iii.

25. Sturgis EM, Potter BO. Sarcomas of the head and neck region. Curr Opin Oncol 2003;15:239–52.

26. Wanebo HJ, Koness RJ, MacFarlane JK, et al. Head and neck sarcoma: report of the Head and Neck Sarcoma Registry. Society of Head and Neck Surgeons Committee on Research. Head Neck 1992;14:1–7.

27. Hariya Y, Yuasa K, Nakayama E, et al. Value of computed tomography findings in differentiating between intraosseous malignant tumors and osteomyelitis of the mandible affecting the masticator space. Oral Surg Oral Med Oral Pathol Oral Radiol Endod 2003;95(4):503–9.

28. Carneiro E, Vibute P, Montazem A, et al. Bisphosphonate-associated mandibular osteonecrosis. AJNR Am J Neuroradiol 2006;27:1096–7.

29. Phal PM, Myall RW, Assael LA, et al. Imaging findings of bisphosphonate-associated osteonecrosis of the jaws. AJNR Am J Neuroradiol 2007;28:1139–45.
30. Shatzkes DR, Meltzer DE, Lee JA, et al. Sclerosis of the pterygoid process in untreated patients with nasopharyngeal carcinoma. Radiology 2004;239:181–6.
31. Curtin H. Detection of perineural spread: fat is a friend. AJNR Am J Neuroradiol 1998;19:1385–6.
32. Curtin H, Williams R, Johnson J. CT of perineural tumor extension: pterygopalatine fossa. AJR Am J Roentgenol 1984;5:731–7.
33. Woodruff WW Jr, Yeates AE, McLendon RE. Perineural tumor extension to the cavernous sinus from superficial facial carcinoma: CT manifestations. Radiology 1986;161:395–9.
34. Parker GD, Harnsberger HR. Clinical-radiologic issues in perineural tumor spread of malignant diseases of the extracranial head and neck. Radiographics 1991;11:383–99.
35. Laine FJ, Braun IF, Jensen ME, et al. Perineural tumor extension through the foramen ovale: evaluation with MR imaging. Radiology 1990;174:65–71.
36. Petri WH, Zoldos J, Wilson TM. Surgical management of basosquamous carcinoma with perineural invasion: report of case. J Oral Maxillofac Surg 1995;53:951–4.
37. Caldemeyer KS, Mathews VP. Imaging features and clinical significance of perineural spread or extension of head and neck tumors. Radiographics 1998;18:97–110.
38. Marler JJ, Mulliken JB. Current management of hemangiomas and vascular malformations. Clin Plast Surg 2005;32:99–116.
39. Hein KD, Mulliken JB, Kozakewich HP, et al. Venous malformations of skeletal muscle. Plast Reconstr Surg 2002;12:1625–35.
40. Ohlms LA, Forsen J, Burrows PE. Venous malformation of the pediatric airway. Int J Pediatr Otorhinolaryngol 1996;37:99–114.
41. Perkins JA, Manning SC, Tempero RM, et al. Lymphatic malformations: review of current treatment. Otolaryngol Head Neck Surg 2010;142:795–803.
42. Robertson RL, Robson CD, Barnes PD, et al. Head and neck vascular anomalies of childhood. Neuroimaging Clin N Am 1999;9(1):115–32.
43. Jeong HS, Baek CH, Son YI, et al. Treatment for extracranial arteriovenous malformations of the head and neck. Acta Otolaryngol 2006;126:295–300.

Parotid Space: Anatomic Imaging

Sangam G. Kanekar, MD[a,c,d,*], Kyle Mannion, MD[b],
Thomas Zacharia, MD[a], Martha Showalter, MD[a]

KEYWORDS

• Parotid • Neck spaces

KEY POINTS

• Most of the pathologies related to parotid space arise from the parotid gland, which may be involved by various neoplastic or non-neoplastic pathologies.
• Cross-sectional examinations are very helpful in localizing the mass, characterizing the parotid tumor, differentiating neoplastic from non-neoplastic lesions, and evaluating the contralateral gland for nonpalpablemass.
• Ultrasonography can be helpful in differentiating cystic lesions from solid lesions, localizing intraglandular from extraglandular masses and providing image guidance for fine needle aspiration biopsy.
• From the surgeon's point of view, the most vital information received from imaging is the evaluation of the extent of the mass as well as invasion of adjacent facial nerve.
• To improve diagnostic accuracy, dynamic contrast-enhanced computed tomography/magnetic resonance imaging (MRI), diffusion weighted MRI, positron emission tomography, proton magnetic resonance spectroscopy imaging, and Tc-99 m pertechnetate scintigraphy may be used.

INTRODUCTION

The parotid space extends from the external auditory canal and mastoid tip superiorly to the angle of mandible inferiorly and is confined within the superficial layers of the deep cervical facia. In addition to the parotid gland, this space also contains intraparotid and extraparotid lymph nodes, the retromandibular vein, the external carotid artery, and extracranial branches of facial nerve. The late encapsulation of the gland and close intimacy of the developing lymphatic system explain the presence of intraparotid lymph nodes and epithelial salivary gland inclusions within periparotid and intraparotid lymph nodes.[1]

[a] Department of Radiology, Penn State University and Hershey Medical Center, 500, University Drive, Hershey, PA 17033, USA; [b] Department of Otolaryngology/Head & Neck Surgery, Vanderbilt University Medical Center, Medical Center East, South Tower 1215 21st Avenue South, Suite 7209, Nashville, TN 37232-8605, USA; [c] Department of Neurology, Penn State University and Hershey Medical Center, 500, University Drive, Hershey, PA 17033, USA; [d] Department of Otolaryngology, Penn State University and Hershey Medical Center, 500, University Drive, Hershey, PA 17033, USA
* Corresponding author. Department of Radiology, Neurology and Otolaryngology, Penn State University and Hershey Medical Center, 500, University Drive, Hershey, PA 17033.
E-mail address: skanekar@hmc.psu.edu

Otolaryngol Clin N Am 45 (2012) 1253–1272
http://dx.doi.org/10.1016/j.otc.2012.08.011
0030-6665/12/$ – see front matter © 2012 Elsevier Inc. All rights reserved.

Abbreviations: Parotid Gland	
1H-MRS	Proton magnetic resonance spectroscopy imaging
ACC	Acinic cell carcinoma
AdCC	Adenoid cystic carcinoma
BCC	Branchial cleft cyst
BLEL	Benign lymphoepithelial lesion
MALT	Mucosa-associated lymphoid tissue
MALTOMA	MALT-type lymphoma
MEC	Mucoepidermoid carcinoma
PA	Pleomorphic adenoma
PNI	Perineural invasion
SCC	Squamous cell carcinoma
SS	Sjögren syndrome
WT	Warthin tumor

Most of the pathologies related to parotid space arise from the parotid gland, which may be involved by various neoplastic or non-neoplastic pathologies. Physical examination of these pathologies is often nonspecific, and therefore imaging plays a vital role in the evaluation of parotid space pathologies. Cross-sectional examinations such as computed tomography (CT) and magnetic resonance imaging (MRI) are very helpful in differentiating neoplastic from non-neoplastic lesions, localizing the mass (intraglandular vs extraglandular), evaluating the contralateral gland for nonpalpable mass, and characterizing the parotid tumor.[2] From the surgeon's point of view, the most important information these modalities provide is the evaluation of the extent of the mass, such as superficial or deep lobe involvement, as well as invasion of adjacent facial nerve. Another imaging modality commonly used in evaluation of parotid pathologies is ultrasonography (US). US is noninvasive and cost-effective and can be helpful in differentiating cystic lesions from solid lesions, localizing intraglandular from extra-glandular masses, and providing image guidance for fine needle aspiration biopsy. Limitations of US include operator dependence and poor evaluation of the deep parotid lobe, parapharyngeal region, and pedunculated parotid tumors.[3]

The conventional imaging characteristics of parotid tumors are nonspecific. Margins, bilateral occurrence or multiplicity, signal intensity or density, intratumoral calcifications, and internal hemorrhage do not definitively distinguish malignant tumors from benign tumors. To improve diagnostic accuracy, alternative methods, such as dynamic contrast-enhanced CT/MRI, diffusion weighted MRI (DWMRI), positron emission tomography (PET), proton magnetic resonance spectroscopy imaging (1H-MRS), and Tc-99 m pertechnetate scintigraphy are used.[4,5]

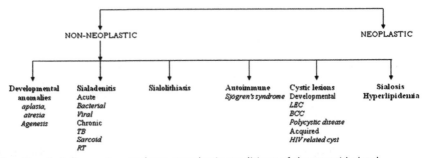

Algorithm 1. Inflammatory and non-neoplastic conditions of the parotid gland.

NON-NEOPLASTIC PAROTID LESIONS

Inflammatory and non-neoplastic conditions of the parotid gland far outnumber the neoplastic lesions (**Algorithm 1**). Etiologies include developmental anomalies, sialoadenitis, sialolithiasis, autoimmune, cystic lesions (developmental or acquired) and sialoadenosis.

Developmental Anomalies

Developmental disorders of the parotid gland are rare. Anomalies like aplasia, atresia, or agenesis may be either unilateral or bilateral and are mostly associated with other facial anomalies.[1,6,7] Clinically, they present with xerostomia, sialoadenitis, and dental caries. Parotid gland agenesis has been reported with hemifacial microstomia, mandibulofacial dysostosis, cleft palate, and anophthalmia. CT or MRI will show absence of normal gland. Glandular absence needs to be confirmed with the clinicians and/or patient for any prior surgery of parotidectomy. In cases of unilateral agenesis of the parotid gland, the existing unilateral gland may be palpated as a mass and referred for imaging. Ectopic gland tissue may be seen in soft tissues or the skin of the anterior neck.[1] This finding is most commonly seen along the anterior border of the sternocleidomastoid muscle. Other rare sites include the middle ear, posterior triangle of the neck, mandible, and maxilla. Non-neoplastic ectopic (choristomatous) masses can be treated with simple excision, while neoplastic lesions should be treated as per their histology.

Sialadenitis

Infection of the salivary gland is called silitis. Primary infection of the gland is termed sialadenitis, while infection of the ducts is known as sialoditis. Infectious sialadenitis may be caused by a variety of microbial agents such as bacteria, viruses, mycobacteria, fungi, parasites, and protozoa. Acute parotitis is most commonly due to bacterial or viral infections.[8]

Most of the bacterial infections are retrograde via the oral cavity. One of the most common precipitating factors is decrease in the salivary flow. Ascending infections are common in the parotid gland because of the wider orifice of the Stensen duct and serous secretions of the parotid gland, which lack antibacterial elements such as lysosomes and immunoglobulin (Ig)A antibodies.[8] Bacterial infections present with acute painful enlargement of gland. Purulent exudates may be seen at the orifice of Stensen duct. Sialadenitis in adults is associated in approximately 50% of cases with sialolithiasis. The most common offending agents are *Staphylococcus aureus, Streptococcus viridans, Streptococcus pneumoniae,* and *Haemophilus influenza.*

US reveals diffusely enlarged hypoechoic gland with duct dilatation. There may be enlarged intraglandular lymph nodes. CT scan is rarely indicated and if performed shows diffuse enlargement and enhancement of the gland[1] (**Fig. 1**). There may be dilatation of the central ducts with wall enhancement. A stone may be seen within the parotid gland duct with resultant either partial or complete blockage of flow of secretions. Hydration and antibiotic therapy are the treatments of choice. Delayed treatment may result in intraglandular abscess formation (**Fig. 2**). These cases require surgical drainage with adequate antibiotic therapy.[1,8]

Mumps, caused by paramyxovirus, is the most common viral infection affecting the salivary gland. The parotid gland is the salivary gland most commonly affected by mumps. Clinically, patients present with prodromal symptoms followed by an acute, painful swelling of the bilateral glands that may persist for 1 week or more. Unilateral involvement is seen in about 20% to 33.3% of the cases. Clinical presentation is

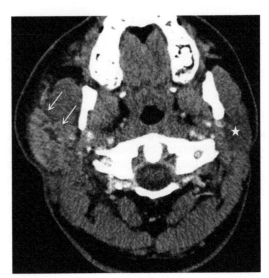

Fig. 1. Bacterial sialoadenitis. Axial contrast-enhanced CT scan shows diffuse enlargement of the right parotid gland with dilatation of the intraparotid ducts. Note the normal left parotid gland (*star*).

sufficient for definitive diagnosis, and imaging findings are nonspecific. Imaging is therefore rarely obtained. Several other viruses including coxsackie virus, lymphocytic choriomeningitis virus, herpes virus, influenza A, parainfluenza, cytomegalovirus, and adenovirus have been associated with sialadenitis. Treatment is predominantly symptomatic.

Chronic sialadenitis of the parotid gland may be either due to obstructive or nonobstructive diseases.[1] Imaging is most commonly performed to differentiate between these 2 etiologies. Chronic sialadenitis may be due to infection (eg, bacteria, mycobacteria, syphilis, toxoplasmosis, and actinomycosis) or noninfectious processes like sarcoidosis, prior irradiation, or autoimmune disease. Chronic inflammation

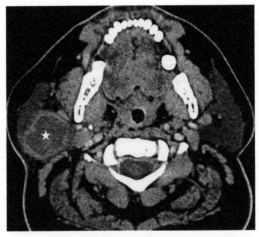

Fig. 2. Parotid abscess. Axial contrast-enhanced CT scan shows a large necrotic lesion (*star*) with thick enhancing capsule in the right parotid gland.

results in shrinkage of the gland, which is inhomogeneous on US. Ductal ectasia may occasionally be seen. Sialadenitis is a common complication of radiotherapy, a common treatment modality for head and neck cancers as well as neck lymphoma. The serous acini of the glands are particularly sensitive to radiation injury, leading to atrophy with xerostomia.

Sarcoidosis, a noncaseating granulomatous infection, involves the parotid glands in 10% to 30% of the cases. Clinically it presents as nontender, nonpainful, chronic enlargement of the gland. On palpation, the gland is often multinodular and may mimic a malignancy. Parotid gland enlargement with sarcoid uveitis and facial nerve paralysis (Heerfordt syndrome) should not be confused with a parotid gland malignancy.[1] On CT or MRI, sarcoid may either present as a solitary parotid mass (indistinguishable from malignancy) or multiple, benign-appearing, noncavitating masses (**Fig. 3**). There may be associated cervical lymphadenopathy and/or associated pulmonary and mediastinal findings.

Sialolithiasis

Sialolithiasis is more common in the submandibular gland/duct (80% and 90%) due to the increased viscosity of submandibular saliva and the upward curved path of the submandibular duct.[9,10] The parotid gland is involved in 20% of cases. Stones are rarely encountered in the sublingual gland. Symptoms are mainly due to ductal obstruction, leading to episodic swelling and postprandial pain. CT is very sensitive in detection of parotid stones. Sialolithiasis may cause mechanical obstruction, resulting in acute or chronic sialoadenitis. They may lead to focal stricture or central dilatation (sialectasia) of the ducts.

Autoimmune

Sjögren syndrome

Sjögren's syndrome (SS) is a systemic autoimmune disorder of the exocrine glands that occurs either as a solitary finding (primary SS) or as a conglomerate of connective tissue diseases (secondary SS).[1,11,12] SS is characterized by periductal lymphocytic and plasma cell infiltration, leading to destruction of exocrine glands, which causes decreased secretions and dryness. When SS involves the parotid gland, the lymphoid

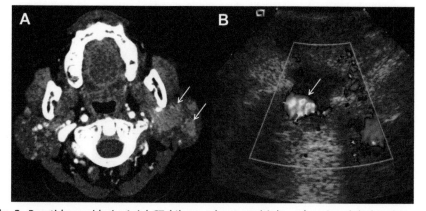

Fig. 3. Parotid sarcoidosis. Axial CT (*A*) scan shows multiple, enhancing, lobulated masses (*arrows*) in the left parotid gland. Doppler US (*B*) showed moderate vascularity (*arrow*) with areas of necrosis. Patient had pulmonary sarcoidosis.

infiltrate produces a localized parenchymal mass referred to as a benign lymphoepithelial lesion (BLEL) or Godwin tumor.[11] SS is most commonly seen between 40 to 60 years of age, with a striking female predominance (90% to 95%). Clinically, SS presents with exocrinopathy involving the lacrimal and salivary glands, leading to keratoconjunctivitis sicca and xerostomia. There may be associated extrasalivary involvement with articular, neurologic, pulmonary, and hepatic manifestations.[12] Although the gland is usually diffusely affected, in some patients a localized area may be more involved, clinically simulating a solitary mass. This finding needs to be further evaluated with biopsy to exclude lymphoma, especially since the risk of developing non-Hodgkin lymphoma in the setting of SS is estimated to be about 44 times greater than in the general population.[13,14]

The primary site of disease in SS is the most peripheral intraglandular ducts and acini. Therefore in the early stages of SS, a sialogram may be more sensitive to early changes than cross-sectional imaging. During this early stage, the sialogram shows a normal central ductal system and numerous peripheral punctate collections of contrast throughout the gland.[1] On CT and MRI, the gland appears normal in early stages. As the disease progresses to acinar destruction, sialogram may show dilatation of the central ducts and changes of sialoadenitis. In the later stages, CT demonstrates glandular enlargement with diffuse high attenuation value.[1,15] As the stages progress, a honeycomb glandular appearance develops on CT, and MRI shows globular enlargement of the parotid ducts with speckled high T2-weighted collections reflecting saliva collections within the dilated ducts (**Fig. 4**). In the advanced stages, the parotid gland shows low signal on T2 WI (weighted image) due to focal accumulation of lymphocytes and fibrous tissue.

Premature deposition of fat associated with SS is easily diagnosed on CT or MRI. Some authors have concluded that monitoring of fat deposition might be useful in diagnosing SS and assessing its progression. MRI sialogram (heavily T2-weighted, fast spin echo sequence with spectral fat suppression) has been shown to be useful in the diagnosis of SS, which shows punctate, globular, cavitary, or destructive appearance within the parotid glands.

Cystic lesions

Primary cystic disease of the parotid gland accounts for 2% to 5% of all the parotid lesions. These cystic lesions can be classified into: developmental (lymphoepithelial cyst, branchial cleft cyst, polycystic dysgenetic disease, epidermoid inclusion cyst,

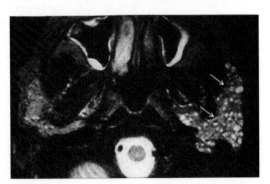

Fig. 4. Sjögren syndrome. Axial T2-weighted image shows multiple punctate high signal intensity areas in both parotid glands (*arrows*). These are suggestive of mucous retention in the dilated ducts.

cystic hygroma and congenital sialectasis), or acquired cysts (eg, ductal sialocyst, acquired immunodeficiency syndrome [AIDS]-related parotid cysts, inflammatory cyst, or neoplastic lesions).[1]

DEVELOPMENTAL CYST
Lymphoepithelial Cyst

The probable origin of these lesions is from the intraparotid lymph nodal system. Cysts show predilection for men and present in adults (40–50 years) as painless masses. Most of these cysts are unilateral, and they may rarely present with facial nerve paralysis. The cysts are well circumscribed and predominantly unilocular, with contents ranging from fluid to mucoid to caseous appearance. On imaging they may be indistinguishable from cystic Warthin tumor (WT), low-grade mucoepidermoid carcinoma (MEC), and true branchial cleft cyst.

Branchial Cleft Cyst

Branchial cleft cyst (BCC) within the parotid glands is very rare. First, BCCs in the parotid space are classified into 1 subtypes (1 and 2).[1] The most common subtype of first BCC is type 2, which is found in the preauricular region of the parotid gland with a fistulous tract extending up toward the membranous and cartilaginous external auditory canals (**Fig. 5**). Type 1 first BCCs are intraparotid and rare. On CT or MRI, they are seen as single fluid-filled masses with thick enhancing walls. These cysts may get infected and clinically present as abscesses and may be difficult to differentiate both clinically and via imaging. Histologically, they are lined by squamous epithelium, ciliated columnar epithelium, or a mixture of both with admixture of skin appendages and cartilage.[1,15]

Polycystic (dysgenetic) disease is a rare developmental abnormality of the salivary gland duct system that has histologic similarity to polycystic disease of the kidney. It is a benign process with female predominance. The entire glandular tissue is replaced by

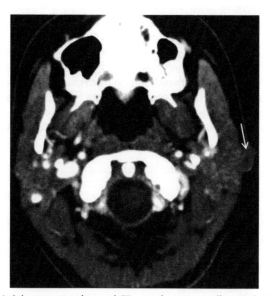

Fig. 5. First BCCs. Axial contrast-enhanced CT scan shows a small cystic lesion in the left preauricular region (*arrow*) with midinflammation of the gland.

cysts, usually bilaterally. This condition needs to be differentiated from cystadenoma and cystadenocarcinoma, both of which are localized masses and, unlike polycystic disease, do not involve the entire gland.

ACQUIRED CYSTS

Salivary duct cysts, or sialocysts, develop as a consequence of duct obstruction. Ductal obstruction may be due to variety of causes like postinflammatory stricture, a calculus, trauma, a postsurgical stenosis, or a mass.[14] Clinically, they present as slowly enlarging, painless masses. Rarely a sialocyst may be filled with air and termed as a pneumocele. Pneumoceles are more common in patients with occupations such as glass blowing and trumpet playing, which lead to increase in intrabuccal pressure.

Human Immunodeficiency Syndrome-Related Parotid Cysts

Kaposi sarcoma, candidal or herpetic oropharyngitis, and cervical lymphadenopathy are the 3 most common presentations of human immunodeficiency virus (HIV) infection in the head and neck.[1] Cystic and solid intraparotid lesions are rare in HIV patients and are called cystic BLEL or BLEL in AIDS.[16,17] These patients present with unilateral or bilateral painless, enlarging parotid masses. On histiopathology, the cystic spaces are lined with squamous epithelium, accompanied by abundant reactive lymphoid stroma. Imaging shows bilateral multiple cysts of varying sizes or a combination of cystic and solid intraparotid lesions causing enlargement of parotid gland. There may be associated Waldeyer lymphatic ring and adenoidal hyperplasia with cervical reactive lymphadenopathy.

NEOPLASTIC PAROTID LESIONS

About 1% of all head and neck malignant tumors arise in the salivary glands, with rule that the smaller the salivary gland involved, the greater the likelihood that a tumor is malignant. As compared with the sublingual gland, where only 15% to 20% of tumors are benign, 70% to 80% of parotid gland tumors are benign.[18] Increased risk of malignancy is seen in Eskimos, survivors of atomic bomb blasts, and persons exposed to previous radiation.

Tumors of the parotid gland can arise from diverse tissue elements such as fat, lymph node, glandular, vascular, and neural tissues.[19] These tumors are mainly classified into 2 major categories: epithelial, arising from glandular and ductal epithelium, and nonepithelial, arising from other tissue elements.[19,20] Tumor stage and grade are more significant predictors than actual histologic subclassification. The presence of metastatic regional lymph node disease indicates a poor prognosis.

Parotid space lesions

NON-NEOPLASTIC		NEOPLASTIC	
EPITHELIAL >90%		NON-EPITHELIAL <5%	
Benign	Malignant	Benign	Malignant
Pleomorphic adenoma	Carcinoma ex Pleomorphic Adenoma	Hemangiomas	Lymphoma
Warthin's Tumor	Mucoepidermoid carcinoma	Lymphangioma	Metastasis
Benign Oncocytic Tumors	Adenoid Cystic Carcinoma	Lipomas	
	Acinic Cell Carcinoma	Neurogenic tumors	
	Malignant Oncocytic Tumors		

Algorithm 2. Epithelial parotid gland tumors.

EPITHELIAL TUMORS

Epithelial parotid gland tumors to be discussed in this article include: pleomorphic adenoma, WT, mucoepidermoid carcinoma, adenoid cystic carcinoma, acinic cell carcinoma, and benign and malignant oncocytic tumors (**Algorithm 2**).

Pleomorphic Adenoma and Carcinoma ex Pleomorphic Adenoma

Pleomorphic adenoma (PA, benign mixed tumor) is the most common (70% to 80%) benign tumor of the major salivary glands. Of all PAs, 84% occur in the parotid gland, 90% of which arise lateral to the plane of the facial nerve.[19–21] Clinically, PA is a very slow growing, painless mass tumor. Histologically, this tumor contains epithelial elements, which may be glandular, ductal, or solid, hence the name pleomorphic. This tumor also contains mesenchyma-like tissue, derived from the myoepithelial cells, which may contain chondroid and fibromyxoid tissue. Sites of necrosis, hemorrhage, hyalinization, calcification, and rarely ossification may be present.[22]

On CT, PA is a smoothly marginated, spherical tumor that has a higher attenuation than the surrounding parotid parenchyma (**Fig. 6**). Tumor contour is often lobulated. At times, PA may be totally cystic due to mucoid contents mimicking a cyst on CT.[1] Almost all the PAs enhance on contrast-enhanced CT. The smaller lesions show homogeneous enhancement, while larger masses may show nonhomogeneous appearance, with sites of lower attenuation representing areas of necrosis, old hemorrhage, and cystic change. Lobulated margin and dystrophic calcifications or ossifications within a parotid mass are highly suggestive of PA. On MRI, these lesions are low on T1-weighted images and high on T2-weighted images.[1] A low signal intensity capsule is often seen on T2-weighted images. Larger masses show heterogeneous signal intensity due to calcification, hemorrhage, necrosis, and ossification (**Fig. 7**). Treatment of the choice is parotidectomy, as the recurrence rate is much higher with enucleation. PA with high stromal chondroid/myoid content has a greater recurrence rate than predominant cellular epithelial tumors.

Three types of malignancies are associated with pleomorphic adenomas: carcinoma ex pleomorphic adenoma, true malignant mixed tumor (carcinosarcoma), and metastasizing benign mixed tumor.[1,23] Carcinoma ex pleomorphic adenoma arises either in an existing PA or develops as a malignant tumor in a previously resected pleomorphic adenoma. If left untreated, nearly 25% of all pleomorphic adenomas may undergo malignant change. Histologically, it is an adenocarcinoma. Classic presentation is rapid growth in a long-existing benign parotid mass. There may be associated pain and facial nerve paralysis. It may metastize to the regional lymph nodes, lungs,

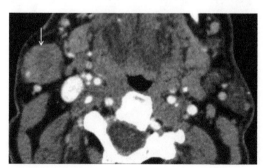

Fig. 6. Pleomorphic adenoma. Axial contrast-enhanced CT scan shows a lobulated, well-defined mass in the right parotid gland (*arrow*).

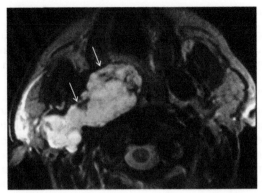

Fig. 7. Pleomorphic adenoma of the deep lobe of the parotid gland. Axial T2-WI shows a lobulated predominately hyperintense mass (*arrows*) arising from the deep lobe of the parotid gland and extending through the stylomandibular canal into the parapharyngeal space.

bones, and brain. Imaging appearance of carcinoma ex pleomorphic adenoma is variable on CT or MRI. The lesion may appear similar to pleomorphic adenoma as a well-defined benign-appearing mass, a focally aggressive lesion, or an aggressive appearance with necrosis, thick, irregular walls, and infiltrating margins (**Fig. 8**). On MRI, this malignant transformation is seen as an area of low signal intensity within the hyperintense mass on T2-WI.

Carcinosarcoma is extremely rare, and it is composed of a mixture of carcinomatous and sarcomatous elements.[1] Metastasis (to lungs, bones, and the central nervous system) from carcinonsarcoma is much more common than in carcinoma ex pleomorphic adenoma. Almost 60% of patients die of local recurrence and/or metastatic disease within 3 years.

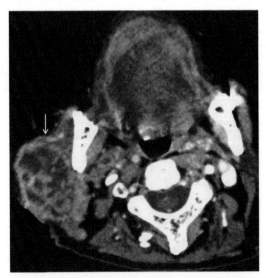

Fig. 8. Carcinoma ex pleomorphic adenoma. Axial contrast-enhanced CT scan shows a large right nonhomogeneous parotid mass (*arrow*) with ill-defined margins.

The metastasizing "benign" mixed tumor is the most rare form of malignancy associated with PA. Metastases may be multiple; involve lungs, bones, and soft tissues; and occur over many decades.

Warthin Tumor

WT (papillary cystadenoma lymphomatosum) is the second most frequent benign tumor arising in the parotid gland, comprising around 4% to 10% of all parotid tumors.[1] They are slow growing, often cystic neoplasms that arise frequently in the lower portion of the parotid gland over the angle of the mandible. They are the most common multifocal or bilateral parotid gland tumor; 25% of them are synchronous, and 75% are metachronous. WTs are well-circumscribed, encapsulated masses with brown to a tan-white color surfaces on pathology specimen. Histologic appearance is distinctive and pathognomonic, composed of varying proportions of lymphoid stroma and epithelium.

On CT, WTs are ovoid, smoothly marginated masses most commonly in the posterior aspect of the superficial lobe of the parotid gland. Tumors often show cystic component (**Fig. 9**). Exophytic WT with cystic component may sometimes mimic lesion branchial cleft cyst or a necrotic node.[1] On MRI, solid WT may be difficult to differentiate from pleomorphic adenomas. They are well defined and show low signal on T1-WI and are hyperintense on T2-WI. Cystic component is very hyperintense on T2-WI. WTs also accumulate ^{99m}Tc-pertechnetate on radionuclide scans due to presence of mitochondrion-rich oncocytes cells. Superficial parotidectomy, with preservation of the facial nerve, is the treatment of choice. Malignancy developing in WT is extremely rare.

Mucoepidermoid Carcinoma

MEC is the most common salivary gland malignancy. More than 80% of these occur in the parotid gland.[1] MEC is most frequently seen in fifth decade of life. It is also the most common salivary malignant tumor in children. The most commonly implicated etiologic factor is radiation (44%). Histologically, MEC is composed of varying proportions of epidermoid and mucus-secreting cells. Clear cells, many of which contain glycogen and/or mucin, are present in most MECs and are a prominent feature. Pathologic grades include low, intermediate, and high.[24,25]

Imaging appearance varies depending on grade of the tumor. On CT, low-grade MEC may mimic appearance of benign tumor. They have well-delineated, smooth margins with cystic areas and rarely focal calcification. On CT and MRI, the high-grade lesions have indistinct infiltrating margins with invasion of salivary ducts.[1] These cellular tumors tend to have low to intermediate signal intensities on both T1- and T2-weighted images (**Fig. 10**). T2-weighted images may show cystic high signal foci.

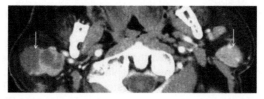

Fig. 9. Bilateral WTs. Axial contrast-enhanced CT scan shows bilateral parotid masses (*arrows*). The largest lesion on the right side is partially cystic. Tumor in the left parotid gland is a well-defined, solid mass in the superficial lobe.

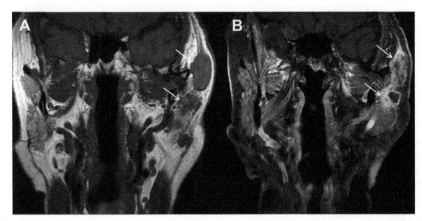

Fig. 10. Mucoepidermoid carcinoma. Coronal T1-weighted (*A*), and coronal (*B*) T1-weighted, fat-suppressed, contrast-enhanced MRI showing an ill-defined mass (*arrows*) in the superficial left parotid gland. Mass is hypointense on T1-WI and shows intense enhancement with necrotic areas.

Gadolinium-enhanced scan shows heterogenous enhancement of the mass. High-grade tumor may show perineural spread along the facial nerve.

Complete surgical excision is the treatment of choice for MEC. The recurrence rate is highest with positive surgical margin, which is up to 50% for low- and intermediate-grade tumors and higher than 80% for high-grade tumors. Adjuvant radiation therapy is added for high-grade tumors. Prognosis is a function of the histologic grade, adequacy of excision, and clinical staging.

Adenoid Cystic Carcinoma

Adenoid cystic carcinoma (AdCC) arises from peripheral parotid ducts and is the second most common major salivary gland malignancy.[26] AdCC is a slow-growing, widely infiltrative tumor with a tendency for perineural spread. It accounts for 2%–6% of parotid gland and 30% of minor salivary gland tumors. It occurs predominately in the fourth to seventh decades of life with female-to-male ratio is approximately 3:2. Clinically it presents as a slow growing mass with symptoms of pain. Among all the head and neck cancers, AdCC has the greatest propensity for the perineural spread. Due to its proximity, the facial nerve is most commonly involved with parotid gland AdCC. Patients present with facial pain and paralysis. The WHO classifies AdCC into three microscopic patterns: tubular, cribriform (most frequent), and solid (least frequent).

The imaging appearance widely depends on the site of the origin of tumor. The parotid lesions tend to appear as benign, well-delineated tumors, whereas the minor salivary gland neoplasms usually have malignant infiltrative margins. Lesions show high signal intensity on T2-WI due to higher water contents. Retrograde tumor extension (perineural invasion) to the skull base often occurs via the facial nerve or the mandibular nerve. CT is less sensitive than MRI in diagnosis of perineural invasion (PNI). CT findings of PNI include nerve thickening, widening of the bony neural canal, and obliteration of the fat in the stylomastoid foramen. On MRI, fat-saturated, contrast-enhanced T1-WI images are most sensitive to diagnose PNI. This sequence demonstrates enhancement of the affected nerve (facial ± trigeminal) with mild thickening of the nerve. Skip lesions may be seen at considerable distances away from the main mass. MRI is equally sensitive in initial diagnosis of PNI or recurrence following total parotodectomy despite anatomic distortion.

Wide surgical resection with negative margins is the standard primary therapy. Adjuvant radiotherapy is usually indicated in most of the cases. Neutron therapy and adoptive immunotherapy in combination with chemoradiotherapy have recently shown to be promising. Generally, major salivary gland sites have a more favorable outcome than minor salivary gland sites. Close follow-up of AdCC is very important, since it has a greater local recurrence rate compared with other malignant salivary tumors.[27] This propensity for local recurrence is highest within the first 5 years, but recurrences have been reported after 20 years.

Acinic Cell Carcinoma

Acinic cell carcinoma (ACC) is a malignant epithelial neoplasm with tumor cells demonstrating differentiation toward (serous) acinar cells. ACC is the second most common malignant salivary gland neoplasm of childhood and is the third most common bilateral salivary gland tumor after WT and pleomorphic adenoma in adult. Most cases are seen in middle age (38–46 years), nearly a decade younger than the ages of patients with other parotid malignancies.

The imaging features are nonspecific, and diagnosis is often established on FNAC (fine needle aspiration and cytology) or surgery (**Fig. 11**). Surgical excision with clear margins is the preferred treatment. Either superficial lobectomy or total parotidectomy is performed, depending on the size and extent of the tumor. Most studies suggest that radiation therapy is of little use in the treatment of ACC.

Benign and Malignant Oncocytic Tumors

Oncocytic tumors are rare primary epithelial salivary gland tumors.[1,9,22] Eighty-five percent of these are found in the major salivary glands and are clinically present with unilateral painless mass. They are most commonly seen in the seventh to ninth decades. Oncocytic tumors can be benign or malignant. Benign tumors are 5 to 16 times more common than their malignant counterparts. Histopathology shows

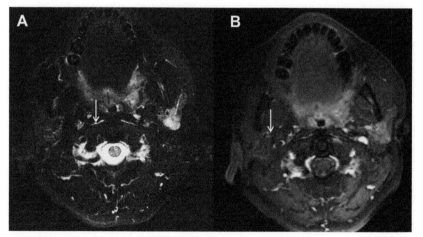

Fig. 11. Acinic tumor. Axial T2 (*A*) and axial (*B*) T1-weighted, fat-suppressed, contrast-enhanced MRI showing an infiltrating mass (*arrows*) in the superficial left parotid gland. This mass is hyperintense on T2-WI and shows moderate enhancement on postcontrast scan.

oncocytes (which are predominantly light cells) as well as a smaller number of dark cells (pyknocytes) that form organoid nests and trabeculae with occasional ducts.[28,29] The glycogen accumulation is responsible for this clear cell change. Malignant oncocytoma shows large and round or polyhedral tumor cells with finely granular cytoplasms. When the distinction is difficult, increased Ki-67 immunostaining may be useful in separating malignant and benign oncocytic tumors.

Imaging findings are nonspecific and present as a solitary or multiple solid masses with sharp, well-delineated margins (**Fig. 12**). These lesions accumulate ^{99m}Tc pertechnetate on salivary radionuclide scans.[1] Oncocytic carcinomas should be treated by wide local excision. Adjuvant radiation therapy with appropriate neck dissection is considered for malignant oncocytoma.

NONEPITHELIAL PAROTID LESIONS

Nonepithelial tumors comprise 50% of pediatric salivary gland tumors and only 5% of salivary gland tumors in adults. Several of the more commonly encountered nonepithelial benign lesions are hemangioma, lymphangioma, lipoma, neurogenic, and fibrous tissue tumors. The 2 most common nonepithelial malignant tumors involving parotid space are lymphoma and metastasis.

Hemangioma

Hemangiomas are the most frequent salivary gland neoplasm in children. These lesions are classified according to their pathology.[30] Capillary hemangiomas are composed of small capillary-sized vessels with plump endothelial cells, and cavernous hemangiomas are made of large, thin-walled vessels with flattened endothelial cells. The diagnosis of capillary hemangiomas is usually made clinically at or immediately after birth. They represent 90% of parotid gland tumors in this age.[22,30] Clinically they are nonencapsulated, lobulated, compressible, bluish-colored, soft masses. Most regress spontaneously. Imaging is typically only performed on deep-seated lesions. Cavernous hemangiomas are well-circumscribed extralobular parotid masses seen in older children and adults. Surgery is the treatment of choice for this type of hemangioma, as these hemangiomas do not regress spontaneously. On US, hemangiomas usually appear as ill-defined, hyperechoic, compressible lesions, or

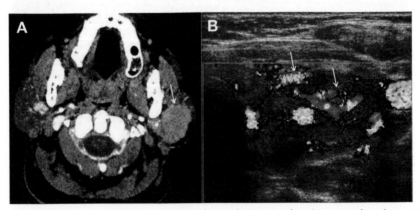

Fig. 12. Oncocytoma. Axial (*A*) contrast-enhanced CT scan showing an enhancing, well-defined mass (*arrow*) in the left parotid gland. This mass showed increased vascularity on the Doppler US (*arrows, B*).

as hypoechoic lesions with a typical lobular pattern. Color Doppler shows hypervascularity. Contrast-enhanced CT demonstrates a intensely enhancing lobulated mass that extends to the overlying skin. Speckled calcifications, (phleboliths) are seen within the mass.[1] On MRI, the lesion is low to intermediate on T1-WI and is hyperintense on T2-WI (**Fig. 13**). There may be areas of high signal intensity on T1- and T2-weighted images, due to prior hemorrhage and slow flow.

Lymphangioma

Approximately 75% of lymphangiomas occur in the neck, most commonly in the posterior compartment. Histologically, they consist of thin-walled spaces with flattened endothelium. A combination of cystic hygroma, cavernous, capillary, and vascular–lymphatic malformations may be present within a single lesion.[30] Eighty percent to 90% of these lesions are diagnosed by the age of 2 years, which corresponds to the period of greatest lymphatic growth. These lesions can invade the parotid gland and surrounding spaces. Patients present with soft and painless masses. Sudden enlargement of lymphangioma is seen with infection or hemorrhage. This sudden increase in size may present with facial palsy secondary to nerve compression.

On US, they are predominantly cystic with septae of variable thickness. When hemorrhage or infection is present, the cysts contain floating debris. On color Doppler, lymphangiomas appear avascular or hypovascularized. On CT, lymphangiomas are thin-walled cystic masses filled with homogeneous low-attenuation (10–20 HU) material. Areas of higher attenuation within the cysts or dependent potion usually correspond to sites of hemorrhage. Infected cysts may show thickened walls and increased attenuation in the surrounding soft tissues. MRI shows fluid levels within the cyst (**Fig. 14**). The multiple, intercommunicating nature of the cysts is better appreciated on T2-WI. Lymphangiomas are often treated either surgically or with sclerotherapy.

Lipoma

Lipomas represent about 1% of parotid space lesions, most of which are simple lipomas. They may be either within the parotid gland or in the periparotid space.[31] Simple lipomas are discrete lesions with homogeneous low attenuation (−65 to −125 HU) on CT (**Fig. 15**). Hemorrhage and fibrotic changes are not uncommon, but if present alter their classical attenuation value on CT. The infiltrating lipoma has

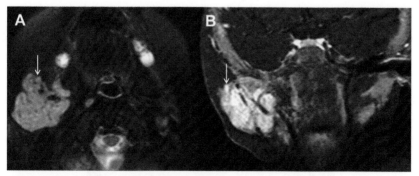

Fig. 13. Parotid hemangioma. Axial T2-weighted (*A*) and coronal (*B*) T1-weighted, fat-suppressed, contrast-enhanced MRI showing lobulated mass (*arrow*) in the right parotid gland showing intense enhancement on the postcontrast scans.

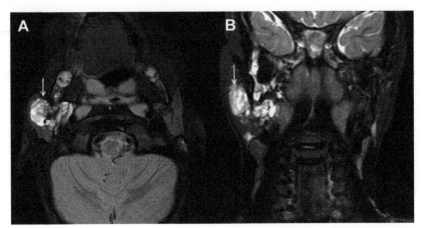

Fig. 14. Parotid lymphangioma. Axial T2-weighted (*A*) and coronal (*B*) T2-weighted MRI showing an infiltrative mass (*arrow*) in the right parotid gland with fluid–fluid level. This mass is seen infiltrating the deep lobe as well as the superficial lobe of the gland.

similar attenuation value to simple lipoma but demonstrates poorly defined margins. On MRI, lipomas have high T1-weighted and intermediate T2-weighted signal intensity. No contrast enhancement is seen in simple or infiltrative lipomas. Any heterointensity or focal enhancement within the lesion should cause suspicion for sarcomatous changes.

Neurogenic Tumors

Neurogenic tumors (schwannomas or neurofibromas) are the second most common benign mesenchymal neoplasm of the parotid space.[32] Schwannomas are solitary, whereas neurofibromas often are multiple and are seen in association with NF1 (Neurofibromatosis 1). Plexiform neurofibromatosis can also involve the parotid space diffusely. Neurofibroma arises from actual neuronal and perineuronal tissue and shows uniform distribution of spindle cells. Schwannoma arises from supporting neural elements and is located eccentric to the nerve. Differentiating neurofibroma and schwannoma may be difficult to differentiate on imaging. However, this distinction is vital, since excision of neurofibroma requires a sacrifice of the nerve; schwannoma can be resected with minimal damage to the nerve (due to its eccentric location).[1] On CT, these tumors are isodense to muscle with cystic changes and show enhancement on postcontrast scan. The cystic changes usually are small and multiple. Neurofibromas may have a low, almost fatty attenuation that may simulate a lipoma. On

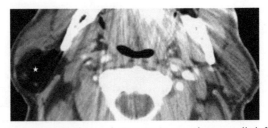

Fig. 15. Lipoma axial contrast-enhanced CT scan image shows well-defined fatty density mass (*star*) in the right parotid gland.

MRI, these tumors usually have low-to-intermediate T1-weighted and high T2-weighted signal intensity (**Fig. 16**). Nonhomogeneous regions of higher and lower signal intensity can occasionally occur, thus making these lesions indistinguishable from a pleomorphic adenoma on MRI.

Lymphoma

Primary lymphoma of the salivary glands is rare.[1,33] The parotid gland is affected in 80% of the reported cases. The diagnosis of the primary lymphoma is considered only if there is histologic proof of involvement of the parotid gland without involvement of the extraparotid lymph node. The most common primary lymphoma is MALT (mucosa-associated lymphoid tissue) type (MALTOMA). MALTOMAS show infiltration of small centrocytes and monocytoid B cells in the parotid ductal and acinar tissue.[33] MALT is more common in patients with autoimmune disease (such as SS and rheumatoid arthritis) and on immunosuppressant therapy. Primary parotid lymphoma usually has a nodular, diffuse infiltrative pattern with inhomogenous signal intensity on MRI. As such, it is nonspecific and can mimic chronic sialadenitis. Diagnosis is established by fine needle aspiration. Systemic workup and bone marrow examination are necessary for staging. Due to the indolent nature of the disease, the overall prognosis of salivary MALTOMAS is favorable.

Secondary lymphomas of the parotid gland (parotid involvement by systemic lymphoma) are more common than primary. Parotid involvement occurs in 1% to 8% of lymphomas and is most commonly seen with high-grade, diffuse large-cell lymphoma. The prognosis is usually poor because of the high-stage and high-grade tumor. The CT appearance of secondary lymphoma of the parotid gland varies with the pathologic distribution of the disease. Usually, each lymph node is homogeneous and may enhance slightly on postcontrast CT scans (**Fig. 17**). On MRI, lymph nodes show homogenous intermediate signal intensity on T1-WI and mildly increased or decreased signal on T2-WI. If the parotid gland parenchyma is involved, a diffuse infiltration will be seen either with poorly defined margins or involving the entire gland.

Metastasis

Metastases to the major salivary glands comprise around 4% of salivary gland neoplasms.[34] The parotid glands contain intraglandular lymph nodes that drain the

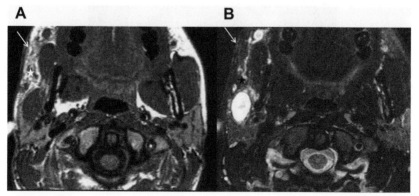

Fig. 16. Neurofibroma. Axial T1-weighted (*A*), and T2-weighted (*B*), MRI showing lobulated mass (*arrow*) in the right parotid gland and in the periparotid space (*star*). This was a plexiform neurofibroma in a patient with NF1.

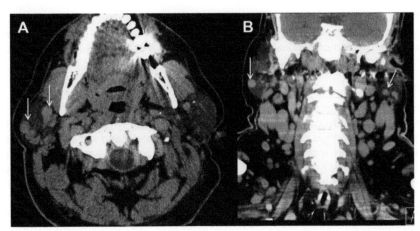

Fig. 17. Secondary lymphoma. Multiple enlarged lymph nodes are seen at multiple levels in the neck bilaterally. Enlarged lymph nodes are also seen within the parotid gland bilaterally (*arrows*).

ipsilateral skin of the upper face and midface. Basal cell cancer, squamous cell carcinoma, and malignant melanoma are the most common neoplasms that metastasize to the parotid gland. Most of them (84% to 89%) arise from the skin (**Fig. 18**). Very rarely non-head and neck cancers from the lung, kidney, and breast may metastasize to the parotid gland. On imaging, it is very difficult to differentiate benign enlarged lymph nodes from metastatic. Therefore persistently enlarged lymph nodes require biopsy. If a metastasis to the parotid gland is solitary, it is indistinguishable from a primary high-grade salivary tumor. MRI may show single or multiple intraparotid masses

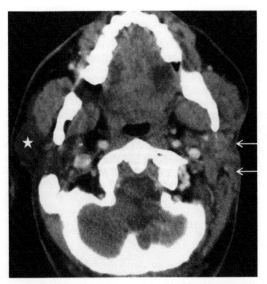

Fig. 18. Axial contrast-enhanced CT scan image shows infiltrative mass lesion extending from the skin–subcutaneous fat into the left parotid gland. This was a basal cell carcinoma of the skin directly infiltrating into the parotid gland. Note the normal left parotid gland (*star*).

with or without central nodal inhomogeneous signal. PET scan is very useful in diagnosis as well as staging of the occult melanoma of the scalp and head and neck. Appropriate treatment depends on the site and stage of the primary. Treatment consists of complete surgical resection and cervical lymph node dissection if there is clinical or radiographic evidence of adenopathy. The prognosis for facial skin primaries that have metastasized to the parotid gland is better if the metastasis is confined to lymph nodes than if the metastatic disease infiltrates the parotid parenchyma.

REFERENCES

1. Peter M Som, Brandwein-Gensler MS. Chapter 40 Anatomy and pathology of the salivary gland. In: Som P, Curtin H, editors. Head and neck Imaging. 5th edition. Mosby-Elsevier; 2011. p. 2449–609.
2. Casselman J, Mancuso A. Major salivary gland masses: comparison of MR imaging and CT. Radiology 1987;165:183–9.
3. Mann W, Wachter W. Ultrasonic diagnosis of the salivary glands. Laryngol Rhinol Otol (Stuttg) 1988;67:355–61.
4. Lee YY, Wong KT, King AD, et al. Imaging of salivary gland tumours. Eur J Radiol 2008;66:419–36.
5. Okamura T, Kawabe J, Koyama K, et al. Fluorine-18 fluorodeoxyglucose positron emission tomography imaging of parotid mass lesions. Acta Otolaryngol Suppl 1998;538:209–13.
6. Mason D, Chisholm D. Salivary Glands in Health and Disease. London: WB Saunders Co; 1975. p. 3–18.
7. Johns M. The salivary glands: anatomy and embryology. Otolaryngol Clin North Am 1977;10:261–71.
8. McQuone SJ. Acute viral and bacterial infections of the salivary glands. Otolaryngol Clin North Am 1999;32:793–811.
9. Batsakis J. Tumor of the Head and Neck: Clinical and Pathological Considerations. 2nd ed. Baltimore: Williams and Wilkins; 1979. p. 1–120.
10. Rabinov K, Weber A. Radiology of the Salivary Glands. Boston: G Hall; 1985. p. 1–221.
11. Work W, Hecht D. Inflammatory diseases of the major salivary glands. In: Paparella M, Shumrick D, editors. Otolaryngology, vol. 3. Philadelphia: WB Saunders; 1973. p. 258–65.
12. Hudson N. Manifestations of systemic disease. In: Cummings C, Fredrickson J, Harker L, et al, editors. Otolaryngology-Head and Neck Surgery, vol. 2. St. Louis: CV Mosby; 1986. p. 1007–13.
13. Selva O'Callaghan A, Angel Bosch Gil J, SolansLaque R, et al. Primary Sjögren's syndrome: clinical and immunological characteristics of 114 patients. Med Clin (Barc) 2001;116:721–5.
14. Mason D, Chisholm D. Salivary Glands in Health and Disease. London: WB Saunders; 1975. 167–206.
15. Som P, Shugar J, Train J, et al. Manifestations of parotid gland enlargement: radiologic, pathologic and clinical correlations, part I: the autoimmune pseudo-sialectasias. Radiology 1981;141:415–9.
16. Sperling N, Lin P, Lucente F. Cystic parotid masses in HIV infection. Head Neck 1990;12:337–41.
17. Olsen W, Jeffrey RJ, Sooy C, et al. Lesions of the head and neck in patients with AIDS: CT and MR findings. AJNR Am J Neuroradiol 1988;151:785–90.

18. Thackray A, Lucas R. Tumors of major salivary glands. Atlas of Pathology. Washington, DC: Armed Forces Institute of Pathology; 1974.
19. Thackray A, Sobin L. Histological typing of salivary gland tumors. International Histological Classification of Tumors. Geneva: World Health Organization; 1972.
20. Lack E, Upton M. Histopathologic review of salivary gland tumors in children. Arch Otolaryngol Head Neck Surg 1988;114:898–906.
21. Rankow R, Polayes I. Surgical treatment of salivary gland tumors. In: Rankow R, Polayes I, editors. Diseases of the Salivary Glands. Philadelphia: WB Saunders; 1976. p. 239–83.
22. Peel R, Gnepp D. Diseases of the salivary glands. In: Gnepp LB, editor. Surgical Pathology of the Head and Neck. New York: Marcel Dekker; 1985. p. 533–645.
23. Tortoledo M, Luna M, Batsakis J. Carcinoma ex pleomorphic adenoma and malignant mixed tumors. Histomorphologic indexes. Arch Otolaryngol Head Neck Sur 1984;110:172–6.
24. Brandwein M, Ivanov K, Wallace D, et al. Mucoepidermoid carcinoma: a clinicopathologic study of 80 patients with special reference to histological grading. Am J Surg Pathol 2001;25:835–45.
25. Plambeck K, Friedrich R, Heller D. Mucoepidermoid carcinoma of the salivary glands. Clinical data and follow-up of 52 cases. J Cancer Res Clin Oncol 1996;122:177–80.
26. Conley J, Dingman D. Adenoid cystic carcinoma in the head and neck (cylindroma). Arch Otolaryngol 1974;100:81–90.
27. Fordice J, Kershaw C, El-Naggar A, et al. Adenoid cystic carcinoma of the head and neck: predictors of morbidity and mortality. Arch Otolaryngol Head Neck Surg 1999;125:149–52.
28. Shellenberger TD, Williams MD, Clayman GL, et al. Parotid gland oncocytosis. CT findings with histopathologic correlation. AJNR Am J Neuroradiol 2008;29:734–6.
29. Ellis G, Auclair P. Atlas of Tumor Pathology: Tumors of the Salivary Glands. Washington, DC: Armed Forces Institute of Pathology; 1996. p. 103–114, 318–24.
30. Touloukian R. Salivary gland diseases in infancy and childhood. In: Rankow R, Polayes I, editors. Diseases of the Salivary Glands. Philadelphia: WB Saunders; 1976. p. 284–303.
31. Som P, Scherl M, Rao V, et al. Rare presentations of ordinary lipomas of the head and neck: a review. AJNR Am J Neuroradiol 1986;7:657–64.
32. Tsutsumi T, Oku T, Komatsuzaki A. Solitary plexiformneurofibroma of the submandibular salivary gland. J Laryngol Otol 1996;110:1173–5.
33. Cankaya H, Ugras S, Dilek I. Head and neck granulocytic sarcoma with acute myeloid leukemia: three rare cases. Ear Nose Throat J 2001;80:224–6.
34. Gnepp D. Metastatic disease to the major salivary glands. In: Ellis G, Auclair P, Gnepp D, editors. Surgical Pathology of the Salivary Glands. Philadelphia: WB Saunders; 1991.

Imaging of the Carotid Space

Clinton Kuwada, MD[a], Kyle Mannion, MD[a,*],
Joseph M. Aulino, MD[b], Sangam G. Kanekar, MD[c,d,e]

KEYWORDS

- Carotid • Head and neck • Anatomy • Imaging • Neck spaces

KEY POINTS

- The carotid space is a complex fascial space spanning the neck from the skull base to the thoracic inlet, encompassing many of the major neurovascular structures of the neck.
- Lesions of the carotid space may arise from asymmetry of normal vasculature, inflammatory or infectious processes, and benign or malignant tumors including metastatic disease processes.
- Cross-sectional imaging plays a key role in identifying particular abnormalities and in planning surgical and nonsurgical therapies.

INTRODUCTION

The carotid space is encircled by the 3 layers of the deep cervical fascia (superficial, middle, and deep), which is often referred to as the carotid sheath and extends from the skull base to the aortic arch. The carotid space is a paired space bordered by the visceral space medially, the prevertebral space posteriorly, and the sternocleidomastoid muscle anterolaterally. In the suprahyoid portion of the neck, the carotid space is often synonymous with the poststyloid compartment of the parapharyngeal space.

The carotid space contains several neurovascular elements, including the carotid artery, internal jugular vein (IJV), vagus nerve (CN X), ansa cervicalis, and sympathetic plexus. Superiorly, the carotid space also contains the glossopharyngeal nerve (IX), the accessory nerve (XI), and the hypoglossal nerve (XII), which all pierce the fascia of the carotid sheath. Within the carotid space, the carotid artery lies medial to the IJV, and the vagus nerve is typically found on the posterior aspect of the 2 vessels. The cervical

[a] Department of Otolaryngology/Head & Neck Surgery, Vanderbilt University Medical Center, Medical Center East, South Tower 1215 21st Avenue South, Suite 7209, Nashville, TN 37232-8605, USA; [b] Neuroradiology Section, Department of Radiology and Radiological Sciences, Vanderbilt University Medical Center, DD-1100 MCN, 1161 21st Avenue South, Nashville, TN 37232-2675, USA; [c] Department of Radiology, Penn State University and Hershey Medical Center, 500 University Drive, Hershey, PA 17033, USA; [d] Department of Neurology, Penn State University and Hershey Medical Center, 500 University Drive, Hershey, PA 17033, USA; [e] Department of Otolaryngology, Penn State University and Hershey Medical Center, 500 University Drive, Hershey, PA 17033, USA
* Corresponding author.
E-mail address: kyle.mannion@vanderbilt.edu

Otolaryngol Clin N Am 45 (2012) 1273–1292
http://dx.doi.org/10.1016/j.otc.2012.08.012
0030-6665/12/$ – see front matter © 2012 Published by Elsevier Inc.
oto.theclinics.com

sympathetic plexus is found embedded in the posterior portion of the carotid sheath and the ansa cervicalis is embedded in the anterior portion of the carotid sheath.

Lesions involving the carotid space may arise from any of these constituents. Therefore, radiographic imaging often helps in the diagnosis of lesions involving the carotid space. Lesions of the carotid space may arise from asymmetry of normal vasculature, inflammatory or infectious processes, and benign or malignant tumors, including metastatic disease processes.[1] The most common of these are discussed in relation to their radiographic diagnosis and clinical implications.

PSEUDOTUMOR

The anatomy and radiologic imaging appearance of the carotid artery and IJV can vary significantly, and this can lead to confusion when evaluating lesions within the carotid space. An ectatic carotid artery and more commonly an asymmetrically enlarged IJV are most commonly an incidental finding on computed tomography (CT) or magnetic resonance imaging (MRI).[1] However, either can also present as a lateral neck mass originating in the carotid space. The right IJV is usually larger than the left IJV and can be several times larger when compared with the left.[2] In addition to being an ectatic vessel, the internal or common carotid artery can have a retropharyngeal course, which may present as a pulsatile retropharyngeal or retrotonsillar mass (**Fig. 1**).[1] This has clear clinical significance when the artery itself is thought to be a mass and may prompt a life-threatening biopsy. In addition, knowledge of a retropharyngeal carotid artery may be crucial to surgical planning for resection of tonsillar or hypopharyngeal tumors. A thorough understanding of the normal arterial and venous anatomy and common variants is important to differentiate a focally dilated artery or vein properly from lymphadenopathy or other disease process. CT, MRI, and ultrasonography can all be helpful for identifying vascular structures in the lateral neck, but ultrasonography becomes less helpful for retropharyngeal anomalies. Multiplanar reformatted CT imaging, in conjunction with rapid scrolling of images while viewing, can clearly define the nature of retropharyngeal structure if it is an aberrantly located carotid artery.[1]

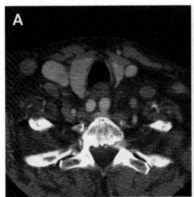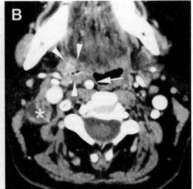

Fig. 1. Tortuous carotid arteries: axial enhanced CT images in 2 patients. (*A*) Tortuous common carotid arteries located near the midline in the retropharyngeal region, at the level of the thyroid gland. (*B*) The tortuous right internal carotid artery (ICA) (*arrow*) impresses on the posterior oropharynx, adjacent to oropharyngeal squamous cell carcinoma primary tumor (*arrowheads*), clinically mimicking submucosal disease. Involved right level IIA necrotic node (*asterisk*).

VASCULAR LESIONS

Vascular lesions, including jugular vein thrombophlebitis, venous and arterial thrombosis, arterial dissection, and arterial aneurysms, present as processes involving the carotid space.

Thrombosis, either arterial or venous in nature, may be diagnosed with contrast-enhanced CT, MRI, or ultrasonography. On contrast-enhanced CT, venous thrombosis appears as a tubular intraluminal filling defect with or without associated mass effect with enhancing vessel wall from the dilated vasa vasorum.[3] In addition, there is usually a distended IJV proximal to the thrombus. MRI can be used when exposure to intravenous contrast needs to be avoided. MRI produces greater soft-tissue contrast and can delineate altered rates of blood flow more sensitively than CT. On T2-weighted MR, acute thrombus of the IJV will have a bright lumen, whereas subacute IJV thrombus will have a low signal.[1] Ultrasonography is an easy, safe, noninvasive, and widely available test. Findings on ultrasonography include a dilated and incompressible vein, intraluminal clot, and no response to the Valsalva maneuver. IJV thrombosis is thought to be an underdiagnosed condition that usually occurs as an associated complication of head and neck infections or surgery, central venous access, malignancy, polycythemia, or intravenous drug abuse.[4] Signs and symptoms of IJV thrombosis can often be subtle but usually include cervical pain and/or neck swelling. A more specific finding is a palpable cord beneath the sternocleidomastoid muscle. Anticoagulant therapy is typically the initial treatment for isolated IJV thrombosis, assuming there is no contraindication for anticoagulation.

IJV may become thrombosed from surrounding soft tissue inflammation or lymphadenopathy. Alternatively, an IJV thrombosis may become secondarily infected, resulting in an IJV thrombophlebitis. IJV thrombophlebitis is radiographically diagnosed in the same manner as a thrombosis with similar findings. There may be significant soft-tissue swelling or other inflammatory changes surrounding the IJV on neck imaging in these cases (**Fig. 2**). An IJV thrombophlebitis caused by an extension of oropharyngeal or odontogenic infection is referred to as Lemierre syndrome. This is classically an anaerobic suppurative process that can produce septic emboli (**Fig. 3**).[5] The treatment of IJV thrombophlebitis requires treating the infectious process with an appropriate antibiotic. Although anticoagulation is not always necessary in the

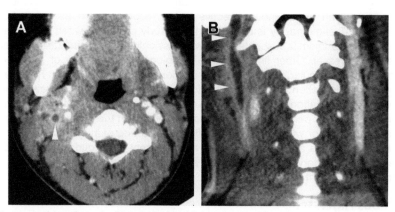

Fig. 2. Internal jugular vein (IJV) thrombophlebitis in a 14-year-old. Axial (*A*) and reformatted coronal (*B*) postcontrast CT images demonstrate nonenhancing thrombus within the right IJV (*arrowheads*) and adjacent partially necrotic adenopathy.

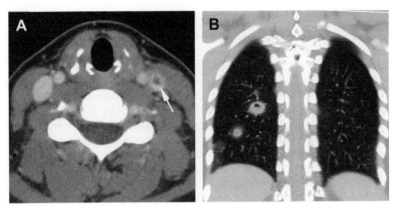

Fig. 3. Lemierre syndrome in a 16-year-old woman. Axial postcontrast CT image (*A*) through the level of the larynx shows a central area of absent enhancement within the left IJV (*arrow*). The patient presented with symptoms of pneumonia, and CT of the chest (*B*, coronal reformatted image) shows multiple cavitary abscesses. MRI of the head revealed additional brain abscesses (not shown).

treatment of IJV thrombophlebitis, systemic anticoagulation is usually recommended if there is any sign of septic emboli or clot propagation.

ARTERIAL DISSECTION

Carotid artery dissection and aneurysms begin as a tear in the intimal lining of the artery, allowing blood under arterial pressure to enter the wall of the artery. This can result in an intramural hematoma leading to a thrombus, which causes narrowing of the lumen. If the tear extends beyond the intima of the vessel, a pseudoaneurysm develops. In either case, the dissected intima or pseudoaneurysm can become a source of distal emboli. Carotid artery dissection and/or pseudoaneurysm can present with symptoms ranging from headache to hemiparesis. A pseudoaneurysm can present as a pulsatile neck mass or cause mass effect on adjacent structures, causing neurologic symptoms such as a Horner syndrome (**Fig. 4**). Carotid artery dissection most commonly presents with ipsilateral face or neck pain. Although rare, the cause of carotid artery dissection or aneurysm is usually from either mechanical trauma or an underlying connective tissue disorder, such as Ehlers-Danlos syndrome.[6] CT angiography is considered the study of choice when carotid artery dissection or aneurysm is suspected, and will classically reveal a change in the caliber of the blood vessel. Other findings on CT angiography indicative of a dissection include an oval, irregular, or slit-like cross section of the vessel lumen. Treatment of carotid artery dissection with anticoagulation is usually performed to prevent thromboembolic complications. More invasive treatment is considered when cerebral ischemic symptoms persist despite anticoagulation, when there is a contraindication to anticoagulation, or when clinically significant narrowing of lumen diameter occurs (**Fig. 5**). Surgery has a limited role in the management of carotid artery dissection. However, carotid artery aneurysms can be surgically repaired with a vein bypass graft or endovascular stent if needed.

INFECTIOUS PROCESSES

Infectious processes from the surrounding parapharyngeal space can spread directly into the carotid space. The parapharyngeal space communicates with all of the deep

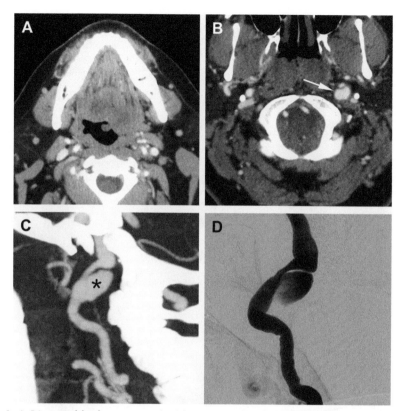

Fig. 4. A 34-year-old who presented with acute onset of dysarthria. (*A*) Axial CT image through the tongue and oropharynx shows swelling of the left tongue, related to acute hypoglossal nerve palsy. (*B*) Axial CT image through the level of the foramen magnum shows a pseudoaneurysm of the left ICA (*arrow*). The enhancing vessel appears enlarged, and there is compression of the adjacent lumen anteriorly. (*C*) Oblique reformatted CT angiography neck image clearly shows the relationship of the pseudoaneurysm (*asterisk*) to the parent vessel, and to adjacent structures, a limitation of catheter angiography (*D*).

neck fascial spaces, therefore there is the potential for all deep neck infections to spread to the carotid space. The most common source of parapharyngeal infections with subsequent carotid space involvement is from odontogenic source, but infections may originate from numerous sources, including the tonsils/oropharynx, nasopharynx, parotid or submandibular glands, trauma, or intravenous drug use.[7] Inflammatory processes involving the carotid space typically present with neck pain, swelling, fever, trismus, or torticollis. More ominous signs include neural deficits such as a Horner sign or palsies of CN IX to XII.[8] Regular spiking fevers may be suggestive of IJV thrombophlebitis and septic embolization (discussed previously). CT scanning with contrast is the imaging modality of choice and is helpful in identifying which fascial compartments are involved. Surgical drainage is usually required, and the approach to drainage depends on the fascial compartments involved as well as the relationship of the abscess and carotid space. In selected cases where the abscess lies medial to the carotid space, the approach to drainage may be through a transoral approach. If there is any concern for damage to the carotid artery of IJV, an external transcervical approach should be used.

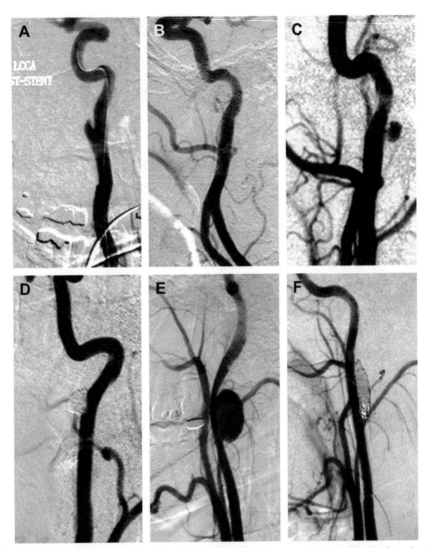

Fig. 5. Carotid artery pseudoaneurysm (PSA) endovascular treatment options in 3 patients. Digital subtraction catheter angiogram images in various stages of treatment. Image immediately poststenting (*A*) shows filling of the pseudoaneurysm with contrast. Follow-up study (*B*) shows subsequent thrombosis of the PSA. Small ICA PSA in another patient (*C*) treated with detachable coils (*D*). Relatively large pseudoaneurysm in a third patient (*E*) was treated with both stenting and coiling (*F*).

BENIGN TUMORS

Benign tumors arising within the carotid space are either neurogenic in origin or associated with the paraganglia of the carotid body, jugulotympanic region, or vagus nerve. At their institution, the authors have also found paragangliomas of both the hypoglossal nerve and the cervical sympathetic trunk within the carotid space.

Paraganglia are collections of cells of neuroectoderm origin that secrete catecholamines and help the autonomic nervous system respond to physiologic stressors.

Tumors of the paraganglia, or "paragangliomas," are richly vascular, slow-growing tumors that are typically benign, with fewer than 10% being malignant. These tumors themselves are rarely secretory. Although most paragangliomas are sporadic in nature, roughly 10% are associated with an autosomal-dominant inheritance pattern or are part of a multiple endocrine neoplasia syndrome (MEN-II or MEN-III). Synchronous or metachronous paragangliomas are fairly common in inherited cases, but rare in patients with sporadic tumor development.[9] These synchronous or metachronous paragangliomas result in roughly 10% of patients overall having multicentric lesions, so all areas for potential paraganglioma development should be closely examined on MRI, particularly in patients with a family history.[10] Paragangliomas are typically diagnosed based on radiologic features and clinical examination. Although CT scan and angiography can aid in the diagnosis of paragangliomas, MRI is considered to be the most helpful imaging modality. Larger paragangliomas may have a characteristic "salt-and-pepper" appearance on T1-weighted and T2-weighted MR images. These hyperintense and hypointense foci are related to slow-flowing and fast-flowing intravascular blood and to intratumoral hemorrhage. The T1-hyperintense foci of slow moving blood were more commonly visible with older MR techniques. Paragangliomas typically have avid enhancement on both MR and CT images. Contrast-enhanced MR angiography (MRA) has been shown to aid in the diagnosis of these hypervascular lesions, and may also be used to identify additional subtle paragangliomas (**Fig. 6**).[11–13]

Carotid body tumors are the most common paraganglioma of the head and neck, and develop from paraganglia within the adventitia at the carotid bifurcation. Carotid body tumors most commonly present as painless, slow-growing neck masses. These tumors are typically mobile horizontally, fixed vertically, and associated with a bruit or vascular thrill. As carotid body tumors enlarge, they may cause cranial nerve or sympathetic chain neuropathies.[14] Enhanced MR and CT imaging typically demonstrate a hypervascular tumor located between the internal and external carotid arteries (**Fig. 7**). Using catheter angiography or cross-sectional imaging, carotid body tumors classically demonstrate the "lyre sign" or splaying of the internal and external carotid arteries.[10] With contrasted CT imaging, the presence of a lucent "halo" around the carotid artery indicates a low likelihood of carotid wall involvement. Loss of this evidence of normal mural thickness should increase the surgeon's anticipation that carotid artery resection may be necessary. The external carotid artery can be sacrificed without impact on the patient, but these surgeries should only be undertaken at institutions with easy access to a vascular surgeon, should the internal carotid artery (ICA) require resection. Carotid body tumors are either treated with surgical excision or radiotherapy, or are simply monitored if they are asymptomatic. The preferred treatment option for carotid body tumors is typically surgical excision, although inherent risks are associated with this option, particularly if the tumor is greater than 5 cm in size. Risks of surgery include temporary or permanent damage to the vagus, hypoglossal, or superior laryngeal nerve, injury to the sympathetic chain resulting in Horner syndrome, and cerebrovascular complication including damage to the carotid artery. Although these risks are rare, first-bite syndrome is a common effect after carotid body tumor resection, caused by loss of autonomics to the parotid gland closely associated with the carotid artery.[14] Although radiotherapy has fewer inherent risks, the primary goal of radiotherapy is to slow or halt the growth of these tumors, not eradicate the tumor. Therefore this option is usually reserved for elderly patients with significant comorbidities or recurrent tumors.

Vagal paragangliomas are rare, accounting for fewer than 5% of all head and neck paragangliomas. These tumors arise from paraganglionic tissue associated with 1 of

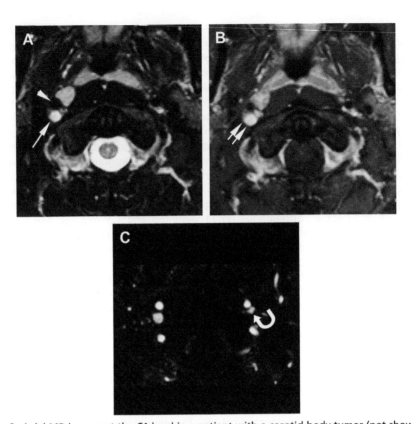

Fig. 6. Axial MR images at the C1 level in a patient with a carotid body tumor (not shown). A small right vagal paraganglioma is apparent on the fat-suppressed T2-weighted image (*A, arrow*), posterior to the ICA flow void (*arrowhead*). The fat-suppressed postcontrast T1-weighted image (*B*) shows avid enhancement of this lesion (*double arrows*). Axial reformatted image (*C*) from contrast-enhanced MRA examination of the neck shows additional small left vagal paraganglioma (*curved arrow*).

the 3 ganglia of the vagus nerve. Vagal paragangliomas tend to present similarly to carotid body tumors but have increased incidence of hoarseness, dysphagia, and/or pharyngeal fullness.[15] Such tumors typically originate high along the extracranial course of the vagus nerve and therefore can be firmly attached to the skull base or even extend intracranially. MRI sometimes demonstrates the classic "salt-and-pepper" appearance on T1-weighted and T2-weighted images seen with all types of paragangliomas. Vagal paragangliomas tend to displace the common or ICA anteromedially (**Fig. 8**) and do not widen the carotid bifurcation like carotid body tumors. If skull base involvement is suspected, CT may be helpful because it provides superior detail in terms of bony changes. The bony margins will appear "moth eaten," in contrast to a high carotid space schwannoma. Contrast-enhanced MRA may be useful to distinguish vagal paraganglioma from other, less vascular tumors such as schwannoma. Surgical treatment involves sacrifice of the vagus nerve and resulting vocal cord paralysis. In addition, because of the typical close proximity to the skull base and occasional intracranial extension, removal of these lesions can be challenging and can result in injury to the glossopharyngeal, spinal accessory, and hypoglossal nerves. Patients with preexisting paralysis of the contralateral vagus or hypoglossal nerves or those

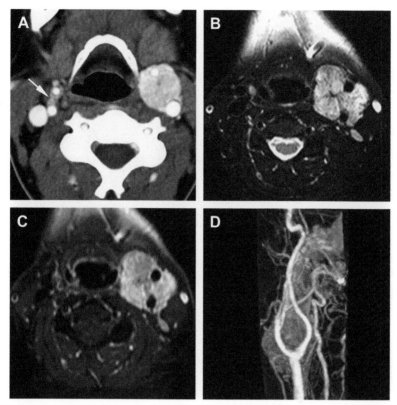

Fig. 7. Typical carotid body tumors. Enhanced axial CT image (*A*) in a patient with bilateral carotid body tumors shows obvious left and subtle right (*arrow*) prominently enhancing tumors within the carotid bifurcations. A lucent halo surrounding the left ICA suggests absent vascular invasion. In another patient with left carotid body tumor (and vagal paraganglioma and glomus jugulare), axial fat-suppressed T2-weighted (*B*) and postcontrast fat-suppressed T1-weighted (*C*) images show a mass centered in the left carotid bifurcation. Enhanced MRA maximum-intensity projection (MIP) image (*D*) shows tumoral enhancement and proximal splaying of the ICA and external carotid artery (ECA). Contiguous but anatomically distinct vagal and jugular foramen paragangliomas enhance prominently as well.

with bilateral vagal paragangliomas are not good surgical candidates. Radiation therapy is typically recommended if there is documented tumor growth.

Paragangliomas can also rarely originate from the sympathetic chain. These types of paragangliomas present similarly to those that arise from the carotid body and vagus nerve. Sympathetic paragangliomas can present with ipsilateral Horner syndrome. Although vagal paragangliomas typically displace the carotid artery anteromedially, sympathetic paragangliomas tend to displace the carotid artery anterolaterally (**Fig. 9**). Because of the normal course of the sympathetic trunk behind the carotid bifurcation, sympathetic tumors (paragangliomas or neurogenic) are misdiagnosed as carotid body tumors more often than any other neoplasm. Because these tumors enlarge, they not only displace the carotids anterolaterally but often splay the bifurcation as well. Splaying of the carotid bifurcation by a lesion whose greatest bulk is medial to both carotids on imaging should increase suspicion for a sympathetic tumor. This distinction becomes important in planning surgery because of the

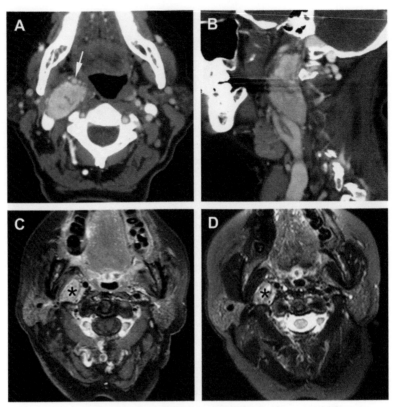

Fig. 8. Typical vagal paragangliomas. Axial (*A*) and sagittal reformatted (*B*) postcontrast CT images in a patient with an isolated right vagal paraganglioma. The markedly enhancing tumor displaces the right ICA (*arrow*) anteriorly and medially. In a different patient, a prominently enhancing (*C*) and relatively T2-hyperintense (*D*) right vagal paraganglioma (*black asterisks*) similarly displaces the dark right ICA flow void anteriorly and medially.

cosmetic and functional impact of a Horner syndrome having much greater patient morbidity than any aftereffects of carotid body tumor excision.

Unlike carotid body tumors and vagal paragangliomas, jugular foramen paragangliomas do not typically present as a neck mass but may secondarily extend inferiorly into the carotid space (**Fig. 10**). Jugular paragangliomas (also referred to as glomus jugulare) typically present with otologic symptoms such as pulsatile tinnitus, conductive hearing loss, or aural fullness. Because these tumors originate within the jugular foramen, the skull base can erode in the region of the jugular fossa and posteroinferior petrous bone with subsequent erosion into the mastoid bone. Significant intracranial and extracranial extension can occur, causing cranial nerve deficits, most commonly involving CN IX to XI.[16] A combination of temporal bone CT scan and temporal bone MR examination is best for evaluating jugular paragangliomas, because CT is ideal for evaluating the extent of bony destruction and MRI is better for delineating tumor limits. The goal of imaging is to identify the extent of tumor and must include the inferior extent within the upper neck, often requiring MRI of the face in addition to the MRI study of the internal auditory canal. High-resolution MR and CT images are required to delineate clearly involvement of the hypoglossal canal, intracranial extension, and proximity to the facial nerve. Contrast-enhanced MRA neck examination is useful to

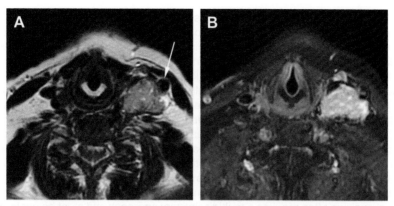

Fig. 9. Sympathetic paraganglioma, axial MR images. The T2-weighted image (*A*) shows an-terolateral displacement of the common carotid artery flow void (*arrow*). Postcontrast fat-suppressed image (*B*) shows marked, homogeneous enhancement. The sympathetic trunk was intimately involved with the tumor at surgery and the vagus nerve was not.

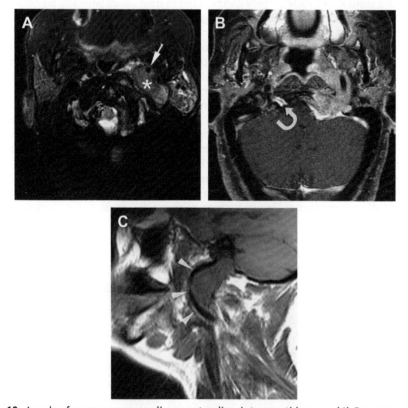

Fig. 10. Jugular foramen paraganglioma extending into carotid space. (*A*) Fat-suppressed T2-weighted image through level C1 to C2 shows anterior displacement of the left ICA flow void (*arrow*) by a mildly T2-hyperintense mass (*white asterisk*). (*B*) Axial postcontrast T1-weighted image at a slightly higher level shows prominent enhancement of the tumor, which involves the left jugular foramen and the left hypoglossal canal. Normal enhance-ment is seen in the right hypoglossal canal (*curved arrow*). (*C*) Sagittal T1-weighted image shows the anterior displacement of the ICA flow void (*arrowheads*) by the paraganglioma.

identify additional subtle paragangliomas, and may help to differentiate jugular foramen paraganglioma from schwannoma. High-resolution CT imaging will show permeative destruction of the bony margins of the jugular foramen from paraganglioma, and sharp sclerotic margins from bony remodeling due to schwannoma. The floor of the hypotympanum must be identified to discern glomus jugulare from glomus jugulotympanicum; often determined by clinical examination, both high-resolution CT and dedicated temporal bone MRI may be useful in this regard (**Fig. 11**).

Similar to other paragangliomas, treatment consists of observation, surgery, or radiation, and the treatment should be individualized based on tumor growth rates, associated symptoms, and patient's age and health status.[10] Observation is recommended when the projected growth rate is not anticipated to cause significant morbidity or mortality over the patient's lifespan. This is established with serial imaging of asymptomatic tumors on an initial yearly basis until stability of the tumor size is confirmed. Surgical excision often requires a multidisciplinary approach and must be customized to match the extent and location of each individual tumor. Surgery for larger tumors often requires a combined otologic and neurosurgical approach, and focuses on preserving the facial nerve and controlling the carotid artery.[16] Both external beam radiation and stereotactic radiosurgery can be used to treat cases whereby surgery is not recommended, and, as with other paragangliomas, this typically results in stabilization of tumor size, but rarely a decrease in tumor volume.

Schwannomas are the most common solitary neurogenic tumor found in the head and neck. Schwannomas in the carotid space can involve any of the nerves found within this space, including the glossopharyngeal, vagus, accessory, hypoglossal, and sympathetic chain nerves.[17] Smaller tumors are typically asymptomatic. As schwannomas grow, they typically present as asymptomatic neck masses, cause motor dysfunction of the involved nerve, or cause pain in the distribution of a sensory nerve (**Fig. 12**, hypoglossal).[18] Schwannomas are usually better visualized on MR than CT imaging. They are enhancing lesions that will often demonstrate areas of cystic degeneration most evident on T2-weighted MR images. These tumors may be hypodense on CT, approaching the attenuation of simple fluid. Contrast-enhanced MRA may help distinguish a schwannoma from a hypervascular paraganglioma (**Fig. 13**, sympathetic schwannoma). Schwannomas involving the vagus or sympathetic chain

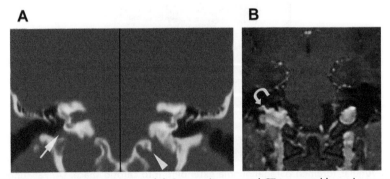

A **B**

Fig. 11. Glomus jugulotympanicum. (*A*) Composite coronal CT temporal bone image of the right and left temporal bones shows erosion of the floor of the right hypotympanum, and abnormal soft tissue within the middle ear inferiorly (*arrow*). The right jugular tubercle is eroded, reflecting hypoglossal canal invasion; compare this with normal left jugular tubercle (*arrowhead*). (*B*) Postcontrast coronal T1-weighted MR image shows prominent enhancement of the paraganglioma and a "tongue" of tumor involving the hypotympanum (*curved arrow*).

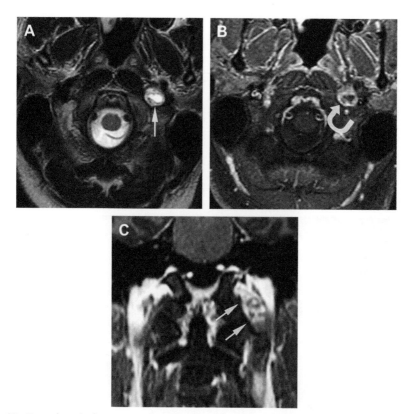

Fig. 12. Hypoglossal schwannoma in a 38-year-old presenting with slurred speech and hypoglossal palsy on examination. (*A*) Axial fat-suppressed T2-weighted MR image through the level of the nasopharyngeal carotid space shows a hyperintense lesion on the left (*arrow*). (*B*) Corresponding fat-suppressed postcontrast T1-weighted image shows rim enhancement and central hypoenhancement (*curved arrow*), reflecting cyst formation or necrosis. (*C*) Coronal fat-suppressed postcontrast T1-weighted image shows the fusiform tumor abuts the hypoglossal canal (*double arrows*).

will displace the internal and external carotid arteries anteriorly. Vagal schwannomas typically push the carotid artery anteromedially (**Fig. 14**), and sympathetic chain schwannomas will push the carotid artery anterolaterally. These relationships are well preserved superiorly in the carotid space for both paragangliomas and schwannomas; however, lower in the neck, the direction of carotid displacement is a less reliable indicator of a tumor's origin. Treatment typically involves either observation or surgery. Because the axonal fibers themselves often course over the surface of the tumor, the involved nerve can often be preserved by separating these fibers longitudinally and enucleating the tumor, particularly if the tumor is small. This approach can often preserve nerve function in the long term but carries a greater risk of tumor recurrence when compared with complete resection of the involved nerve. If nerve function is already absent preoperatively, it will likely not regain function even after enucleation of the tumor.

Neurofibromas are another neurogenic tumor found in the carotid space. Roughly 50% of all neurofibroma cases are sporadic, whereas the remaining 50% are

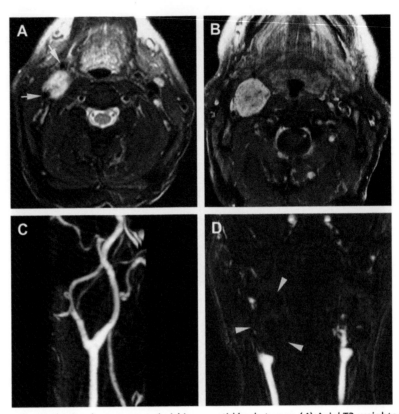

Fig. 13. Sympathetic schwannoma mimicking carotid body tumor. (*A*) Axial T2-weighted MR image just above the carotid bifurcation shows bright signal between the right ICA and ECA flow voids (*arrows*). (*B*) Axial postcontrast T1-weighted image slightly superior to (*A*) reveals prominent enhancement of the tumor. Contrast-enhanced MRA neck MIP image (*C*) and coronal source image (*D*) show splaying of the ICA and ECA, but no tumor enhancement (*arrowheads* mark schwannoma margins).

associated with von Recklinghausen disease (neurofibromatosis type 1 [NF-1]). Sporadic neurofibroma cases typically present with an asymptomatic neck mass. Multiple neurofibromas are seen in the setting of NF-1.[1] Sporadic neurofibromas are visualized on CT as a fluid-dense mass with variable contrast enhancement, and demonstrate hyperintense T2 signal on MRI. Solitary neurofibromas in the setting of NF-1 tend to be large (**Fig. 15**). When nerve trunks and multiple branches are involved, the term plexiform neurofibroma is used. These tumors are typically poorly marginated, fluid-dense masses on CT scan and have a confluence of multiple high signal foci on T2-weighted MR images (**Fig. 16**). Without a history of neurofibromatosis, it is difficult to distinguish between a schwannoma and a neurofibroma by imaging, and plexiform neurofibromas are difficult to resect surgically. Because the nerve fibers typically pass through the tumor in neurofibromas, surgery usually involves sacrificing the involved nerve. These fibers often involve multiple nerve roots of the cervical plexus, which are not technically within the carotid sheath but can surround these structures extensively.

Meningiomas involving the carotid space are rare. These meningiomas emanate from the jugular foramen and may present with a complex lower cranial neuropathy

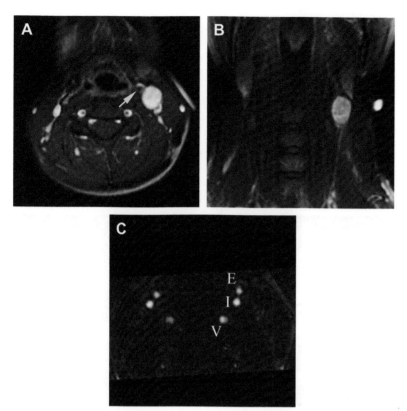

Fig. 14. Vagal schwannoma within the left carotid sheath. (*A*) Axial postcontrast T1-weighted MR image shows a prominently enhancing tumor lateral and posterior to the left proximal ICA flow void (*arrow*). (*B*) Hyperintense signal is present within the tumor on T2-weighted fat-suppressed coronal image. (*C*) Axial reformatted image from postcontrast neck MRA, same imaging plane as (*A*), shows no tumor enhancement, helping to exclude atypical lateral paraganglioma. I, ICA; E, ECA; V, vertebral artery.

involving CN IX to XII. The best diagnostic clue is a connection to the jugular foramen above with jugular foramen margins showing sclerotic or hyperostotic changes on bone CT scan (**Fig. 17**). Meningiomas of the carotid space can be treated with surgical resection, but there is significant risk to the ICA and lower cranial nerves.[1]

MALIGNANT TUMORS

Malignant tumors involving the carotid space are typically the result of an extracapsular spread of deep cervical parajugular lymph nodes involved by metastatic disease. Most cervical metastases are squamous cell carcinomas that originate from primary sites in the upper aerodigestive tract.[19] Other sources of deep cervical metastasis include skin, salivary gland, or thyroid neoplasms. Parajugular lymph nodes that invade the carotid space must have extracapsular spread because the lymph nodes do not lie within the carotid sheath (**Fig. 18**, carotid invasion). The extracapsular spread of these involved lymph nodes makes them inherently more advanced and/ or aggressive.[19] Metastatic squamous cell carcinoma involving the parajugular lymph nodes may present as palpable neck masses with no other symptoms if they are from

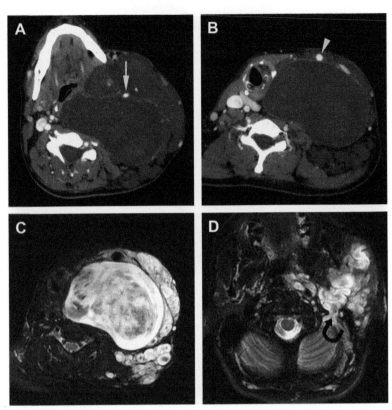

Fig. 15. Large, dominant carotid sheath neurofibroma in a patient with NF-1. (*A*) Axial post-contrast CT image shows a low-density, multilobular left neck mass surrounding the enhancing left ICA (*arrow*). (*B*) As seen on axial CT image more inferiorly, the common carotid artery is displaced anteriorly (*arrowhead*). (*C*) Extensive associated plexiform neurofibroma is well visualized on axial fat-suppressed T2-weighted images. (*D*) Axial T2-weighted image through the C1 level shows tumor extending into the left jugular foramen (*curved arrow*).

a small primary lesion or, in some cases, even unidentified or unknown primary lesions. However, most lymph nodes with extracapsular growth involved by metastatic squamous cell carcinoma are associated with larger primary tumors that cause localized symptoms. Metastatic lymph nodes that invade the carotid space may be adherent to the IJV, carotid artery, and/or CN IX to XII. Direct tumor invasion into the carotid space can also occur in very large primary tumors. CT is the most common imaging modality to evaluate and assess lymph node involvement in squamous cell carcinoma.[19] CT findings suggestive of nodal metastases include ill-defined or irregular bordered masses, rounded shape, central necrosis, and nodal grouping. In addition, the periphery of the nodes is typically thickened and enhances with contrast. Obliteration of the fat plane around the carotid sheath is a sign of carotid space infiltration. IJV involvement by metastatic disease is difficult to assess radiographically. The IJV has a thin wall that is not distinct on imaging and is easily obstructed by compression from adjacent masses. This often results in loss of a visible lumen on cross-sectional imaging, but this rarely indicates involvement by a nodal mass. More commonly, when a mass has obvious extranodal extension into surrounding

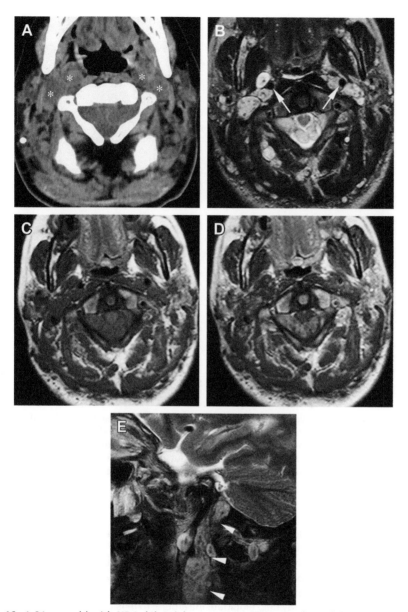

Fig. 16. A 21-year-old with NF-1. (*A*) Axial noncontrast CT image shows bilateral parapharyngeal region lobular, relative hypodensity (*asterisks*). (*B*) Axial T2-weighted image shows hyperintense signal within innumerable scattered nodules. Lesions are located within the carotid spaces bilaterally, intimately associated with the ICA flow voids (*arrows*). Precontrast and postcontrast MR images through the C1 level (*C, D*) show mild enhancement of the neurofibromas. (*E*) Sagittal T2-weighted image through the right nasopharyngeal carotid space shows fusiform tumor (*arrowheads*) posterior to the ICA flow void.

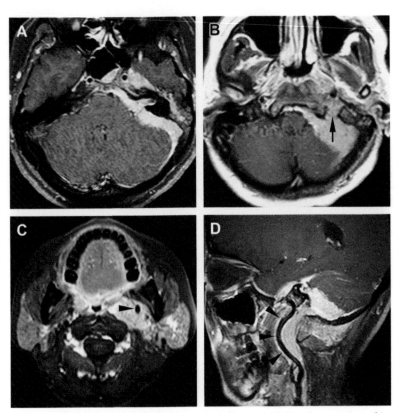

Fig. 17. Postcontrast T1-weighted MR images showing carotid sheath extension of intracranial meningioma. (*A*) There is extensive tumor involvement of the dura of the left posterior fossa. (*B*) Enhancing tumor extends through the left jugular foramen (*black arrow*). Extensive bony involvement is difficult to discern without fat suppression. Axial (*C*) and sagittal (*D*) images show enhancing tumor encasing and anteriorly displacing the left ICA flow void (*black arrowheads*).

soft tissue structures such as the sternocleidomastoid or strap muscles, one should be suspicious of vascular involvement as well. The jugular vein typically provides a barrier between these lymph nodes and the carotid artery, such that carotid involvement is rare. When the patient has had a prior neck surgery with IJV sacrifice or if the metastatic node is posterolateral to the jugular vein, it may be seen to abut the carotid artery on CT scan. MRI may help elucidate intramural extension of disease when there is complete loss of tissue planes between the carotid artery and the metastatic node. Treatment options for metastatic squamous cell carcinoma involving the carotid space are either radiation therapy with or without adjuvant chemotherapy or surgery involving a modified radical or radical neck dissection. The treatment of metastatic neck disease is obviously influenced by the treatment options of the corresponding primary tumor. Involvement of the carotid artery is a relative contraindication to surgical resection; however, when surgery is the only available treatment option, the carotid artery may be resected and replaced with a vein graft. Even with encouraging results on preoperative balloon occlusion tests, carotid replacement is preferable to ligation.

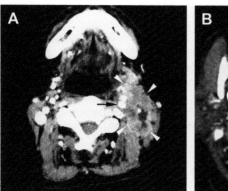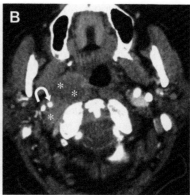

Fig. 18. Carotid space invasion by squamous cell carcinoma nodal disease: axial postcontrast CT images. (*A*) A 62-year-old with a history of right oral tongue T2 cancer resection with left-sided level II regional recurrence. The nodal mass (*white arrowheads*) obliterates the IJV by compression or invasion. The tumor abuts the ICA (*black arrow*) and partially encases the adjacent ECA. At surgery, the vagus nerve, hypoglossal nerve, ECA, and IJV were involved by tumor, and the ICA was spared. (*B*) A 69-year-old with right tonsil cancer presented with partially necrotic right retropharyngeal nodal disease (*asterisks*) that completely encases and mildly narrows the right ICA (*curved arrow*).

SUMMARY

Processes within the carotid space typically originate from the normal neurovascular structures within the space, but occasionally masses outside the carotid space may invade to involve these structures as well. Cross-sectional imaging plays a key role in identifying particular abnormalities and in planning surgical and nonsurgical therapies.

REFERENCES

1. Harnsberger HR, Osborn AG. Differential diagnosis of head and neck lesions based on their space of origin. 1. The suprahyoid portion of the neck. AJR Am J Roentgenol 1991;157:147–54.
2. Eisele DE, Netterville JL, Hoffman HT, et al. Parapharyngeal space masses. Head Neck 1999;21(2):154–9.
3. Albertyn LE, Alcock MK. Diagnosis of internal jugular vein thrombosis. Radiology 1987;162(2):505–8.
4. Chowdhurry K, Bloom J, Black MJ, et al. Spontaneous and nonspontaneous internal jugular vein thrombosis. Head Neck 1990;12(2):168–73.
5. Sinave CP, Hardy GJ, Fardy PW. The Lemierre syndrome: suppurative thrombophlebitis of the internal jugular vein secondary to oropharyngeal infection. Medicine 1989;68(2):85–94.
6. Debette S, Leys D. Cervical-artery dissections: predisposing factors, diagnosis, and outcome. Lancet Neurol 2009;8(7):668–78.
7. Daramola OO, Flanagan CE, Maisel RH, et al. Diagnosis and treatment of deep neck space abscesses. Otolaryngol Head Neck Surg 2009;141(1):123–30.
8. Oliver ER, Gillespie MB. Deep neck space infections. In: Cummings otolaryngology: head and neck surgery. 5th edition. Philadelphia: Mosby; 2010. p. 201–8.

9. Pellitteri PK, Rinaldo A, Myssiorek D, et al. Paragangliomas of the head and neck. Oral Oncol 2004;40(6):563–75.
10. Semaan MT, Megerian CA. Current assessment and management of glomus tumors. Curr Opin Otolaryngol Head Neck Surg 2008;16(5):420–6.
11. Van den Berg R, van Gils AP, Wasser MN. Imaging of head and neck paragangliomas with three-dimensional time-of-flight MR angiography. AJR Am J Roentgenol 1999;172(6):1667–73.
12. Neves F, Huwart L, Jourdan G, et al. Head and neck paragangliomas: value of contrast enhanced 3D MR angiography. AJNR Am J Neuroradiol 2008;29(5): 883–9.
13. Ferre JC, Brunet JF, Carsin-Nicol B, et al. Optimized time-resolved 3D contrast-enhanced MRA at T: appreciating the feasibility of assessing cervical paragangliomas. J Neuroradiol 2010;37(2):104–8.
14. Netterville JL, Reilly KM, Robertson D, et al. Carotid body tumors: a review of 30 patients with 46 tumors. Laryngoscope 1995;105:114–26.
15. Urquhart AC, Johnson JT, Myers EN, et al. Glomus vagale: paraganglioma of the vagus nerve. Laryngoscope 1994;104(4):440–5.
16. Probst LE, Shankar L, Hawke M. Radiological features of glomus tympanicum and glomus jugulare. J Otolaryngol 1991;20(3):225–7.
17. Saito DM, Glastonbury CM, El-Sayed IH, et al. Parapharyngeal space schwannomas: preoperative imaging determination of the nerve of origin. Arch Otolaryngol Head Neck Surg 2007;133(7):662–7.
18. Hamza A, Fagan JJ, Weissman JL, et al. Neurilemmomas of the parapharyngeal space. Arch Otolaryngol Head Neck Surg 1997;123(6):622–69.
19. Don DM, Anzai Y, Lufkin RB, et al. Evaluation of cervical lymph node metastases in squamous cell carcinoma of the head and neck. Laryngoscope 1995;105(7 Pt 1): 669–74.

Retropharyngeal and Prevertebral Spaces: Anatomic Imaging and Diagnosis

J. Matthew Debnam, MD*, Nandita Guha-Thakurta, MD

KEYWORDS

- Retropharyngeal space • Prevertebral space • Imaging • Metastasis • Biopsy

KEY POINTS

- Because of the deep location of the retropharyngeal space and prevertebral space within the neck, lesions arising within these spaces are difficult, if not impossible, to evaluate on clinical examination.
- Cross-sectional imaging plays an important role in the evaluation of the retropharyngeal space and prevertebral space and consists of various modalities: plain radiography, fluoroscopy, multidetector computed tomography, magnetic resonance imaging, ultrasonography, and positron emission tomography/computed tomography.
- Knowledge of the normal anatomy of these spaces, the common lesions affecting them, and the imaging and biopsy techniques used to evaluate such lesions will aid the head and neck surgeon who encounters them in clinical practice.

Abbreviations: RETROPHARYNGEAL AND PREVERTEBRAL SPACES	
AP	Anteroposterior
FDG	Fluorodeoxyglucose
FNA	Fine needle aspiration
MDCT	Multidetector computed tomography
NPC	Nasopharyngeal carcinoma
PVS	Prevertebral space
RPS	Retropharyngeal space

INTRODUCTION

The retropharyngeal space (RPS) extends from the skull base to the upper mediastinum, and the prevertebral space (PVS) extends from the skull base to the coccyx. Diseases of these spaces are uncommon but can result in significant morbidity. As

This work was supported in part by the National Institutes of Health through MD Anderson's Cancer Center Support Grant CA016672.
The authors have no financial information or potential conflicts of interest to disclose.
Section of Neuroradiology, MD Anderson Cancer Center, The University of Texas, 1515 Holcombe Blvd, Houston, TX 77005, USA
* Corresponding author.
E-mail address: matthew.debnam@mdanderson.org

Otolaryngol Clin N Am 45 (2012) 1293–1310
http://dx.doi.org/10.1016/j.otc.2012.08.004
0030-6665/12/$ – see front matter © 2012 Elsevier Inc. All rights reserved.
oto.theclinics.com

these lesions are inaccessible to clinical inspection,[1,2] cross-sectional imaging plays an important role in the evaluation of the RPS and PVS and consists of various modalities. Diseases in the RPS and PVS include primary tumors, direct spread of tumors from adjacent spaces, metastasis, congenital/developmental lesions, inflammation, and infection (**Table 1**).

IMAGING TECHNIQUES

The RPS and PVS can be evaluated by plain radiography, fluoroscopy, multidetector computed tomography (MDCT), magnetic resonance imaging (MRI), ultrasonography, and positron emission tomography/computed tomography (PET/CT). Plain radiographs have been replaced, for the most part, by the more advanced modalities of MDCT and MRI because these provide a more comprehensive evaluation of the neck.

Plain radiographs obtained in anteroposterior and lateral projections may be used to detect radio-opaque foreign bodies and, in the lateral plane, to assess for thickening

Table 1 Lesion of the retropharyngeal and prevertebral spaces	
Primary lesions	Lipoma Liposarcoma Synovial sarcoma

Direct spread	Nasopharyngeal carcinoma
	Squamous cell carcinoma
	   Supraglottic
	   Oropharyngeal
	   Sinonasal
	Lymphoma
	Thyroid, goiter
	Chordoma
	Primary spinal tumors

Nodal metastasis	Squamous cell carcinoma
	   Pharyngeal
	   Larynx
	   Oral cavity
	   Sinonasal
	Non–squamous cell carcinoma
	   Lymphoma
	   Papillary thyroid carcinoma
	   Melanoma
	   Esthesioneuroblastoma

Other	Branchial cleft cyst Foregut duplication cysts Ectopic parathyroid adenoma Nerve sheath tumors Vascular malformations Lymphatic malformations Hemangioma Leiomyoma Disk bulge Edema Osteomyelitis Abscess Calcific tendinitis Tortuous carotid artery

of the PVS soft tissues (**Fig. 1**). On plain radiography, a PVS thickness of less than 6 mm at the level of C3 is considered normal in children[3]; in adults, a PVS of less than 6 mm at C2 and less than 22 mm at C6 is within normal limits. The differential diagnosis of a widened PVS includes edema, hematoma, abscess, tumors, and surgical reconstruction.

Fluoroscopic evaluation of the upper aerodigestive tract after ingestion of contrast material can reveal defects in the posterior pharyngeal wall or fistulous tracts (**Fig. 2**) and also be used to assess the swallowing function.

MDCT provides images in the axial plane at a 1.25-mm thickness. Computer manipulation allows reconstruction of the images in any plane deemed necessary. Different window settings can highlight either the soft tissues or the bony structures of the head and neck, including the skull base and vertebral column. MRI acquires images in axial, coronal, or sagittal planes and, because of better contrast resolution between various tissues, can aid in identifying subtle changes, such as perineural tumor spread. Commonly used MR sequences include T1 weighted without and with contrast, which delineate the anatomy and pathologic conditions; the T2-weighted sequences show the water content of a region and is helpful in the differentiation between various lesions. The administration of intravenous contrast is important for both MDCT and MRI to determine the extent of disease, which is important for staging and treatment planning.

The RPS may be evaluated with ultrasonography by placing a transducer in the oral cavity and oropharynx; this technique is used for fine-needle aspiration (FNA) biopsy to evaluate RPS nodes. PET/CT allows the detection of disease in the RPS and PVS as well as distant disease spread throughout the body (**Fig. 3**). Lesions with increased glucose use, such as tumors, take up fluorodeoxyglucose (FDG) when imaged with PET. Because PET images do not provide adequate anatomic detail, they are fused with a CT scan for lesion localization (ie, the PET/CT study [see **Fig. 3**A]).

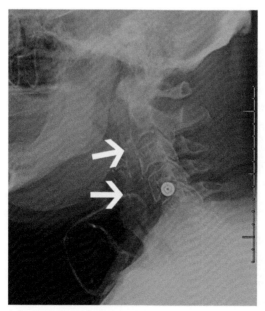

Fig. 1. Thickening of the PVS. Lateral plane radiograph in a patient after total laryngectomy shows thickening of the RPS and PVS (*arrows*) secondary to reconstruction of the larynx and pharynx.

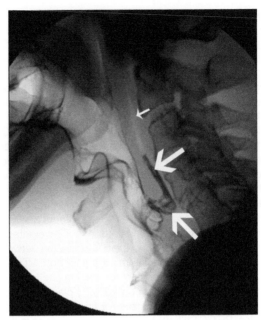

Fig. 2. Fistulous tract between the aerodigestive tract and the RPS. Gastrografin contrast fluoroscopy image in a patient after chemotherapy and radiation therapy for base of tongue carcinoma shows a fistulous tract containing contrast (*large arrows*) between the aerodigestive tract and the RPS. Note presence of air (*small arrow*) superiorly in the RPS.

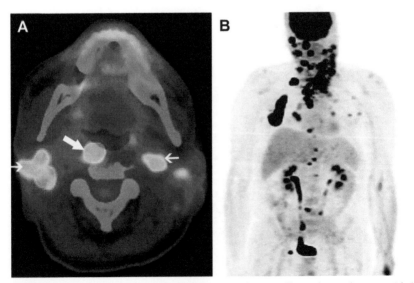

Fig. 3. Metastatic melanoma. (*A*) Axial PET/CT scan shows a fluorodeoxyglucose-avid right lateral retropharyngeal node (*large arrow*) and bilateral neck nodes (*small arrows*). (*B*) PET image shows diffuse metastatic disease.

ANATOMY

The RPS extends from the clivus to the upper mediastinum, lies posterior to the pharynx and esophagus, and is anterior to the prevertebral musculature.[4,5] It is bounded by the buccopharyngeal fascia anteriorly, the prevertebral fascia posteriorly, and the carotid space laterally (**Fig. 4**A). The very thin alar fascia, a part of the deep layer of the deep cervical fascia, extends from the medial border of the carotid space on either side and divides the RPS into 2 components: the anteriorly positioned true or proper RPS and the posteriorly situated danger space. The true RPS extends from the clivus inferiorly to a variable level between the T1 and T6 vertebrae where the alar fascia fuses with the visceral fascia to obliterate the true RPS.[6] The danger space

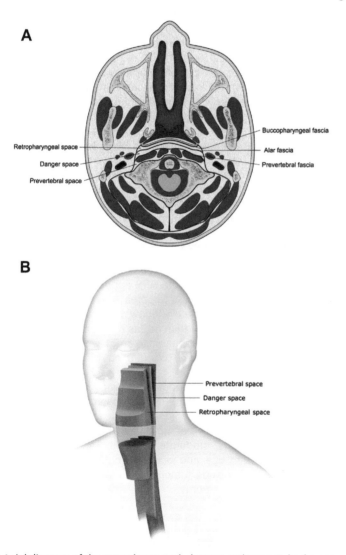

Fig. 4. (*A*) Axial diagram of the retropharyngeal, danger, and prevertebral spaces with associated fascial planes. (*B*) The relationship of the retropharyngeal, danger, and prevertebral spaces.

extends further inferiorly into the posterior mediastinum to the level of the diaphragm and is named as such because it provides a conduit for spread of infection from the pharynx to the mediastinum (see **Fig. 4B**).

The RPS can be further divided into the suprahyoid and infrahyoid RPS, each with different contents. The suprahyoid RPS contains fat and lymph nodes, whereas the infrahyoid RPS contains only fat and, thus, can be involved only by non-nodal disease. The suprahyoid retropharyngeal nodes lie medial to the medial aspect of the internal carotid artery[7] at the level of the transverse process of the atlas and are divided into medial and lateral groups. The medial group of nodes is not consistently present and is located anterior to the medial parts of the longus colli muscles. The lateral group, also known as the nodes of Rouvière, lies ventral to the longus colli muscles.[1,2,4–6,8] Retropharyngeal nodes are normally present in children and then atrophy in puberty. Small nodes may be present in two-thirds of asymptomatic adults and, when present, can be visible on imaging.[8] Normal retropharyngeal nodes should be less than 1 cm in diameter.[8,9]

The PVS is situated between the prevertebral fascia anteriorly and the vertebral bodies posteriorly (see **Fig. 4**); the contents include the prevertebral muscles and fat. Controversy exists in the literature regarding the lateral aspect of the PVS and whether or not the contents of a paravertebral space (ie, the scalene muscles, levator scapulae muscle, splenius capitis and splenius cervicis muscles, brachial plexus nerve roots, and vertebral artery and vein) should be included with the PVS to form a combined perivertebral space.[10] Because the deep layer of the deep cervical fascia attaches to the transverse process for the cervical vertebrae, separating the PVS and the paravertebral space, the term PVS (*pre*vertebral space) is used in this article for identifying the region between the carotid sheaths laterally, the prevertebral fascia anteriorly, and the vertebral bodies posteriorly.[11]

PRIMARY TUMORS OF THE RPS AND PVS

Primary tumors of the RPS are extremely uncommon. Lipoma (**Fig. 5**) is the most common primary neoplasm. Lipomas of the RPS appear elliptical on axial sections, conforming to the shape of the RPS.[4] A lipoma may be differentiated from air (**Fig. 6**) on CT by use of the appropriate window width and window level settings because air is less dense (more black) than fat (as measured on CT with Hounsfield units). On MRI, fat has a hyperintense appearance on T1-weighted images and is suppressed with fat saturation techniques, often used in postcontrast T-weighted sequences.

Malignant neoplasms, such as liposarcoma and synovial sarcoma, are even rarer than lipomas in the RPS.[12,13] Well-differentiated liposarcomas may have homogeneous adipose tissue, characterized by T1 signal hyperintensity, with only several thin septa.[14] Features more suggestive of malignancy include greater than 25% non-adipose tissue, irregular margins, moderate to marked enhancement of thickened septa and nodules, large lesion size, and increased patient age.[14,15]

Primary tumors of the PVS include tumors of the longus colli and longus capitis muscles and are predominantly sarcomas.

DIRECT SPREAD OF TUMOR TO THE RPS AND PVS

Pharyngeal masses, such as nasopharyngeal carcinoma (NPC) and squamous cell carcinoma of the oropharyngeal wall, can spread directly and invade the RPS. NPC involves the mucosal surface of the nasopharynx and its spread is initially limited by the pharyngobasilar fascia. Once this fascia is breached, NPC may extend posteriorly

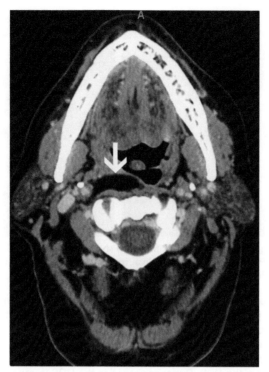

Fig. 5. Lipoma. Axial contrast-enhanced neck CT scan shows fat density (−20 Hounsfield units) in a right RPS lipoma (*arrow*).

and inferiorly into the PVS (**Fig. 7**). A study by King and colleagues[16] demonstrated that involvement of the prevertebral musculature occurred in 58 out of 150 patients (39%) with NPC. On MRI, NPC typically enhances less than normal mucosa and is not as intense on T2-weighted imaging.[17] NPC may also spread superiorly to involve the skull base and the intracranial compartment through direct invasion or perineural

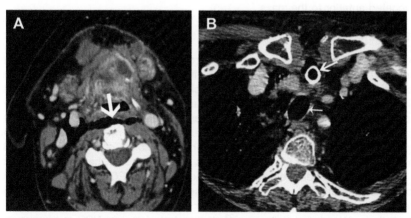

Fig. 6. PVS air collection. (*A*) Axial contrast-enhanced neck CT scan shows air (−920 Hounsfield units) (*arrow*) in the PVS. (*B*) Axial contrast-enhanced neck CT scan shows placement of a tracheostomy cannula (*large arrow*) in the soft tissues anterior to the trachea (*small arrow*).

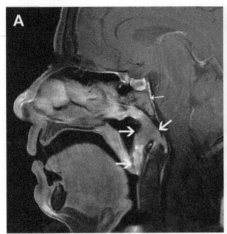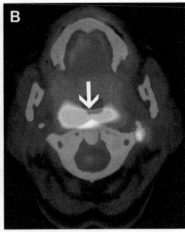

Fig. 7. NPC. (*A*) Sagittal T1 postcontrast MRI scan shows inferior extension of tumor (*large arrows*) into the RPS and PVS. Note the clival involvement (*small arrow*). (*B*) Axial PET/CT scan shows FDG-avid disease (*arrow*) in the RPS and PVS.

spread. The presence of tumor spread into the clivus and intracranial compartment, together with the presence of systemic metastasis, favors a diagnosis of NPC over other pharyngeal carcinomas.[18]

Supraglottic, oropharyngeal, or sinonasal tumors may also grow into the RPS and can extend in a craniocaudal direction after gaining access because there are no fascial barriers within the RPS. Superior spread in the RPS is impeded by the attachment of the buccopharyngeal fascia to the skull base, and disease spread may result in extensive erosion of the clivus.[19]

Lesions of the thyroid, including goiters, can extend posteriorly and medially into the RPS. Primary lesions of the spine and chordoma can invade the PVS and then the RPS from a posterior direction. Chordomas (**Fig. 8**) are midline lesions arising from the clivus, have variable enhancement, and are hyperintense on T2-weighted images.[20,21] Clues to the location of a mass in the PVS include preservation but anterior displacement of RPS fat and effacement of the longus colli and longus capitis muscles, which are located anterior to the mass.

NODAL METASTASIS

NPC and squamous cell carcinoma of the oropharynx and larynx can metastasize to retropharyngeal nodes (**Fig. 9**), especially if there is involvement of the posterior pharyngeal wall. Other primary tumors associated with retropharyngeal nodal metastasis include tumors of the oral cavity and paranasal sinuses and non–squamous cell carcinoma lesions, such as papillary thyroid carcinoma, melanoma, and esthesioneuroblastoma.[6] The imaging features of retropharyngeal nodal metastasis are focal nodal necrosis, ill-defined margins, or 2 or more involved nodes on 1 side of the RPS. A minimal axial diameter of 6 mm or more has been reported to have 87.5% accuracy for identifying malignant retropharyngeal nodes from NPC.[22] Central necrosis or evidence of extracapsular spread should raise concern about metastatic involvement of retropharyngeal nodes, regardless of their size (**Fig. 10**).

A study by Wang and colleagues[23] demonstrated that in NPC, retropharyngeal nodes are involved less commonly than level IIB nodes (72.2% vs 86.5%). However, retropharyngeal nodes are considered N1 disease in the 2010 American Joint

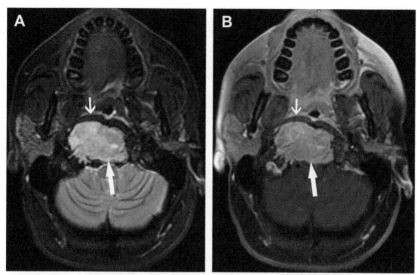

Fig. 8. Chordoma. (*A*) Axial T1 postcontrast and (*B*) axial fast spin echo T2 MRI scans show a heterogeneously enhancing, T2-hyperintense PVS mass (*large arrow*) that is anteriorly displacing the prevertebral musculature (*small arrow*).

Committee on Cancer staging system for NPC because involvement of these nodes increases the risk of distant metastasis and affects prognosis[24]; retropharyngeal nodal metastases are associated with poor treatment response and decreased survival because there is decreased control of disease in the neck.[25,26]

If malignant-appearing nodes are seen in the RPS and there is no known primary tumor, the pharyngeal mucosal space and the nasopharynx should be thoroughly

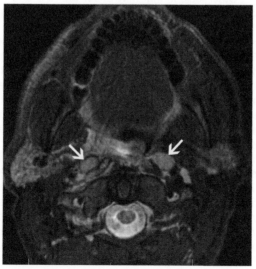

Fig. 9. Retropharyngeal nodal metastasis. Axial T1 postcontrast MRI scan shows enlarged bilateral retropharyngeal nodes (*arrows*).

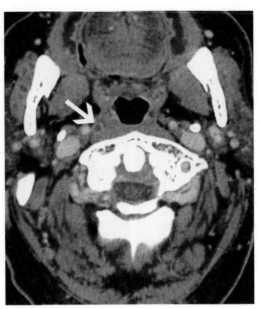

Fig. 10. Retropharyngeal nodal metastasis. Axial contrast-enhanced neck CT scan shows a nonpathologically enlarged, centrally necrotic, right lateral retropharyngeal node (*arrow*).

inspected for submucosal tumor.[27] Retropharyngeal nodes also indicate a poor prognosis in patients with primary lesions arising outside the nasopharynx.[28]

OTHER LESIONS

Congenital lesions of the RPS include branchial cleft cyst (**Fig. 11**) and foregut duplication cysts. Ectopic parathyroid adenoma, or hyperplasia, may occur at the level of the pyriform sinus.[29] Other lesions that may affect the RPS and PVS include nerve sheath tumors (**Fig. 12**), vascular malformations, lymphatic malformations, hemangioma, and leiomyoma.

Radiation therapy is effectively used to treat a variety of head and neck malignancies. Fluid collections (**Fig. 13**) may appear 4 to 6 weeks after radiation therapy and usually disappear by 8 to 12 weeks. This fluid may accumulate in the RPS, conforms to the elliptical shape of the RPS, and does not seem to be under tension as seen in RPS abscess (**Fig. 14**).[30] Soft tissue ulceration is another complication of radiation therapy[31] and may extend from the pharyngeal wall into the RPS or PVS. These ulcerations may be benign (**Fig. 15**) or malignant; lack of associated enhancement suggests benignity.

Nonmalignant lesions arising from the vertebral bodies, including anterior disk bulges (**Fig. 16**) and spinal osteomyelitis (**Fig. 17**), may involve the PVS. Fluid collections, such as edema, suppurative adenitis, and RPS abscess (see **Fig. 14**), can mimic a malignancy. Clinical history and imaging findings, such as peripheral enhancement; soft tissue thickening; and reticulation in the surrounding soft tissues, such as the parapharyngeal or carotid spaces, are suggestive of inflammatory response.

In the case of primary involvement of the RPS by acute prevertebral calcific tendinitis, an inflammatory condition caused by deposition of calcium hydroxyapatite in the superior oblique tendon fibers of the longus colli muscles, there is a fluid collection and soft tissue swelling in the RPS. It is important to distinguish this process from an infectious cause. This differentiation can be achieved by the identification of calcific density in

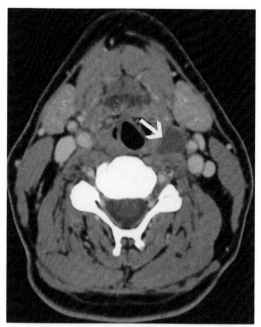

Fig. 11. Retropharyngeal cyst. Axial contrast-enhanced neck CT scan shows a branchial cleft cyst in the left RPS (*arrow*).

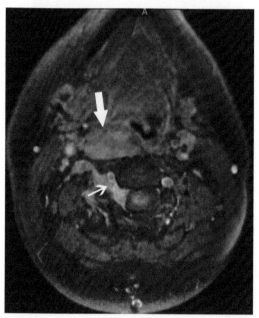

Fig. 12. Schwannoma. Axial T1 postcontrast MRI scan with fat saturation shows a presumed right retropharyngeal schwannoma (*large arrow*) in a patient with neurofibromatosis 1. Nerve sheath tumor is seen extending out of the right neural foramen (*small arrow*).

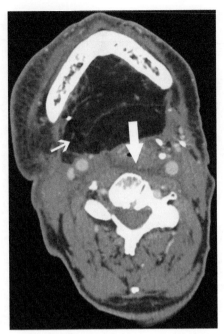

Fig. 13. Retropharyngeal fluid. Axial contrast-enhanced neck CT scan shows fluid in the retropharynx following radiation therapy (*large arrow*). A fat graft is noted in the oral cavity following total glossectomy (*small arrow*).

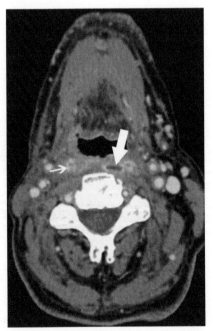

Fig. 14. Retropharyngeal abscess. Axial contrast-enhanced neck CT scan shows a peripherally enhancing left RPS fluid collection (*large arrow*) under tension. Heterogeneous enhancement is present in the right RPS (*small arrow*) consistent with inflammatory change.

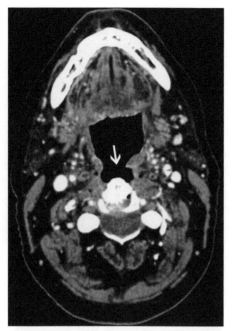

Fig. 15. Soft tissue ulceration. Axial contrast-enhanced neck CT scan shows a radiation-associated ulceration (*arrow*) extending from the pharyngeal wall through the RPS and PVS to the anterior margin of the exposed vertebral body.

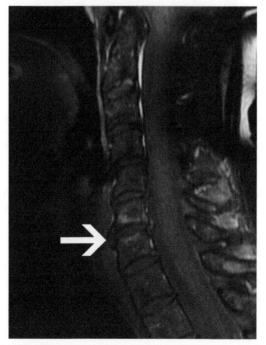

Fig. 16. Anterior disk extrusion. Sagittal T1 postcontrast MRI scan with fat saturation shows an incidentally discovered anterior disk extrusion (*arrow*).

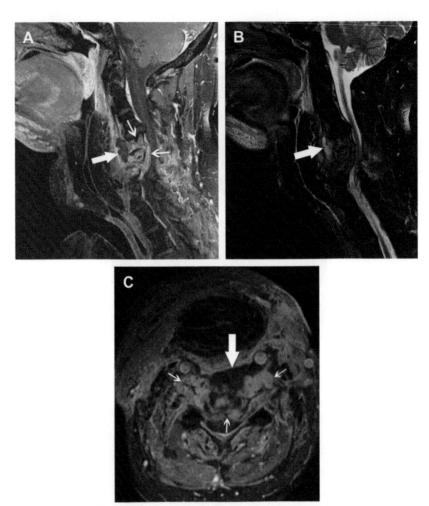

Fig. 17. Prevertebral abscess/osteomyelitis. (*A*) Sagittal T1 postcontrast MRI scan, (*B*) sagittal fast spin echo T2 scan, and (*C*) axial T1 postcontrast MRI scan show infection of the vertebral column, epidural space, and the RPS and PVS (*small arrows*) characterized by soft tissue enhancement and a prevertebral abscess (*large arrows*).

the longus colli (particularly at the C1-2 level) along with the aforementioned imaging features and avoids misdiagnosis, inappropriate medical treatment, and surgical drainage.[32]

A tortuous carotid artery may mimic an RPS mass. In this condition, the vessel is not contained within the RPS but instead bows the alar fascia medially and projects into the RPS (**Fig. 18**). Unilateral jugular vein occlusion or jugular vein compression results in a low-attenuation collection in the RPS. Air in the RPS or PVS (see **Fig. 6**) may result from trauma, assisted ventilation, or foreign body ingestion.[6]

BIOPSY

Suspicious retropharyngeal nodes may be evaluated with FNA biopsy with CT using multiple approaches, including subzygomatic, premaxillary (**Fig. 19**), and

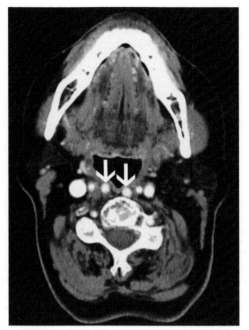

Fig. 18. Axial contrast-enhanced CT scan shows medial positioning of the internal carotid arteries (*arrows*) into the RPS.

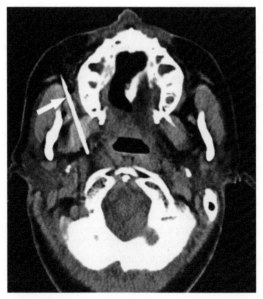

Fig. 19. CT-guided transfacial biopsy. Axial non–contrast-enhanced CT scan shows the biopsy needle (*arrow*) extending toward the right RPS.

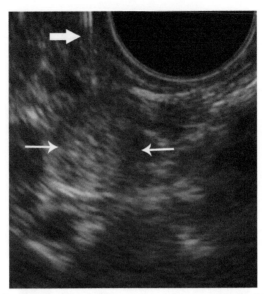

Fig. 20. Ultrasound-guided transoral FNA biopsy. Sonogram shows the biopsy needle (*large arrow*) extending into a right retropharyngeal lymph node (*small arrows*).

retromandibular. A transoral approach through the oropharynx may be selected for ultrasonographic FNA of the RPS or PVS (**Fig. 20**). A high diagnostic yield has been reported when FNA specimens of head and neck lesions are interpreted by an experienced cytologist.[33,34]

SUMMARY

Primary lesions of the RPS and PVS are rare. Most disease involvement of these spaces is the result of direct spread from adjacent sites or metastasis. Knowledge of the normal anatomy of these spaces, the common lesions affecting them, and the imaging and biopsy techniques used to evaluate such lesions will aid the head and neck surgeon who encounters them in clinical practice.

ACKNOWLEDGMENTS

The authors wish to thank David Bier, medical illustrator, MD Anderson Cancer Center, for the wonderful illustrations.

REFERENCES

1. Nyberg DA, Jeffrey RB, Brant-Zawadzki M, et al. Computed tomography of cervical infections. J Comput Assist Tomogr 1985;9(2):288–96.
2. Wong YK, Novotny GM. Retropharyngeal space - a review of anatomy, pathology, and clinical presentation. J Otolaryngol 1978;7(6):528–36.
3. Warner WC. Rockwood and Wilkins' fractures in children. In: Beaty JH, Kasser JR, editors. Cervical spine injuries in children. Baltimore (MD): Lippincott Williams & Wilkins; 2001. p. 809–84.
4. Branstetter BF 4th, Weissman JL. Normal anatomy of the neck with CT and MR imaging correlation. Radiol Clin North Am 2000;38(5):925–40.

5. Chong VF, Fan YF. Radiology of the retropharyngeal space. Clin Radiol 2000; 55(10):740–8.
6. Davis WL, Harnsberger HR, Smoker WR, et al. Retropharyngeal space: evaluation of normal anatomy and diseases with CT and MR imaging. Radiology 1990;174(1):59–64.
7. Som PM, Curtin HD, Mancuso AA. Imaging-based nodal classification for evaluation of neck metastatic adenopathy. AJR Am J Roentgenol 2000;174(3):837–44.
8. Mancuso AA, Harnsberger HR, Muraki AS, et al. Computed tomography of cervical and retropharyngeal lymph nodes: normal anatomy, variants of normal, and applications in staging head and neck cancer. Part II: pathology. Radiology 1983;148(3):715–23.
9. Som PM. Lymph nodes of the neck. Radiology 1987;165(3):593–600.
10. Davis WL, Harnsberger HR. CT and MRI of the normal and diseased perivertebral space. Neuroradiology 1995;37(5):388–94.
11. Som PM, Curtin HD. Fascia and spaces of the neck. In: Som PS, Curtin HD, editors. Head and neck imaging. 5th edition. St. Louis (MO): Mosby; 2011. p. 2203–34.
12. Gundelach R, Ullah R, Coman S, et al. Liposarcoma of the retropharyngeal space. J Laryngol Otol 2005;119(8):651–4.
13. Ozawa H, Soma K, Ito M, et al. Liposarcoma of the retropharyngeal space: report of a case and review of literature. Auris Nasus Larynx 2007;34(3):417–21.
14. Ohguri T, Aoki T, Hisaoka M, et al. Differential diagnosis of benign peripheral lipoma from well-differentiated liposarcoma on MR imaging: is comparison of margins and internal characteristics useful? AJR Am J Roentgenol 2003;180(6): 1689–94.
15. Kransdorf MJ, Bancroft LW, Peterson JJ, et al. Imaging of fatty tumors: distinction of lipoma and well-differentiated liposarcoma. Radiology 2002;224(1):99–104.
16. King AD, Lam WW, Leung SF, et al. MRI of local disease in nasopharyngeal carcinoma: tumour extent vs tumour stage. Br J Radiol 1999;72(860):734–41.
17. Goh J, Lim K. Imaging of nasopharyngeal carcinoma. Ann Acad Med Singapore 2009;38(9):809–16.
18. Glastonbury CM. Nasopharyngeal carcinoma: the role of magnetic resonance imaging in diagnosis, staging, treatment, and follow-up. Top Magn Reson Imaging 2007;18(4):225–35.
19. Chong VF, Fan YF. The retropharyngeal space: route of tumour spread. Clin Radiol 1998;53(1):64–7.
20. Meyers SP, Hirsch WL Jr, Curtin HD, et al. Chordomas of the skull base: MR features. AJNR Am J Neuroradiol 1992;13(6):1627–36.
21. Nishiguchi T, Mochizuki K, Ohsawa M, et al. Differentiating benign notochordal cell tumors from chordomas: radiographic features on MRI, CT, and tomography. AJR Am J Roentgenol 2011;196(3):644–50.
22. Zhang GY, Liu LZ, Wei WH, et al. Radiologic criteria of retropharyngeal lymph node metastasis in nasopharyngeal carcinoma treated with radiation therapy. Radiology 2010;255(2):605–12.
23. Wang XS, Hu CS, Ying HM, et al. Patterns of retropharyngeal node metastasis in nasopharyngeal carcinoma. Int J Radiat Oncol Biol Phys 2009;73(1):194–201.
24. Tham IW, Hee SW, Yap SP, et al. Retropharyngeal nodal metastasis related to higher rate of distant metastasis in patients with N0 and N1 nasopharyngeal cancer. Head Neck 2009;31(4):468–74.
25. McLaughlin MP, Mendenhall WM, Mancuso AA, et al. Retropharyngeal adenopathy as a predictor of outcome in squamous cell carcinoma of the head and neck. Head Neck 1995;17(3):190–8.

26. Chua DT, Sham JS, Kwong DL, et al. Retropharyngeal lymphadenopathy in patients with nasopharyngeal carcinoma: a computed tomography-based study. Cancer 1997;79(5):869–77.
27. Silver AJ, Mawad ME, Hilal SK, et al. Computed tomography of the nasopharynx and related spaces. Part II: pathology. Radiology 1983;147(3):733–8.
28. Harnsberger HR. Handbook of head and neck imaging. 2nd edition. St Louis (MO): Mosby; 1995. p. 89–104.
29. Miller DL, Craig WD, Haines GA. Retropharyngeal parathyroid adenoma: precise preoperative localization with CT and arterial infusion of contrast material. AJR Am J Roentgenol 1997;169(3):695–6.
30. Graber MA, Kathol M. Cervical spine radiographs in the trauma patient. Am Fam Physician 1999;59(2):331–42.
31. Debnam JM, Garden AS, Ginsberg LE. Benign ulceration as a manifestation of soft tissue radiation necrosis: imaging findings. AJNR Am J Neuroradiol 2008; 29(3):558–62.
32. Shin DE, Ahn CS, Choi JP. The acute calcific prevertebral tendinitis: report of two cases. Asian Spine J 2010;4(2):123–7.
33. DelGaudio JM, Dillard DG, Albritton FD, et al. Computed tomography–guided needle biopsy of head and neck lesions. Arch Otolaryngol Head Neck Surg 2000;126(3):366–70.
34. Sack MJ, Weber RS, Weinstein GS, et al. Image-guided fine-needle aspiration of the head and neck: five years' experience. Arch Otolaryngol Head Neck Surg 1998;124(10):1155–61.

Submandibular and Sublingual Spaces: Diagnostic Imaging and Evaluation

Amit K. Agarwal, MD*, Sangam G. Kanekar, MD

KEYWORDS

- Submandibular space • Sublingual space • Cystic lesions • CT • MRI

KEY POINTS

- Computed tomography (CT), magnetic resonance imaging (MRI), or ultrasonography (US) may be necessary for a reliable assessment of lesion extension to deeper structures when diagnosing or evaluating the submandibular space.
- CT is particularly useful for evaluating acute inflammatory processes because it is capable of depicting mandibular cortical bone erosion and destruction, cutaneous changes, and submandibular duct calculi.
- MRI provides better soft tissue resolution than CT and is particularly useful for staging oral cavity malignancies that involve the floor of the mouth and complex disease processes that extend through multiple anatomic spaces.

INTRODUCTION AND OVERVIEW

The mylohyoid muscle divides the lower part of the oral cavity into 2 spaces: the sublingual space, which is located superior to the muscle, and the submandibular space, inferior to the muscle but superior to the hyoid bone. A wide range of pathologic processes may involve these spaces. They include lesions that arise uniquely in this location (eg, ranula, submandibular duct obstruction) as well as inflammatory processes, vascular abnormalities, and various malignancies that may also occur elsewhere in the head and neck. Some lesions that arise in superficial tissues may be easily diagnosed at physical examination. However, computed tomography (CT), magnetic resonance imaging (MRI), or ultrasonography (US) may be necessary for a reliable assessment of lesion extension to deeper structures. This article outlines the radiologic anatomy of the region, describes the various pathologic processes that may affect it, and discusses the use of imaging in their evaluation.

The authors have nothing to disclose.
Division of Neuroradiology, Department of Radiology, Hershey Medical Center, Penn State University, 500 University Drive, Hershey, PA 17033, USA
* Corresponding author.
E-mail address: aagarwal1@hmc.psu.edu

ANATOMY

The mylohyoid muscle is an anterior suprahyoid muscle located deep or superior to the anterior belly of the digastric muscle. The mylohyoid muscle separates the sublingual space from the submandibular space and is a key landmark in imaging of the oral cavity and upper neck (**Fig. 1**A). Surgical approaches are chosen based on the relationship of a lesion to the mylohyoid muscle.

The sublingual space is a potential space without a fascial lining. The sublingual space is superomedial to the mylohyoid muscle and lateral to the genioglossus and geniohyoid muscles in the oral cavity. The major contents of the sublingual space are the sublingual salivary gland; the submandibular duct (Wharton duct); the deep portion of the submandibular salivary gland; and the lingual nerve, artery, and vein. The sublingual space communicates with the submandibular space at the posterior margin of the mylohyoid muscle. However, there can be a defect in the midportion of the muscle (boutonnière). The normal sublingual gland or sublingual lesions can pass through this defect to reach the submandibular space as well. The deep portion of the submandibular gland wraps around the posterior edge of the mylohyoid muscle, so a small part of the gland is cranial to the muscle in the sublingual space. The rest of the gland is located in the submandibular space. Contents of the submandibular space are the anterior belly of the digastric muscle, submandibular nodes, submandibular gland, and facial vein. The platysma forms the superficial margin of the submandibular space. Further, sublingual lesions are classically considered to extend into the submandibular space at the posterior edge of the muscle.

In the United States, CT is the modality of choice for imaging the floor of the mouth because of the widespread availability of CT scanners and the short examination time. CT is particularly useful for evaluating acute inflammatory processes because it is capable of depicting mandibular cortical bone erosion and destruction, cutaneous changes, and submandibular duct calculi. MRI provides better soft tissue resolution than CT and is particularly useful for staging oral cavity malignancies that involve the floor of the mouth and complex disease processes that extend through multiple anatomic spaces.

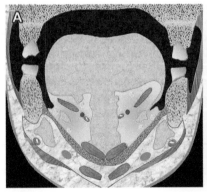 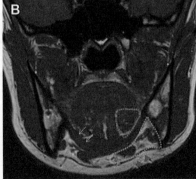

Fig. 1. (*A*) The sublingual (*shaded in green*) and submandibular (*shaded in blue*) spaces with their contents. The mylohyoid muscle (*arrows*) separates the sublingual space from the submandibular space and is a key landmark in imaging of the oral cavity. Coronal T1-weighted magnetic resonance (MR) image (*B*) showing the sublingual and submandibular spaces. The platysma forms the superficial margin of the submandibular space (*arrowhead*).

The mylohyoid muscle and the spaces can be seen on axial, sagittal, and coronal images on CT and MRI. However, the shape of the muscle sling is best seen on CT and MRI in the coronal plane (see **Fig. 1B**).

LESIONS

Although the submandibular and sublingual spaces are a small region, many different pathologic processes may occur there: cystic lesions, inflammatory conditions with various causes (eg, infection, obstruction of the main submandibular duct), rare vascular lesions, and benign and malignant neoplasms (**Box 1**).

CYSTIC LESIONS

Cystic lesions in the sublingual/submandibular region are usually slow growing and often cause signs and symptoms only after they are large. Most often cysts in the floor of the mouth are benign and arise from salivary glands.[1] The more common cystic lesions include ranulas and dermoid or epidermoid cysts and rarer lesions include false sialoceles, branchial cleft cysts, and thyroglossal duct cysts.[2] Vascular anomalies and malignancies may manifest as cystic lesions, and, in these circumstances, specific imaging criteria and contrast-enhanced MRI may provide clues to the diagnosis.[3]

Ranulas

A ranula is a mucous retention cyst or mucocele that arises from a sublingual gland or minor salivary gland and thus has a peripheral epithelial layer. Ranulas are

---

Box 1
Common pathologic processes in the submandibular and sublingual spaces

- Cystic lesions
  - Ranulas (simple or plunging)
  - Dermoid cysts
  - Epidermoid cysts
  - Thyroglossal duct cyst
  - Branchial cleft cysts
- Inflammatory processes (infectious/noninfectious)
  - Cellulitis/abscess
  - Ludwig angina
  - Submandibular duct obstructions (stenosis/calculi)
  - Systemic disorders
- Vascular malformations
  - High-flow arteriovenous malformations
  - Low-flow hemangiomas, venous vascular malformations, lymphatic duct malformations
- Neoplastic lesions
  - Benign neoplasms (eg, lipomas)
  - Malignant neoplasms (eg, squamous cell carcinomas, salivary gland tumors, lymphomas)
- Pseudotumors

characterized as either simple (**Fig. 2**A) or plunging (diving). They typically result from trauma or inflammation of the salivary glands. A plunging or diving ranula (see **Fig. 2**B) develops after a simple ranula ruptures. The ruptured ranula usually extends posteriorly from the sublingual space into the submandibular space. Less commonly, it may extend anteriorly through a mylohyoid defect into the anterior submandibular space. Because the extension lacks an epithelial lining, a plunging ranula is classified as a pseudocyst.[4] The lesion usually measures less than 6 cm at its maximum diameter in the submandibular space, with a narrower tail extending into the floor of the mouth.[2] All ranulas are homogeneous, well-defined masses with fluid density on CT or extremely high T2-weighted signal intensity on MRI. It is essential to differentiate ranulas from other cystic masses before surgery because the surgical approach to ranulas differs from approaches to other types of masses.[3]

Congenital Cysts

Dermoid/epidermoid

Dermoid/epidermoid cysts derive from ectodermal tissue trapped during embryonic development; those with skin appendages on their capsules are termed dermoid, and those without are termed epidermoid. Although these cysts are mostly found in the midline of the floor of the mouth (that is, between the genioglossus muscles), they can occur also in the sublingual or submandibular space. On CT or MRI, dermoid cysts typically look like inhomogeneous masses, reflecting mixtures of keratin or fat with their contents. In contrast, epidermoid cysts are likely to be more homogeneous and, when occurring in the sublingual space, may be indistinguishable from simple ranulas.[5]

Thyroglossal duct and branchial cleft cysts

Thyroglossal duct cysts (**Fig. 3**A) are the most common congenital neck cysts, and occur anywhere along the course of the thyroglossal duct, presenting as midline neck masses. Although they are mostly located at or just below the hyoid bone, they occasionally occur above the hyoid, in the submandibular space.

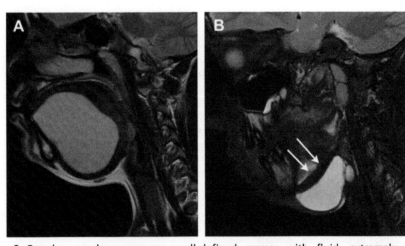

Fig. 2. Ranulas are homogeneous, well-defined masses with fluid, extremely high T2-weighted signal intensity on MRI. Simple ranulas (*A*) are confined to the sublingual space. Plunging ranula (*B*), also known as diving ranula, dissects along facial planes beyond the confines of the sublingual space, around the posterior edge of the mylohyoid muscle (*arrows*).

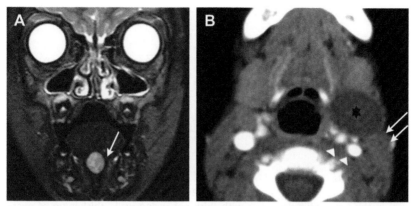

Fig. 3. Thyroglossal duct cysts (*A; arrows*) are the most common congenital neck cysts, present as midline neck masses. Although they are mostly located at or just below the hyoid bone, they occasionally occur above the hyoid, in the submandibular space. Branchial cleft cysts (*B; star*) are lateral neck masses that characteristically displace the sternocleidomastoid muscle posterolaterally (*arrows*), the carotid and jugular vessels posteromedially (*arrowheads*).

Branchial cleft cysts (see **Fig. 3**B), properly called second branchial cleft cysts, arise from the remnant of the second branchial apparatus. On images, they characteristically displace the sternocleidomastoid muscle posterolaterally, the carotid and jugular vessels posteromedially, and the submandibular gland anteriorly. The contents of the cysts are known to vary from watery fluid to a gelatinous, mucoid material.[6]

INFLAMMATORY LESIONS

There are many possible causes of inflammation in the floor of the mouth. One of the most common is the spread of a dental infection, usually from the premolar teeth or the first molar tooth. Other causes include penetrating trauma, obstructing submandibular duct calculi, and intravenous drug use.[7] Noninfectious inflammatory disorders in this region include systemic disorders affecting the salivary glands, such as autoimmune diseases and sarcoidosis. The mandibular teeth and mylohyoid sling have a relationship that determines which space is primarily involved by dental infections. The apices of the second and third molars lie below the mylohyoid ridge such that apical infections tend to involve the submandibular space, primarily, whereas infections of the first or premolar root apices, located above the mylohyoid ridge, involve the sublingual space.

Cellulitis/Abscess

Cellulitis is a diffuse infection that involves cutaneous and subcutaneous tissues.

On imaging studies, thickening of the skin, edematous fat, and enhancement of the fascial planes are all easily identified. If myositis is also present, there is enlargement of the involved muscle. Abscesses are single or multiloculated collections that usually conform to the fascial spaces. On CT, they are typically low-density collections that show peripheral rim enhancement. Signs of surrounding cellulitis may also be present. On MRI, the collections are usually hypointense to isointense on T1-weighted imaging and hyperintense on T2-weighted imaging (**Fig. 4**A, B).

Ludwig Angina

Ludwig angina is a severe form of cellulitis, usually caused by streptococcal or staphylococcal bacteria. Before the development of antibiotics, the infection often spread

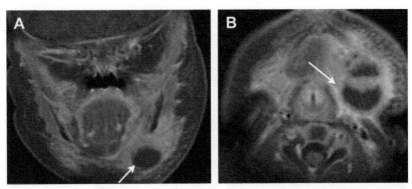

Fig. 4. Cellulitis with abscess. Postcontrast MR images reveal a multiloculated abscess (*arrows*) in the submandibular space with thick enhancing walls, thickening of overlying muscle and fat stranding.

inferiorly along fascial planes into the mediastinum, thus producing chest pain. The diagnosis of Ludwig angina requires that 4 criteria be met: (1) the process always involves both the sublingual and submandibular spaces (**Fig. 5**A) and is frequently bilateral; (2) there is gangrene or serosanguinous phlegmon but little or no frank pus; (3) it involves connective tissue, fascia, and muscle but spares glandular structures (see **Fig. 5**B); and (4) it spreads by contiguity, not by lymphatics. Ludwig angina is typically encountered in association with a 2-day to 4-day history of prior mandibular dental extraction. Infections of the mandibular molars account for up to 90% of reported cases. On imaging studies, Ludwig angina appears as a diffuse cellulitis. The role of imaging is to determine airway patency, document the presence of any gas producing organisms, detect any underlying dental infection, detect osteomyelitis, and identify any drainable abscess.[8] Early recognition and treatment are vital. Treatment is aimed at securing the airway and includes intravenous antibiotics and surgical decompression of the submandibular space. Ludwig angina is associated with a mortality of up to 10%.

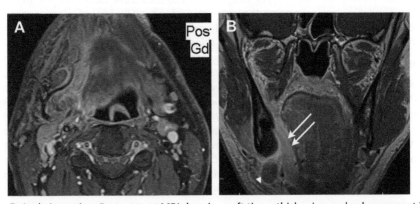

Fig. 5. Ludwig angina. Postcontrast MRI showing soft tissue thickening and enhancement in the right sublingual and submandibular spaces with involvement of mylohyoid (*arrows*) and sparing of the submandibular gland (*arrowhead*). There is gangrene or serosanguinous phlegmon but no frank pus.

Submandibular Duct Obstruction

The main submandibular duct (Wharton duct), which courses through the sublingual space, may become obstructed by calculi or strictures. The submandibular gland, which accounts for 85% of all salivary gland calculi, is prone to calculous disease because of the high mucus content and viscous nature of its secretions. Between 80% and 90% of the calculi are opaque and therefore visible on radiographs.[9] CT has the highest sensitivity for the detection of submandibular gland calculi (**Fig. 6**), particularly when multiple calculi are present.[10] Although US is operator dependent, it can reliably depict ductal obstruction and calculi as small as 3 mm.[11]

Sialography can show the cause of a ductal stricture that is not evident at CT or US. Strictures may be secondary to a calculus, recurrent infection, autoimmune disease, or, more rarely, trauma.[12] Sialography is the traditional reference standard for showing ductal obstruction and its cause, and it is capable of depicting third-order branches of the duct. However, the technique is invasive and has a failure rate of 14%. With a failure rate of only 5%, magnetic resonance (MR) sialography may be a better alternative; it is less invasive and does not require the exposure of patients to ionizing radiation. Several investigators who studied diagnostic performance with MR sialography (performed by using T2-weighted three-dimensional constructive interference in steady state and half-Fourier single-shot turbo spin-echo sequences) found it comparable with conventional sialography for detecting the cause of ductal obstruction.[13]

VASCULAR LESIONS

The classification and nomenclature used to describe endothelial malformations has been a source of confusion. The most widely accepted classification system, by Mulliken and Glowacki,[14] separates endothelial malformations into 2 large groups, hemangiomas and vascular malformations, from their natural history, cellular turnover, and histology.

Hemangiomas tend to be small or absent at birth and often are not initially noticed by parents and caregivers. Shortly after birth they undergo a proliferative phase, with rapid growth that may last several months. They then undergo a stationary period, followed by a period of involution. In contrast, vascular malformations are always present at birth and enlarge in proportion to the growth of the child. They do not involute and

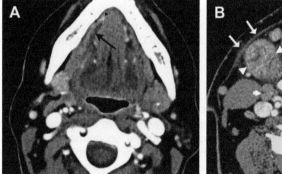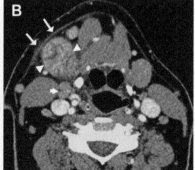

Fig. 6. Submandibular sialadenitis with sialolithiasis: Dilatation of the right Wharton duct (*A; arrows*) with small calculus at tip (*arrowhead*). The submandibular gland is enlarged and shows increased heterogeneous enhancement (*B; arrowhead*). There is thickening of overlying muscle (*thin arrows*) with reactive lymphadenopathy (*thick arrows*).

remain present throughout the patient's life. Vascular malformations are subcategorized as lymphatic, capillary, venous, arteriovenous, and mixed malformations from their histologic makeup. Although MRI has been used to classify vascular malformations into one of these categories, a more pertinent issue is classifying vascular malformations as either low-flow or high-flow lesions. Malformations with arterial components are considered high-flow lesions and those without arterial components are considered low-flow lesions.[15]

Low-Flow Lesions

Infantile hemangiomas (capillary hemangiomas) are true vascular neoplasms that usually manifest by age 3 months, proliferate in the first year, and involute by age 9 years. The diagnosis is based on clinical information, and imaging is not usually required.

Low-flow venous malformations (eg, cavernous hemangiomas) in the head and neck occur most frequently in the buccal space or the floor of the mouth. The lesions are compressible and have a hypoechoic, heterogeneous appearance with multiple anechoic sinusoidal spaces on US images. The slowing of flow in a lesion is often undetectable at power Doppler imaging and conventional angiography. MRI and CT are preferred because they allow a complete evaluation of the extent and transspatial dimensions of the lesions. Depending on the size of the venous channels, low-flow lesions range from predominantly cystic masses with high-signal-intensity venous lakes on T2-weighted fat-saturated MR images to more solid lesions with signal isointense to that of muscle. The lesions may contain calcified phleboliths, which appear as round foci that are devoid of signal on MR images and show high attenuation on CT images.

Lymphatic malformations (lymphangiomas), of which cystic hygromas are the most common, usually manifest as transspatial cystic masses within the first 2 years of life. They are most commonly located in the posterior triangle of the neck and affect the submandibular space (**Fig. 7**A) more frequently than the floor of the mouth. A transspatial, multilocular mass with fluid-fluid levels at MRI and a lack of phleboliths suggests the diagnosis.[2]

High-Flow Lesions

Arteriovenous malformations (high-flow vascular malformations) of the head and neck are rare lesions with unclear pathogenesis. They usually present during childhood, growing proportionately with the child. The lesions are best depicted on MR images, in which they appear as ill-defined masses with multiple flow voids (see **Fig. 7**B), a large feeding artery (see **Fig. 7**C) or draining vein, and, occasionally, intraosseous extension.[16]

NEOPLASTIC LESIONS
Benign Lesions

Benign neoplasms of the submandibular space include lipomas, benign mixed tumors (pleomorphic adenomas) of the salivary glands, and neural sheath tumors. Nerve sheath tumors (schwannomas and neurofibromas) are uncommon in this region. Neurofibromas are mostly associated with neurofibromatosis. Schwannomas (neurilemmomas) tend to occur in the fourth decade of life, arising from peripheral motor, sensory, and sympathetic nerves, most commonly in women. Schwannomas arising from the lingual and hypoglossal nerves in the floor of the mouth have been reported.[17]

Lipomas are common mesenchymal tumors with most occurring in the posterior aspect of the neck. They rarely develop in the anterior aspect of the neck,

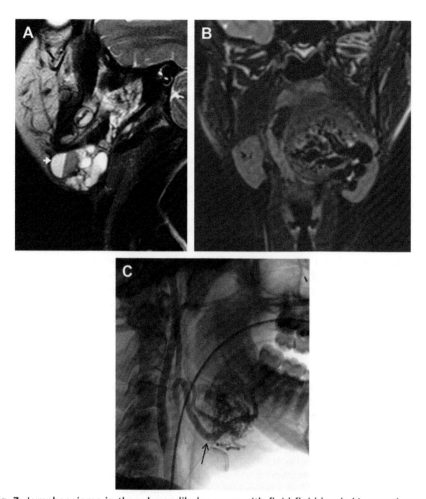

Fig. 7. Lymphangioma in the submandibular space with fluid-fluid levels (*A; arrow*) represents a low-flow vascular lesion. Large arteriovenous malformation involving the left sublingual space (*B*) with multiple flow voids, representing a high-flow lesion. The arterial supply on the angiogram (*C*) is predominantly through the lingual artery (*arrow*).

infratemporal fossa, oral cavity, larynx, tonsil, and parotid region. Lipomas can be differentiated from normal fatty deposits by their internal architecture, their mass effect on adjacent structures, and their metabolic behavior. Most are well-defined encapsulated masses found just beneath the skin or between muscles and other connective-tissue structures. The imaging characteristics of classic lipomas include attenuation equivalent to that of subcutaneous fat on CT images and high signal intensity on both T1-weighted and T2-weighted MR images. On fat-suppressed images, the signal within lipomas drops out completely. Thin septa occasionally can be seen within the tumors, but simple lipomas rarely present a diagnostic challenge.[18]

Benign salivary gland neoplasms

Most benign neoplasms in submandibular space are pleomorphic adenomas (benign mixed tumors).[18] Pleomorphic adenomas rarely occur in the sublingual space. Only

1% of pleomorphic adenomas are found in the sublingual gland. At CT, pleomorphic adenomas typically appear as well-defined homogeneous lesions with attenuation slightly higher than that of muscle. At MRI, the lesions have variable signal intensity depending on the presence and extent of necrosis, hemorrhage, or cystic change.[2] Other rare salivary gland tumors include Warthin tumor/adenolymphoma, onconcytoma, monomorphic adenoma, and benign fibroma.[19]

Malignant Lesions

Squamous cell carcinoma
The most common malignant tumor that occurs in the oral cavity and floor of mouth is squamous cell carcinoma (SCCA), which accounts for more than 90% of malignant oral cavity lesions. When encountered in the sublingual or submandibular space, it usually indicates spread from the tongue base or adjacent oral tongue.[8] SCCA occurs mostly in men aged 45 years and older and is associated with tobacco and alcohol consumption. The typical SCCA is an ulcerated, infiltrative lesion (**Fig. 8**A, B). However, some tumors may be superficial without deep extension. Radiologic staging is often performed and is based on the TNM (tumor, node, metastasis) classification scheme developed by the American Joint Committee on Cancer.[20] MRI, with its superior soft tissue resolution, allows more accurate classification of these tumors and involved nodes than is achievable with CT. In addition, bone marrow involvement and perineural spread are better depicted by MRI. In 20% of cases of SCCA of the floor of the mouth, metastases are identified in submental, submandibular, and upper deep cervical nodal groups.

Malignant salivary gland tumors
Malignancies of the salivary glands in the floor of the mouth are uncommon; less than 10% of all salivary gland tumors arise in the sublingual and minor salivary glands. However, most of these tumors (50%–81%) are malignant. Adenoid cystic carcinoma is the most common such malignancy. It is usually slow growing, has a propensity for perineural spread, and may be indistinguishable from SCCA at imaging. Perineural spread is best shown on contrast-enhanced T1-weighted fat-saturated MR images, in which its typical manifestation is an enlarged, enhancing nerve. On CT images, perineural spread is shown as enlargement of the neural foramen. Mucoepidermoid

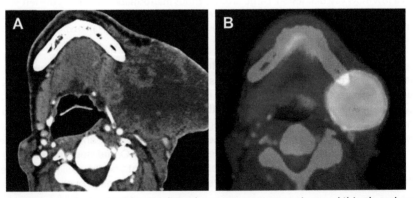

Fig. 8. Contrast-enhanced CT shows a large heterogeneous necrotic mass (*A*) in the submandibular space with overlying skin ulceration. The mass shows intensely increased fluorodeoxyglucose uptake (*B*) on positron emission tomography/CT. SCCA accounts for more than 90% of malignant oral cavity lesions.

carcinoma is the second most common malignant neoplasm of the submandibular gland after adenoid cystic carcinoma. Metastatic cervical lymphadenopathy is more common in cases of mucoepidermoid carcinoma.[2]

Lymphoma/malignant adenopathy

Lymphoma is the most common malignant tumor of the head and neck in children. Hodgkin lymphoma has a predilection for internal jugular chain lymph nodes, often with involvement of contiguous nodal groups in the mediastinum. Non-Hodgkin lymphoma frequently manifests as noncontiguous adenopathy and more commonly shows extranodal disease, frequently involving Waldeyer ring. Enlarged lymph nodes in lymphoma are generally homogeneous, and calcifications are rare in the absence of prior therapy, particularly radiation. No reliable size criteria exist for distinguishing benign, reactive from lymphomatous adenopathy. Nodal biopsy is required for diagnosis. Fluorodeoxyglucose (FDG) positron emission tomography typically shows high FDG avidity for nodal and non-nodal disease.[21] Central necrosis is rare unless treatment has been given, and this may help distinguish lymphoma from metastatic adenopathy, which frequently has central necrosis. Submandibular and jugulodigastric adenopathy of less than 2 cm in diameter is present in 30% of patients with SCCA of the floor of the mouth.[8]

DENERVATION MUSCLE ATROPHY (PSEUDOTUMORS)

Cranial nerves provide motor supply to various muscles and muscle groups in the head and neck. When the innervation is interrupted by neural involvement with tumor or infection, there is a loss of motor function ipsilateral to the lesion. This loss results in muscle wasting, fatty infiltration, and hemiatrophy of involved muscles.[22] On imaging studies, the fatty atrophy is easily appreciated (**Fig. 9**A, B). However, the asymmetry can be mistaken for tumor because the normal side appears enlarged compared with the atrophic side.

The hypoglossal nerve provides motor innervation to the intrinsic and extrinsic muscles of the tongue. Lesions that affect the nerve can produce muscle atrophy and fatty replacement in 2 to 3 weeks. When present, a search for abnormalities must be made along the entire course of the hypoglossal nerve, including the

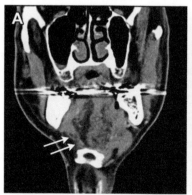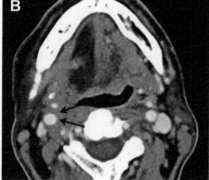

Fig. 9. Coronal (*A*) And axial (*B*) CT images show marked atrophy of the right mylohyoid muscle (*arrows*), submandibular gland, and sublingual gland with fatty replacement of the right half of the tongue caused by denervation atrophy secondary to perineural malignancy along the carotid sheath (*B; arrows*).

brainstem. The mandibular nerve (V3) provides motor innervation to not only the muscles of mastication, tensor tympani, and tensor palatini muscles but also to the anterior belly of the digastric muscle and the mylohyoid muscle via the mylohyoid nerve. Injury to the mandibular nerve results in fatty atrophy of all the muscle bundles, whereas isolated injury to the mylohyoid nerve results in fatty infiltration and atrophy of only the anterior belly of the digastric and mylohyoid muscles. As with hypoglossal injury, a search for neural disorders along the entire course of the nerve, back to the brainstem, is required when V3 atrophy is identified.[23]

SURGICAL APPROACH

Of the surgical approaches for the benign submandibular disorders, the transcervical approach is the most widely accepted and simple, and the salivary gland tissue can be removed without difficulty and without alteration of the salivary system. However, the transcervical procedure has frequently been associated with neurologic complications after surgery, including the marginal mandibular nerve and lingual and hypoglossal nerves.[24] Alternative surgical approaches have been developed to avoid neurologic risks and visible scarring in the upper neck. Hong and Kim[25] reported a new surgical approach for intraoral removal of benign submandibular disorders and suggested that the intraoral approach could be extended as an alternative to the transcervical approach. However, this approach also has problems, such as temporal sensory paresis and limited movement of the tongue, but this resolved spontaneously, and, in the severe adhesion to surrounding tissue, the intraoral dissection of gland is not easily accomplished. For lesions superior to the mylohyoid muscle (sublingual space), an intraoral approach is preferable because it preserves the mylohyoid muscle.[1]

REFERENCES

1. Vogl TJ, Steger W, Ihrler S, et al. Cystic masses in the floor of the mouth: value of MR imaging in planning surgery. Am J Roentgenol 1993;161(1):183–6.
2. La'porte SJ, Juttla JK, Lingam RK. Imaging the floor of the mouth and the sublingual space. Radiographics 2011;31(5):1215–30.
3. Kurabayashi T, Nakamura S, Ogura I, et al. The sublingual and submandibular spaces. Oral Radiol 2003;19(2):28–34.
4. Kurabayashi T, Ida M, Yasumoto M, et al. MRI of ranulas. Neuroradiology 2000; 42(12):917–22.
5. Colt WE, Harnsberger HR, Osborn AG, et al. Ranulas and their mimics: CT evaluation. Radiology 1987;163:211–6.
6. Kurabayashi T, Ida M, Sasaki T. Differential diagnosis of submandibular cystic lesions by computed tomography. Dentomaxillofac Radiol 1991;20:30–4.
7. Wiggins R. Oral cavity. In: Harnsberger HR, editor. Diagnostic imaging: head and neck. Salt Lake City (Utah): Amirsys; 2004. III-4-6–III-4-48.
8. Laine FJ, Smoker W. Oral cavity: anatomy and pathology. Semin Ultrasound CT MR 1995;116(6):527–45.
9. Jäger L, Menauer F, Holzknecht N, et al. Sialolithiasis: MR sialography of the submandibular duct—an alternative to conventional sialography and US? Radiology 2000;216(3):665–71.
10. Yousem DM, Kraut MA, Chalian AA. Major salivary gland imaging. Radiology 2000;216(1):19–29.
11. Rinast E, Gmelin E, Hollands-Thorn B. Digital subtraction sialography, conventional sialography, high-resolution ultrasonography and computed tomography in the diagnosis of salivary gland diseases. Eur J Radiol 1989;9(4):224–30.

12. Becker M, Marchal F, Becker CD, et al. Sialolithiasis and salivary ductal stenosis: diagnostic accuracy of MR sialography with a three-dimensional extended-phase conjugate-symmetry rapid spin-echo sequence. Radiology 2000;217(2): 347–58.
13. Kalinowski M, Heverhagen JT, Rehberg E, et al. Comparative study of MR sialography and digital subtraction sialography for benign salivary gland disorders. AJNR Am J Neuroradiol 2002;23(9):1485–92.
14. Mulliken JB, Glowacki J. Hemangiomas and vascular malformations in infants and children: a classification based on endothelial characteristics. Plast Reconstr Surg 1982;69:412–22.
15. Donnelly LF, Adams DM, Bisset GS. Vascular malformations and hemangiomas: a practical approach in a multidisciplinary clinic. Am J Roentgenol 2000;174: 597–608.
16. Chimona TS, Papadakis CE, Hatzidakis AA, et al. Arteriovenous malformation of the floor of the mouth: a case report. Eur Arch Otorhinolaryngol 2005;262(11): 939–42.
17. Kawakami R, Kaneko T, Kadoya M, et al. Schwannoma in the sublingual space. Dentomaxillofac Radiol 2004;33(4):259–61.
18. Razek AA, Huang BY. Soft tissue tumors of the head and neck: imaging-based review of the WHO classification. Radiographics 2011;31(7):1923–54.
19. Munir N, Bradley PJ. Diagnosis and management of neoplastic lesions of the submandibular triangle. Oral Oncol 2008;44:251–60.
20. Lip and oral cavity. In: Edge SB, Byrd DR, Compton CC, et al, editors. AJCC cancer staging manual. 7th edition. New York: Springer; 2010. p. 29–35.
21. Friedman E, John S. Imaging of pediatric neck masses. Radiol Clin North Am 2011;49:617–32.
22. Harnsberger HR, Dillon WP. Major motor atrophic patterns in the face and neck: CT evaluation. Radiology 1985;155:665–70.
23. Larsson SG. Hemiatrophy of the tongue and floor of the mouth demonstrated by computed tomography. J Comput Assist Tomogr 1995;9:914–8.
24. Hong KH, Yang YS. Surgical results of the intraoral removal of the submandibular gland. Otolaryngol Head Neck Surg 2008;139:530–4.
25. Hong KH, Kim YK. Intraoral removal of the submandibular gland: a new surgical approach. Otolaryngol Head Neck Surg 2000;122:798–802.

Larynx

Anatomic Imaging for Diagnosis and Management

Benjamin Y. Huang, MD, MPH[a],*, Michael Solle, MD, PhD[a,b],
Mark C. Weissler, MD[c]

KEYWORDS

- Diagnostic imaging • Anatomic imaging • Head and neck • Larynx • Vocal cords
- Laryngeal cancer

KEY POINTS

- Radiologic imaging plays a critical role in guiding the diagnosis and treatment of a variety of benign and malignant diseases of the larynx along with the primary tools of laryngoscopy and biopsy.
- Cross-sectional imaging is essential for evaluating the submucosal and deep tissues of the larynx, which are not amenable to direct visualization, and for assessing extension of disease into adjacent spaces in the neck.
- Rapidity of image acquisition in CT is particularly advantageous for general imaging, because it allows CT to be less susceptible to artifacts caused by swallowing and breathing, which frequently result in suboptimal or nondiagnostic magnetic resonance (MR) studies.
- MRI has 2 distinct advantages over CT for head and neck imaging: (1) it does not require exposure to ionizing radiation and (2) it provides superior soft tissue contrast compared with CT.

INTRODUCTION

Although direct laryngoscopy and biopsy remain the primary tools for evaluating patients with suspected laryngeal pathology, radiologic imaging often plays a critical role in guiding the diagnosis and treatment of a variety of benign and malignant diseases of the larynx. Cross-sectional imaging is essential for evaluating the submucosal and deep tissues of the larynx, which are not amenable to direct visualization, and for assessing extension of disease into adjacent spaces in the neck. Questions of when to order radiologic tests and which tests to order may arise, particularly

[a] Department of Radiology, University of North Carolina School of Medicine, 101 Manning Drive, CB #7510, Chapel Hill, NC 27599, USA; [b] VHA National Teleradiology Program, Durham, NC, USA; [c] Division of Head and Neck Oncology, Department of Otolaryngology/Head and Neck Surgery, University of North Carolina School of Medicine, 101 Manning Drive, CB #7070, Chapel Hill, NC 27599, USA
* Corresponding author.
E-mail address: bhuang@med.unc.edu

Otolaryngol Clin N Am 45 (2012) 1325–1361
http://dx.doi.org/10.1016/j.otc.2012.08.006
0030-6665/12/$ – see front matter © 2012 Elsevier Inc. All rights reserved.

when considering the numerous and constantly changing options for laryngeal imaging currently available. Furthermore, interpretation of studies relies on a firm grasp of normal radiologic anatomy and its variability as well as familiarity with the common entities occurring in the larynx and their characteristic imaging features. The goal of this article is to provide an overview of fundamental aspects of laryngeal imaging for otolaryngologists. The initial sections cover commonly used imaging techniques, relevant cross-sectional anatomy of the larynx, and indications for ordering imaging studies, whereas the later sections review the imaging features of commonly encountered diseases of the larynx.

IMAGING TECHNIQUES
CT

At many institutions, including the University of North Carolina (UNC), CT is the preferred imaging modality for initial evaluation of the larynx and the neck due to its widespread availability, familiarity to clinicians, and rapidity of image acquisition. The last feature is particularly advantageous for general imaging, because it allows CT to be less susceptible to artifacts caused by swallowing and breathing, which frequently result in suboptimal or nondiagnostic MR studies. A routine neck CT performed on a modern 64-slice multidetector CT scanner takes approximately 10 seconds to acquire with coverage from the skull base to the carina. Unlike early-generation scanners, current multidetector CT scanners also offer excellent spatial resolution and allow for high-quality multiplanar images to be reconstructed in any orientation. Although the soft tissue contrast of CT does not match that of MRI, it is usually adequate for diagnosis and for guiding treatment decisions. Furthermore, CT surpasses MRI in its ability to identify calcification within lesions and to assess fine bone detail.

Unless there is a clear contraindication, the authors recommend that all routine scans be performed with intravenous iodinated contrast. Patients with a documented allergy to iodinated contrast or a history of renal insufficiency can be scanned without contrast, but the absence of intravenous contrast on CT reduces the ability to detect, delineate, and characterize primary lesions; makes it difficult to differentiate blood vessels from lymph nodes; limits the ability to identify abnormal lymph node morphology; and makes it impossible to assess vascular patency. Routine use of multiphase CT scans performed "with and without" contrast or with early-phase (arterial) and late-phase (venous) postcontrast imaging should be avoided altogether, because the additional scanning multiplies patient radiation exposure, while typically providing little or no additional useful information.

Neck CT protocol
At UNC, the routine neck CT protocol calls for imaging during quiet breathing or with an expiratory breath hold. Scanning is initiated after a postinjection delay of approximately 40 seconds to allow for adequate vascular and soft tissue enhancement. From the acquired data set, 3-mm–thick slices are reconstructed in axial, coronal, and sagittal planes for viewing with both soft tissue and bone windows. In some circumstances, it may be useful to reconstruct the images using thinner sections, in a nonstandard oblique imaging plane, or use a 3-D volume rendered technique to better delineate certain anatomic structures, such as the true vocal cords and laryngeal ventricles.

Considerations in imaging outcomes for diagnosis
The data derived from the combination of direct laryngoscopy and a routine contrast-enhanced neck CT are sufficient for diagnosis and for planning and initiating treatment in the majority of patients; however, in rare instances, the results of this initial work-up

may be inconclusive or may not adequately depict the extent of a lesion or its relationship to nearby structures. This is commonly the case with small lesions, which can be hidden due to apposition of adjacent anatomic structures. Furthermore, on scans performed during apnea or quiet breathing, the true vocal cords and laryngeal ventricles are often poorly delineated, which may make it difficult to assess transglottic tumor spread.[1]

In these instances, additional imaging acquired while a patient performs specific dynamic maneuvers may better define these structures. The most useful of these maneuvers are the modified Valsalva maneuver (blowing through pursed lips or a pursed nose) and phonation (saying "eee" continuously and uniformly). The former technique has the effect of opening the glottis and distending the laryngeal vestibule and piriform sinuses, thus allowing better visualization of lesions of the vestibule and hypopharynx. The true and false cords are abducted with this technique and are, therefore, often difficult to distinguish. Phonation causes the true and false cords to become adducted and provides excellent visualization of these structures and the intervening laryngeal ventricle, thus allowing more accurate determination of tumor spread across the ventricle.[1] This technique can also be useful for confirming suspected vocal cord paralysis.[2]

MRI

MRI has at least 2 distinct advantages over CT for head and neck imaging:

1. It does not require exposure to ionizing radiation.
2. It provides superior soft tissue contrast compared with CT.

The second factor can be particularly advantageous for precisely delineating tumor boundaries and for evaluation of cartilaginous invasion by tumor.[3,4] Nonetheless, MRI is primarily used as a second-line tool for laryngeal imaging at most centers because current imaging protocols take substantially longer to acquire, and the images are more likely to be degraded by motion caused by breathing and swallowing. Furthermore, MR cannot be performed in patients with certain implanted devices and retained metallic foreign bodies.

Neck MRI protocol

Routine neck MRI at UNC is performed with a dedicated multichannel neck coil and takes approximately 20 to 25 minutes to complete. The authors' protocol includes a coronal short tau inversion recovery (STIR) acquisition, axial T1-weighted and T2-weighted images, and sagittal and coronal T1-weighted images acquired before administration of intravenous contrast. T1-weighted images are particularly good for assessing anatomy and fat-containing spaces, which are normally hyperintense (bright) relative to soft tissues, such as muscle. T2-weighted and STIR images are useful for identifying fluid and tissue edema, and most laryngeal tumors also tend to demonstrate increased signal intensity on these sequences. Unless gadolinium is contraindicated, T1-weighted images after intravenous administration of a gadolinium-containing contrast agent are then obtained in all 3 planes, preferably with fat suppression. Contraindications to giving MR contrast include significant renal impairment, which is associated with a risk of developing nephrogenic systemic fibrosis and known allergies to gadolinium chelates.

Fluorodeoxyglucose F 18–Positron Emission Tomography

In the head and neck, fluorodeoxyglucose F 18 (FDG)–positron emission tomography (PET) is primarily used for the staging and post-treatment follow-up of cancers, in particular squamous cell carcinomas. FDG is a glucose analog that is transported across cell membranes and subsequently becomes trapped within cells after phosphorylation. Increased uptake of the radiopharmaceutical is seen in processes in which there is increased cellular metabolism, including malignant tumors and their metastases and inflammatory processes. At UNC, whole-body PET imaging is performed 1 hour after intravenous injection of approximately 12 mCi of FDG. The acquired PET images are coregistered to CT images obtained concurrently on the same dedicated PET/CT scanner, which improves tumor localization.

IMAGING ANATOMY OF THE LARYNX

The larynx is a dynamic organ system that is responsible for maintaining and protecting the airway and allowing phonation. It maintains its shape via a rigid supporting skeleton composed of the hyoid bone superiorly and the epiglottic, thyroid, arytenoid, and cricoid cartilages more inferiorly (**Figs. 1–3**). These osseous and cartilaginous structures are connected by various membranes, ligaments, and joints, and their interior surfaces are covered by laryngeal epithelial mucosa, which extends from the base of the tongue superiorly to the trachea inferiorly.[5]

Epiglottis

The epiglottis is an extremely flexible, leaf-shaped sheet of elastic cartilage, which tapers to a point inferiorly (the petiole) and attaches to the thyroid cartilage just above the anterior commissure. The suprahyoid portion of the epiglottis projects obliquely upward behind the tongue base and functions to protect the larynx during swallowing (see **Fig. 2**).

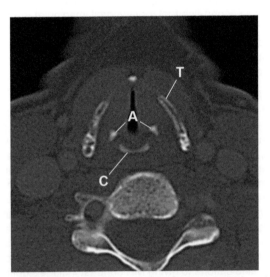

Fig. 1. Axial bone algorithm CT image through the glottis in a 40-year-old woman demonstrates the normal appearance of laryngeal cartilage ossification. Ossified cartilage demonstrates high-attenuation cortex peripherally and a central lower attenuation medullary space, which in this case is best demonstrated in the chevron shaped thyroid cartilage (T). Normal variability of the progression of this ossification process is present, best seen along the left lateral aspect of the thyroid cartilage in this patient, where there is no dense cortex present along a short segment. A, arytenoids; C, cricoid.

Laryngeal Cartilages

The thyroid cartilage spans the length of the true and false vocal folds. On axial CT and MRI, this cartilage has the appearance of a chevron or inverted V (see **Fig. 1**). The cricoid cartilage forms a complete ring, which is taller posteriorly and spans the length of the subglottis. The posterior lamina of the cricoid extends cranially to the level of the arytenoid cartilages with which it articulates to form the cricoarytenoid joints. The paired arytenoid cartilages are pyramidal shaped structures that are perched along the superior edge of the posterior cricoid lamina and span the laryngeal ventricle. At the base of each arytenoid is an anterior projection referred to as the vocal process, which serves as the posterior attachment of the vocal ligament and demarcates the level of the true vocal cord.[6]

In most adults, the laryngeal cartilages are easy to identify on CT because they are, with the exception of the epiglottis, usually ossified. Ossified cartilage demonstrates high-attenuation (calcified) cortex peripherally and a central lower attenuation medullary space (see **Fig. 1**). There is, however, considerable variability in the normal degree of cartilage ossification, both between individuals and across ages. In addition, ossified cortex frequently appears discontinuous or can be asymmetric in normal individuals, which can make it difficult to differentiate tumor invasion from normal cortical discontinuity on CT. Ossification of the laryngeal cartilages typically begins in the second decade of life and increases with age, with men tending to show a greater degree of ossification than women later in life.[7]

On MRI, nonossified cartilage demonstrates intermediate to low signal on both T1-weighted and T2-weighted images. With ossification, the cortex eventually becomes calcified and demonstrates very low signal intensity on all MR sequences, whereas the medullary portion transitions to the signal intensity of fat (high on T1-weighted images).[8]

The larynx is traditionally divided into 3 separate yet contiguous parts:

1. Supraglottis
2. Glottis
3. Subglottis

Supraglottis

The supraglottis extends from the base of the tongue (glossoepiglottic and pharyngoepiglottic folds, specifically) to the apex of the laryngeal ventricle and contains the epiglottis, the anterior aspect of the aryepiglottic folds, the false vocal cords, the laryngeal ventricle, and the arytenoid cartilages. An important midline imaging landmark in the supraglottis is the preepiglottic space, which is a fat-containing space situated between the ventral surface of the epiglottis posteriorly and the hyoid bone, thyrohyoid membrane, and thyroid cartilage anteriorly. Its upper margin is formed by the thyrohyoid ligament and its caudal margin is the thyroepiglottic ligament.[6,9]

Posteriorly, the supraglottis communicates with the hypopharynx, with which it shares a significant continuous mucosal interface and is separated by the aryepiglottic folds. At the base of the supraglottis, demarcating it from the glottis, are the laryngeal ventricles and the upper arytenoid cartilages. Axial images through the supraglottis are useful for visualizing the epiglottis, aryepiglottic folds, false vocal cords, and arytenoids, whereas coronal images nicely demonstrate the false vocal folds and laryngeal ventricles (see **Figs. 2** and **3**).

Glottis

The glottis consists of the soft tissues of the thyroarytenoid musculature and vocal ligament, which are essentially indistinguishable on imaging studies and together make up the true vocal cords. The glottis is defined as extending from the apex of the laryngeal ventricle to 1 cm below that level. The vocal ligaments meet anteriorly at the anterior commissure. Axial and coronal images are most useful for assessing the true vocal folds, with the midcoronal plane best depicting the relationship between the true cords, laryngeal ventricles, and false cords (see **Figs. 2** and **3**). Axial images are most useful for evaluating the anterior commissures, which should normally measure no more than 2 mm in greatest thickness (see **Fig. 2**).[10]

Spanning the lateral supraglottic and glottic regions is a paired compartment known as the paraglottic (or paralaryngeal) space, which resides between the laryngeal mucosa and the inner surface of the thyroid cartilage and is composed of fat, lymphatics, and the intrinsic laryngeal musculature.[5] This space is continuous with

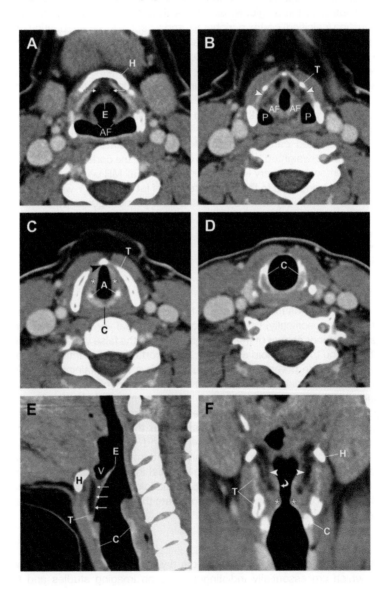

the preepiglottic space superiorly and is bounded inferiorly by the conus elasticus. As in the preepiglottic space, fat in the paraglottic space is often replaced or obscured by pathologic processes, making it an important imaging landmark for detecting submucosal disease spread in the supraglottic larynx. At the glottis, there is generally no fat visible in the paraglottic space, because the thyroarytenoid muscle fills the space at this level.[11] Neither the preepiglottic nor paraglottic spaces are visible endoscopically. Therefore, complete evaluation of these spaces requires cross-sectional imaging, on which they normally demonstrate low density on CT and high signal intensity on T1-weighted MR. The preepiglottic space is generally best viewed on axial and sagittal images, whereas the axial and coronal planes are usually best for depicting the paraglottic spaces (see **Figs. 2** and **3**).

Subglottis

The subglottis contains the inferior part of the cricoid cartilage and extends from the inferior surface of the glottis (as discussed previously, defined by a plane located 1 cm below the apex of the laryngeal ventricle) to the inferior margin of the cricoid cartilage.[11] In the subglottis, the mucosa is closely apposed to the inner surface of the cricoid, so soft tissue is not normally seen between the airway and the cricoid cartilage (see **Fig. 2**).

INDICATIONS FOR IMAGING THE LARYNX
Staging and Surveillance of Squamous Cell Carcinoma

At UNC, the most common indications for laryngeal imaging are initial staging of a suspected or biopsy-proved squamous cell carcinoma and post-treatment surveillance. In the former case, the primary goals of imaging are to evaluate the subsites of the larynx that are involved, to assess the extent of submucosal or extralaryngeal tumor spread, to detect tumor invasion of cartilage, and to identify regional spread to lymph nodes, all of which influence decisions regarding the most appropriate therapy (discussed later).[8]

◄───

Fig. 2. Normal laryngeal anatomy on CT. Axial soft tissue algorithm CT images through the supraglottis at the level of the hyoid bone (A) and false cords (B) nicely depict the low density, fat-containing preepiglottic (arrows) and paraglottic spaces (arrowheads). The aryepiglottic folds (AF) separate the laryngeal airway from the piriform sinuses (P) which reside in the hypopharynx. Axial image at the level of the glottis (C) demonstrates the soft tissue density true vocal cords (asterisks) and the anterior commissure (arrowhead). Fat is not visualized at the level of the true cords because this space is filled primarily by the thyroarytenoid muscle. Note also how there is little or no soft tissue between the symphysis of the thyroid cartilage and the airway at the anterior commissure, which should be less than 2 mm in thickness. On an axial image obtained at the level of the subglottis (D), note how there is no soft tissue visualized between the inner margin of the cricoid cartilage and the airway. Midsagittal image (E) depicts the fat-containing preepiglottic space (arrows) situated between the epiglottis posteriorly and the hyoid, thyroid cartilage, and thyrohyoid membrane anteriorly. In this patient, the cartilages are not well ossified but are still slightly hyperdense relative to muscle. Coronal image (F) through the middle of the laryngeal airway again clearly demonstrates the fat-containing paraglottic spaces (arrowheads), deep to the mucosa of the supraglottis. The curved arrow points to the right false vocal fold, and the muscular true vocal folds are indicated by the asterisks. The slight concavities seen between the true and false vocal folds represent the laryngeal ventricles. As this image was obtained in quiet respiration, the laryngeal ventricles are not as well defined as they would be if the scan was obtained during phonation. A, arytenoids; C, cricoid; E, epiglottis; H, hyoid bone; T, thyroid cartilage; V, vallecula.

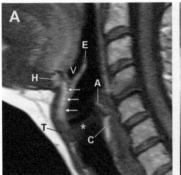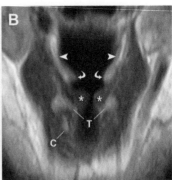

Fig. 3. Normal laryngeal anatomy on MRI. Sagittal T1-weighted image (*A*), obtained just off of the midline nicely depicts the fat-containing preepiglottic space (*arrows*) as a high intensity region situated between the epiglottis posteriorly and the hyoid, thyroid cartilage, and thyrohyoid membrane anteriorly. In this image, one of the intermediate signal intensity true vocal cords (*asterisk*) can also be seen. Coronal T1-weighted image (*B*) through the middle of the laryngeal airway clearly demonstrates the fat-containing paraglottic spaces (*arrowheads*), deep to the mucosa of the supraglottis. The false vocal folds (*curved arrows*) and true vocal folds (*asterisks*) are also well depicted, and in this case the laryngeal ventricles are easily identified as concavities seen between the true and false vocal folds. A, arytenoids; C, cricoid; E, epiglottis; H, hyoid bone; T, thyroid cartilage; V, vallecula.

Evaluation of Submucosal Masses

Occasionally, patients present with an entirely submucosal mass with normal overlying mucosa by direct visualization. These lesions are more likely due to processes other than squamous cell carcinoma, and, in these cases, imaging is indicated to confirm the presence of a mass, to determine the deep structures involved, to characterize the potential etiology of the lesion, and, when necessary, to direct the endoscopist to the optimal site(s) from which to obtain deep biopsies.[8] Although the imaging characteristics of submucosal tumors are often nonspecific, certain lesions may demonstrate typical imaging features that allow a specific diagnosis to be made or guide the differential diagnosis.

Evaluation of Hoarseness and Vocal Cord Paralysis

Laryngoscopy remains the primary diagnostic tool for evaluating patients with dysphonia, and in most cases imaging studies are not indicated because a cause can be identified via direct assessment. Indications in which imaging is warranted include (1) vocal cord paralysis or paresis, (2) presence of a mass or lesion of the vocal fold or larynx that suggests malignancy or airway obstruction, and (3) the need to exclude a potentially reducible arytenoid subluxation or dislocation.[4,12] If a true vocal fold palsy is identified and recent surgery can explain the paralysis, then imaging studies are not usually useful. If the cause of vocal fold paralysis is not evident by history or on laryngoscopy, however, then imaging should be performed rule out a lesion along the course of the vagus or recurrent laryngeal nerve (discussed later). In general, the authors prefer CT for this purpose and reserve MRI for evaluation of pathology suspected at or above the skull base.

Evaluation of Laryngeal Trauma

CT is the imaging study of choice for the initial evaluation of blunt or penetrating laryngeal trauma. It is typically performed in conjunction with direct fiberoptic laryngoscopy and is useful for demonstrating fractures of the laryngeal cartilages and hyoid bone, joint dislocations, submucosal hematomas, and the degree of airway obstruction.[13,14] Whether imaging is indicated in all cases of laryngotracheal injury or only on a selective basis remains an area of debate. Some investigators suggest that CT is not indicated in patients with mild, isolated injuries or in those with severe injuries requiring immediate surgical intervention,[15] whereas other investigators routinely order CT for cases of known or suspected laryngeal trauma once a patient has been stabilized and can be safely transported from an emergency department or operating room.[13]

Evaluation of Laryngotracheal Stenosis

At many centers, CT imaging is routinely performed in the preoperative assessment of patients with laryngotracheal stenosis. The combination of unlimited multiplanar reformatting capabilities and 3-D viewing techniques available with modern multislice scanners and viewing software allows CT to accurately demonstrate the site, length, and severity of stenoses in a noninvasive fashion (**Fig. 4**). Although endoscopy remains the gold standard for endoluminal evaluation of the upper airways, particularly with regards to assessment of the airway mucosa, CT often provides valuable complementary information, because it can demonstrate the presence and distribution of airway thickening, the overall length of the stenotic segment, the presence of associated cartilage fractures, multifocal stenoses, and whether a stenosis is due to external compression from an extraluminal process.[16,17] Furthermore, CT imaging may be better at characterizing high-grade and total stenoses (Cotton grades III and IV), which often cannot be negotiated with a rigid endoscope.[17]

IMAGING OF SPECIFIC LARYNGEAL PATHOLOGIES
Squamous Cell Carcinoma

Approximately 12,760 new cases of laryngeal cancer are diagnosed in the United States annually, with an estimated 3560 deaths caused by the disease every year.[18] Of these, more than 90% are squamous cell carcinomas.[8] Proper interpretation of imaging studies performed for known or suspected carcinomas of the larynx depends on

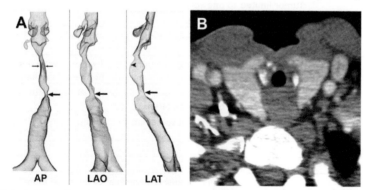

Fig. 4. Subglottic and tracheal stenosis in a 26-year-old man who previously underwent emergent cricothyroidotomy with prolonged intubation for trauma, now with persistent dyspnea since being decannulated. (*A*) Anteroposterior (AP), left anterior oblique (LAO), and lateral (LAT) projections from a 3-D CT surface shaded reconstruction of the airway demonstrate a long segment stenosis of the subglottis and trachea, with a focal area of severe proximal tracheal narrowing (*large arrows*). (*Arrowhead*) Anterior commissure; (*small arrows*) true vocal fold level. Axial CT image through the subglottis (*B*) Demonstrates circumferential soft tissue thickening along the airway wall and fragmentation of the cricoid cartilage.

knowledge of typical patterns of spread of disease based on the site of origin of the tumor, with particular attention to the findings that change the staging of the cancer and can, therefore, affect treatment planning and outcomes. Malignancies of the larynx are staged by the TNM system defined by the International Union Against Cancer and the American Joint Commission on Cancer, which is used to help determine patient treatment and prognosis and to facilitate clinical research. The clinical or pretherapeutic

Tumor (T) Stage	Description
Table 1 T staging for laryngeal carcinoma	
TX	Primary tumor cannot be assessed
T0	No evidence of primary tumor
Tis	Carcinoma in situ
Supraglottis	
T1	Tumor limited to one subsite of supraglottis with normal vocal cord mobility
T2	Tumor invades mucosa of more than one adjacent subsite of supraglottis or glottis or region outside the supraglottis without fixation of the larynx
T3	Tumor limited to larynx with vocal cord fixation and/or invades any of the following: postcricoid area, preepiglottic space, paraglottic space, and/or inner cortex of thyroid cartilage
T4a	Tumor invades through the thyroid cartilage and/or invades tissues beyond the larynx
T4b	Tumor invades prevertebral space, encases carotid artery, or invades mediastinal structures
Glottis	
T1	Tumor limited to the vocal cord(s) with normal mobility (may involve anterior or posterior commissure)
T1a	Tumor limited to one vocal cord
T1b	Tumor involves both vocal cords
T2	Tumor extends to supraglottis and/or subglottis, and/or with impaired vocal cord mobility
T3	Tumor limited to the larynx with vocal cord fixation and/or invasion of paraglottic space, and/or inner cortex of the thyroid cartilage
T4a	Tumor invades through the outer cortex of the thyroid cartilage and/or invades tissues beyond the larynx
T4b	Tumor invades prevertebral space, encases carotid artery, or invades mediastinal structures
Subglottis	
T1	Tumor limited to the subglottis
T2	Tumor extends to vocal cord(s) with normal or impaired mobility
T3	Tumor limited to larynx with vocal cord fixation
T4a	Tumor invades cricoids or thyroid cartilage and/or invades tissues beyond the larynx
T4b	Tumor invades prevertebral space, encases carotid artery, or invades mediastinal structures

Adapted from Larynx. In: American Joint Committee on Cancer, editor. AJCC cancer staging manual. 7th edition. New York: Springer; 2010. p. 57–67; with permission.

classification of the primary tumor (summarized in **Table 1**) is based on site of origin of the original lesion and the extent of invasion into the adjacent structures.[19]

Supraglottic cancers

Supraglottic cancers account for 30% of all carcinomas of the larynx[8] and can arise from any subsite within the supraglottis, including the suprahyoid epiglottis, infrahyoid epiglottis, laryngeal surface of the aryepiglottic folds, laryngeal ventricles, and false cords. Depending on their subsite of origin, they have typical patterns of spread. Lesions arising from the infrahyoid epiglottis, which normally contains numerous perforations, typically invades the preepiglottic fat early on or may extend to the anterior commissure, and then invades the glottis and subglottis. Lesions arising more superiorly in the epiglottis can spread to adjacent sites such as the base of tongue. Tumors arising from the false cords, aryepiglottic fold, or laryngeal ventricle often invade the adjacent paraglottic fat, and submucosal extension of disease can be extensive.

Glottic cancers

Glottic squamous cell cancers account for 65% of laryngeal cancers and usually arise from the anterior portion of the vocal cord.[8] Their typical route of spread is to the anterior commissure. Once tumor reaches the anterior commissure, spread to the thyroarytenoid muscle, contralateral vocal cord, paraglottic spaces, and supraglottis or subglottis can occur. The term, *transglottic*, applies to any tumor that involves both the supraglottis and glottis at the time of diagnosis. These tumors often traverse the laryngeal ventricle, and because there is a gap at this level between the conus elasticus below and the quadrangular ligament above, which each form a barrier to deep tumor invastion, transglottic tumors can spread freely into the paraglottic space.

Subglottic cancers

Tumors arising primarily from the subglottis are less common than subglottic extension of glottic and supraglottic tumors. These primary tumors account for approximately 5% of laryngeal cancers and tend to spread to the cricoid ring and trachea, with further invasion then extending to the superior thyroid gland and cervical esophagus.

Staging and treatment for laryngeal cancers

Over the past decade, the paradigm for initial treatment of early to moderately advanced squamous cell cancers of the larynx has shifted away from open partial or total laryngectomy in favor of organ-preserving modalities, such as radiation therapy (RT) alone, combined concurrent chemoradiotherapy (CRT), and transoral endoscopic laser microsurgery with or without adjuvant postoperative RT or CRT. Still, open laryngectomies continue to be performed both primarily for advanced-stage disease and for salvage of initial treatment failures. The radiologic survey should, therefore, focus on findings that affect the overall staging and prognosis of a given cancer, determine the resectability of a tumor, and, finally, affect the feasibility of subtotal surgical options. In addition to the location and absolute volume of tumor, important features to assess on staging scans should include[8,9,20]

1. Preepiglottic and/or paraglottic space invasion
2. Anterior or posterior commissure involvement
3. Transglottic tumor extension
4. Subglottic extension
5. Neoplastic cartilage invasion
6. Involvement of the carotid artery and/or prevertebral soft tissues
7. Regional nodal disease

Supraglottic and glottic carcinomas demonstrating preepiglottic or paraglottic space invasion are staged as at least T3 tumors, regardless of whether vocal cord fixation is evident clinically (see **Table 1**). Because these spaces communicate, there is no barrier to prevent spread of tumor between them once one is invaded. Furthermore, tumor involvement of these spaces is associated with a greater likelihood of nodal metastases[21] and has been reported to be associated with poorer cure rates after RT.[11,22,23] Preepiglottic space invasion also affects reconstruction options for supracricoid laryngectomies, because minor preepiglottic invasion is a contraindication for supracricoid laryngectomies with cricohyoidoepiglottopexy, whereas massive preepiglottic space even precludes supracricoid laryngectomies with cricohyoidopexy.[24] Submucosal tumor spread into the preepiglottic and paraglottic spaces can be impossible to appreciate on clinical examination, and, therefore, imaging is necessary to exclude its presence. On both CT and MR, tumor invasion can be identified as soft tissue replacement of the normal fat within these spaces (**Figs. 5** and **6**).

Anterior or posterior commissure involvement by a glottic tumor does not actually affect T staging but can drastically affect options for treatment and overall prognosis.[25] Endoscopic exposure of the anterior commissure can be problematic, making complete transoral resection more difficult, and outcomes for laser excision of tumors involving the anterior commissure tend to be poorer compared with those confined to the membranous cord.[20] The lack of submucosal tissue overlying the commissures places the mucosa in nearly direct contact with the subjacent thyroid cartilage anteriorly and between the medial aspects of the arytenoid cartilages posteriorly. Therefore, on endoscopy or imaging, the presence of soft tissue thickening (>2 mm) in either the anterior or posterior commissure should be viewed with suspicion, whereas, conversely, the absence of soft tissue in these locations generally excludes tumor involvement (**Fig. 7**).[10]

Transglottic tumors cross the laryngeal ventricle or anterior commissure to involve both the supraglottis and glottis. Extension of a supraglottic tumor below the laryngeal

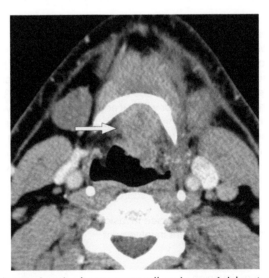

Fig. 5. Preepiglottic space invasion by squamous cell carcinoma. Axial postcontrast CT image at the level of the hyoid bone in a patient with an epiglottic cancer demonstrates enhancing tumor extending from the epiglottis into the normally fat-containing preepiglottic space (*arrow*).

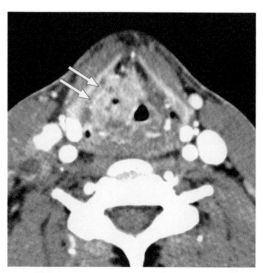

Fig. 6. Paraglottic space invasion by squamous cell carcinoma. Axial contrast-enhanced CT image demonstrates an enhancing tumor of the right false vocal fold with deep extension in the right paraglottic space (*arrows*). Compare this with the normal-appearing fat in the paraglottic space on the left.

ventricle to the glottis is a contraindication to performing a standard horizontal supraglottic partial laryngectomy.[25] Coronal imaging can be particularly useful for demonstrating transglottic tumor spread (**Fig. 8**).

Subglottic extension of tumor can be difficult to evaluate endoscopically, and cross-sectional imaging plays a useful role in its identification. The normal subglottis features

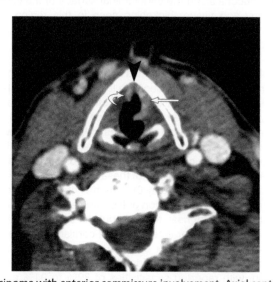

Fig. 7. Glottic carcinoma with anterior commissure involvement. Axial contrast-enhanced CT image through the glottis demonstrates an enhancing lesion originating on the left true vocal fold (*arrow*) extending across the anterior commissure (*arrowhead*) to involve the anterior third of the right true vocal fold (*curved arrow*). The anterior commissure should normally measure no more than 2 mm in thickness.

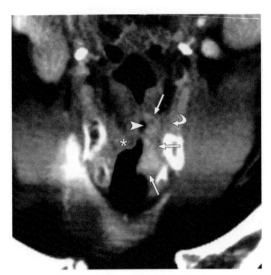

Fig. 8. Glottic carcinoma with transglottic and subglottic tumor spread. Coronal contrast-enhanced CT image demonstrates a left glottic carcinoma (*arrows*), which extends across the laryngeal ventricle (*arrowhead*) to involve the supraglottis, as well as inferiorly into the subglottis. The fat of the paraglottic space on the left is infiltrated (*curved arrow*), raising the possibility of paraglottic space invasion (compare with the contralateral paraglottic fat). Note also the presence of asymmetric sclerosis of the right thyroid and cricoid cartilage, which is a suggestive but nonspecific finding of possible cartilage invasion. (*Asterisk*) Right true vocal fold.

only a thin layer of mucosa along the endoluminal surface of the cricoid and tracheal cartilages. Thus, any soft tissue thickening seen in this region is suspicious for possible extension of tumor (see **Fig. 8; Fig. 9**). Subglottic extension generally precludes any type of partial laryngectomy, leaving only total laryngectomy as a surgical option.

The presence of neoplastic cartilage invasion can have a dramatic influence on prognosis and therapeutic approach, because it is associated with higher recurrence rates after partial laryngectomy and, therefore, often limits the treatment options to total laryngectomy or CRT. Furthermore, cartilage invasion in advanced laryngeal tumors is associated with poorer local responses to RT compared with laryngectomy and with a higher likelihood for developing subsequent chondroradionecrosis.[9,26]

CT findings of cartilage invasion include sclerosis, erosion, lysis, and frank extralaryngeal tumor spread. The presence of any of these signs taken together has a reported sensitivity of 91% but a specificity of only 68%. If the criterion of sclerosis is excluded and only the presence of cartilage erosion or lysis and extralaryngeal spread of tumor is used (**Fig. 10**), the specificity rises to 92%, but the sensitivity falls to only 61%.[27] Unfortunately, because the appearance of normal cartilage ossification varies, it can be difficult to distinguish inner cortex erosion by an adjacent tumor from normal discontinuous ossification on CT. MR is widely considered superior to CT for detection of cartilage invasion, with reported sensitivities of 89% to 94% and specificities of 74% to 88%.[3,8] Invaded cartilage demonstrates low to intermediate signal on T1-weighted images, higher signal on T2-weighted images, and enhancement after intravenous contrast administration. If all these features are absent on MR, then cartilage infiltration can be ruled out with a high degree of certainty.

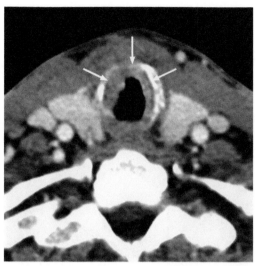

Fig. 9. Subglottic tumor extension. Axial contrast-enhanced CT through the subglottis in a patient with a transglottic cancer demonstrates soft tissue thickening of the mucosal surface of the airway (*arrows*), indicative of subglottic tumor extension. There should normally be no soft tissue visible between the airway and the inner cortex of the cricoid cartilage.

Extralaryngeal spread of tumor with carotid artery or prevertebral soft tissue involvement represents very advanced local disease (stage T4b) and is generally considered unresectable. Unfortunately, it can be difficult to determine whether these structures are involved by imaging. Tumor abutment of the carotid does not necessarily mean that the tumor has invaded the carotid adventitia. Conventionally, if a tumor contacts less than 180° of the circumference of the carotid, then the likelihood of invasion is low, whereas encasement of greater than 270° of the vessel's circumference is associated with a high probability of invasion (**Fig. 11**). When the interface is between 180° and 270°, the likelihood of carotid invasion cannot be determined reliably with imaging.[28]

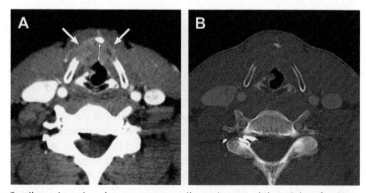

Fig. 10. Cartilage invasion by squamous cell carcinoma. (*A*) Axial soft tissue window contrast-enhanced CT image at the level of the glottis demonstrates a large enhancing tumor extending through both thyroid laminae into the prelaryngeal soft tissues (*arrows*), making this a T4a tumor. Note the marked thickening of the anterior commissure (*double arrow*). (*B*) Corresponding bone algorithm image demonstrates complete lysis of the thyroid laminae by the tumor.

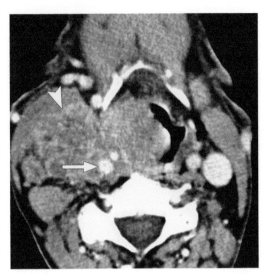

Fig. 11. Carotid encasement by squamous cell carcinoma. Axial contrast-enhanced CT image through the supraglottis demonstrates a large right-sided supraglottic tumor extending into the extralaryngeal soft tissues posteriorly. The mass surrounds the entire circumference of the right common carotid artery (*arrow*), making this a T4b lesion. The tumor also obliterates the normal fat plane that resides between the pharynx and prevertebral muscles, but this finding alone is not a reliable predictor of prevertebral involvement. A large nodal conglomerate is also evident in the right neck straddling levels II and III (*arrowhead*).

In these situations, direct neck exploration is generally necessary to determine resectability.

Involvement of prevertebral fascia is difficult to definitively diagnose by imaging, and intraoperative assessment remains the best method of determination. In normal individuals, there is typically a thin plane of retropharyngeal fat anterior to the prevertebral space that can be identified on both CT and T1-weighted MRI. Complete visualization of the retropharyngeal fat plane virtually rules out prevertebral involvement; however, obliteration of this plane does not reliably predict invasion of the prevertebral space unless obvious tumor bulk is evident in the prevertebral soft tissues, because tumor can compress the fat without violating the prevertebral fascia.[29]

The presence of regional nodal disease greatly affects outcome, and even the presence of a solitary ipsilateral nodal metastasis (N1 disease) is reported to reduce survival by approximately 50%.[30] Nodal spread is more common in supraglottic cancers relative to glottic and subglottic cancers, because of the rich lymphovascular network within the paraglottic tissues. Supraglottic tumors typically metastasize to jugular chain nodes at levels II, III, and IV (see **Fig. 11**), whereas subglottic tumors may spread to the visceral nodes (pretracheal and paratracheal nodes, nodal level VI), level IV, and superior mediastinal nodes. Glottic cancers limited to the endolarynx rarely spread to nodes. When they do metastasize regionally, they tend to follow the dominant direction of tumor growth. That is, if there is predominantly supraglottic spread, then nodal disease tends to be in jugular chain nodes, whereas if there is infraglottic spread, nodal disease occurs at levels VI and IV.[31] The sensitivity and specificity of CT and MRI for detecting nodal disease are good, but there remains a role for nodal dissections for patients with N0 staging depending on the risk for nodal metastases and the practice preferences of the surgeon and the informed decision of the patient.[9]

Staging outcomes with CT, MRI, and FDG-PET

When combined with CT, FDG-PET generally improves the accuracy of N staging by 15% to 20%, because it may identify small nodal metastases not be considered positive by CT criteria alone. The utility of FDG-PET to detect nodal disease is greatest in patients with more advanced tumors, in whom the likelihood of lymphatic spread is higher. In patients staged clinically and with conventional imaging as N0, however, FDG-PET has not been shown as consistently useful for refining the N stage.[32]

Due to its intrinsically limited spatial resolution, even when coregistered with CT images (which is standard at most centers), FDG-PET does not seem to improve initial T-staging over CT or MRI alone[9,32]; however, some centers routinely perform a pretreatment FDG-PET on head and neck squamous cell carcinomas to use for comparison at post-treatment follow-up. It has been reported that the pretreatment tumoral standard uptake value (SUV) can have prognostic implications, with lower pretreatment SUV correlating with a lower rate of local recurrence and improved disease-free survival.[33] FDG-PET in the pretreatment setting, however, is most useful clinically for nodal staging and detection of distant metastases.

Imaging After Treatment of Squamous Cell Carcinoma

The normal imaging features of the larynx after therapy depend on many factors, including the location and pretreatment size of the tumor, the treatment modality used, and the patient's anatomy. Therefore, it is of critical importance to know this information beforehand and to have any pretreatment imaging available for comparison when evaluating a post-treatment scan.

RT or CRT treatment

For patients undergoing primary RT or CRT, the normal post-treatment protocol at UNC is to perform a baseline neck CT 6 weeks after completion of therapy, with periodic clinical and imaging follow-up thereafter. From patient to patient, generally consistent tissue changes are evident on scans performed after radiation, but these changes are at times confusing. Radiation induces edema and fibrosis, which may involve any of the tissues contained within the treated portals. In the larynx, mucositis and submucosal edema typically occur and result in thickening of the epiglottis, aryepiglottic folds, and false vocal folds; stranding of the preepiglottic and paraglottic fat; and prominent mucosal contrast enhancement. Symmetric subglottic thickening also develops in approximately 80% of patients.[34] Typical extralaryngeal CT changes, which are evident, include thickening of the skin and platysma muscle, reticulation of the subcutaneous and deep fat, and edema of the carotid sheath.[34,35]

Complete resolution of a mass on a study performed after RT suggests successful local control, whereas absence of significant change in the appearance of a mass suggests treatment failure. Partial resolution of a mass on imaging should be considered indeterminate, and patients showing a partial treatment response on CT should undergo further FDG-PET imaging or close clinical and serial radiologic observation. Stability of a mass over a 2-year period suggests that the radiographic findings represent fibrosis and scarring, but interval growth of a lesion or development of new lesion should be considered highly suspicious for local recurrence.[34,35]

Total laryngectomy

In patients undergoing curative partial or total laryngectomies, the role of imaging for surveillance is not well defined. Because the postoperative larynx is easily evaluated endoscopically, many investigators suggest that serial imaging not be performed in asymptomatic patients with clear surgical margins but be reserved for newly symptomatic patients or patients with endoscopically proved recurrences.[36]

Post-treatment imaging outcomes with CT, MRI, and FDG-PET

The utility of FDG-PET in post-treatment surveillance is well established. It has been shown that FDG-PET is superior to both CT and MRI alone for detecting recurrent head and neck cancer, particularly at the primary site (**Fig. 12**).[32] In one meta-analysis, the pooled sensitivity and specificity of FDG-PET for detection of laryngeal cancer recurrence after RT were 89% and 74%, respectively.[37] In general, the optimal timing for FDG-PET imaging after combined chemotherapy and radiation therapy is at 2 to 3 months. Scanning before then results in a higher rate of false-positive results due to the inflammatory changes typically seen with RT.[38]

Complications of Cancer Therapy

Many complications can occur as a consequence of cancer treatment in the larynx. The most common complications of radiation to the larynx are[39]

- Laryngeal edema
- Skin breakdown
- Perichondritis
- Chondronecrosis

Complications related to surgery include

- Pharyngocutaneous fistula formation
- Wound infection
- Chyle leak
- Swallowing and airway problems

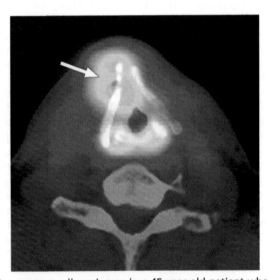

Fig. 12. Recurrent squamous cell carcinoma in a 45-year-old patient who completed definitive RT for a T3 glottic carcinoma 6 months earlier, now presenting with several weeks of new hoarseness and dysphagia. Axial fused PET CT image at the level of the glottis demonstrates avid FDG uptake in the right anterior glottis (*arrow*), indicating local tumor recurrence. Symmetric FDG uptake seen in the posterior larynx is physiologic.

Chondroradionecrosis

Chondroradionecrosis is a delayed complication of RT, usually presenting after a latent period of up to a year after completion of treatment.[40] The incidence of chondroradionecrosis has declined over the past several decades from 5% to approximately 1%, due to improved irradiation techniques and quality control measures.[39] Tumor invasion of the laryngeal cartilages predisposes to this complication, with up to 27% of advanced (T3 and T4) cancers developing chondronecrosis compared with 2% of tumors initially staged as T1 or T2.[40]

Chondroradionecrosis can be difficult to diagnose because it may present with nonspecific symptoms that often mimic symptoms of cancer recurrence, including dysphagia, odynophagia, hoarseness, and stridor. Symptoms of more severe (grade IV) radiation necrosis can include respiratory distress, severe pain, fistula formation, and airway obstruction. The imaging features of laryngeal chondroradionecrosis may also mimic those of tumor recurrence, particularly when the primary finding is soft tissue thickening surrounding the cartilage, but certain CT findings, such as progressive cricoarytenoid sclerosis, anterior dislocation or sloughing of the arytenoid cartilage, thyroid cartilage fragmentation and collapse, and/or the presence of gas bubbles around the cartilage, strongly suggest the diagnosis of chondronecrosis **(Fig. 13)**.[41] These findings are absent in up to half of cases, however.[39] When imaging and biopsy results are equivocal for differentiating radionecrosis from tumor recurrence, repeat imaging may be helpful, because development of these findings or unchanged findings make the diagnosis of chondroradionecrosis more likely.

Local surgical complications

Local complications related to primary or salvage total laryngectomy occur in approximately 25% of patients and occur more frequently in patients undergoing salvage after CRT compared with those undergoing primary laryngectomies. Among surgical complications, pharyngocutaneous fistula is the most common (approximately 15%), followed by wound infection and skin necrosis.[42,43]

Pharyngocutaneous fistulae occur when there is breakdown or inadequate closure of the suture line, eventually allowing salivary flow through a cutaneous orifice. These

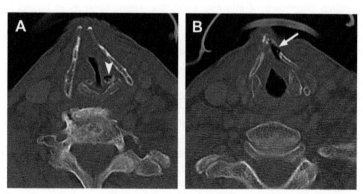

Fig. 13. Chondroradionecrosis in a 69-year-old man with a history of 2 separate laryngeal squamous cell carcinomas, both treated with radiation in the past, now with respiratory distress requiring tracheotomy. Axial bone algorithm CT image through the level of the arytenoids (*A*) demonstrates gas within the left arytenoid cartilage (*arrowhead*). An image slightly caudal to this (*B*) demonstrates fragmentation of the anterior thyroid cartilage lamina on the left with adjacent gas (*arrow*). Cartilage fragmentation and gas are highly suggestive of chondronecrosis.

usually become clinically evident 7 to 11 days after surgery.[44] Fluoroscopic swallowing studies, in which videofluoroscopic or rapid fluoroscopic spot imaging is performed as a patient swallows boluses of water-soluble contrast media, are frequently conducted after surgery to evaluate the neopharynx and to confirm or to exclude anastomotic complications before resumption of oral intake. Abnormalities on swallowing studies can include minimal extravasation into a small blind-ending tract, extravasation into larger contained collections in the neck, or a frank fistulous tract extending through the skin. Most cases resolve spontaneously, but more severe leakages (ie, large contrast extravasations or frank fistula formation) are associated with prolonged healing and longer delays in initiation of oral intake after surgery. Contrast-enhanced CT or MRI may be required to rule out loculation or formation of an abscess, which appear as a peripherally enhancing fluid collection near the anastomotic site. In up to one-third of cases, fluoroscopic swallow studies may be negative even when a fistula is clinically apparent. False-negative results are usually due to small fistulae, and in these instances the clinical signs and symptoms should take precedence over radiologic findings.[44]

Nonsquamous Cell Neoplasms

Benign tumors

Hemangioma Hemangiomas of the larynx are generally subdivided into infantile and adult types. Infantile laryngeal hemangiomas have generally received greater attention because they are more likely to result in significant airway obstruction due to their subglottic predilection, and they are the most common subglottic airway lesions in newborns and young infants. They occur primarily during the first few months of life and are twice as common in female infants than in male infants.[36] Infants with subglottic hemangiomas are usually asymptomatic during the first several weeks of life but classically develop symptoms of stridor or respiratory distress mimicking croup at approximately 1 to 3 months of age, due to rapid tumor proliferation. Up to 50% of infants with subglottic hemangiomas also have cutaneous lesions, which are often found in a beard-like distribution.[45]

The definitive diagnosis of infantile subglottic hemangiomas is based on direct laryngoscopy, but imaging can provide crucial additional information about the airway and assess the total volume of the tumor.[46] Hemangiomas can cause localized or concentric airway narrowing and on contrast-enhanced CT usually show intense contrast enhancement. On MRI, subglottic hemangiomas demonstrate characteristically high signal intensity on T2-weighted images and intermediate signal intensity on T1-images and enhance avidly after gadolinium administration (**Fig. 14**).[47]

Adult hemangiomas are more common among men and their development is believed related to factors, including vocal abuse, cigarette smoking, and laryngeal trauma. They are usually found in the supraglottis or glottis, but their imaging characteristics are otherwise similar to those of the infantile subtype.[48] In addition to hemangioma, the differential for a circumscribed, intensely enhancing tumor of the larynx includes paraganglioma as well as metastases from highly vascularized tumors, such as renal adenocarcinoma, both of which are rare.[36]

Lipoma Lipomatous tumors arising in the larynx are uncommon but are among the few entities for which CT and MRI can provide a definitive diagnosis in virtually all cases. They most often arise in the supraglottic region with the aryepiglottic folds the most common site. Laryngeal lipomas are usually pedunculated and may prolapse into the esophagus or trachea resulting in a globus sensation or airway obstruction.[36,49]

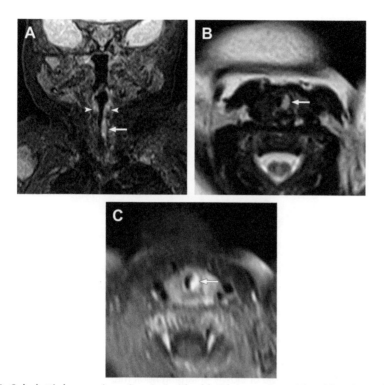

Fig. 14. Subglottic hemangioma in a 2-month-old girl presenting with stridor. Coronal STIR image (*A*) Through the larynx and trachea demonstrates a hyperintense lesion (*arrow*) extending along the left lateral wall of the subglottic larynx and trachea. The arrowheads indicate the true vocal cords. (*B*) Axial T2-weighted MRI also demonstrates the lesion (*arrow*) to have high signal intensity and to narrow the subglottic airway. (*C*) Fat-suppressed T1-weighted image with gadolinium demonstrates strong homogenous enhancement (*arrow*).

Simple lipomas are typically well-circumscribed, homogeneous masses that demonstrate fat density on CT (usually between −65 HU and −125 HU). On MRI, they are nearly isointense to subcutaneous fat on all MR pulse sequences and should suppress with fat-suppression techniques. No enhancement is seen on either modality after contrast administration. It is not uncommon for lipomas to contain strands of fibrous or soft tissue elements (so-called fibrolipomas) **(Fig. 15)**; in these cases, it can be impossible to distinguish a benign lipoma from a well-differentiated liposarcoma radiographically.[36,49] Fortunately, liposarcomas of the larynx are rare, with approximately 30 cases reported to date in the English literature.[50]

Chondroma Cartilaginous tumors, which include chondroma and its malignant counterpart chondrosarcoma, account for less than 1% of all laryngeal tumors.[51] Nearly all these slow-growing tumors arise from the laryngeal cartilages, although rare soft tissue chondromas of the larynx have also been reported.[52] The cricoid cartilage is the most common location for laryngeal chondromas (70%–78%), with the thyroid cartilage giving rise to 15% to 20% and the arytenoids and epiglottis each accounting for a small percentage.[51]

The mean age at presentation for laryngeal chondromas is in the sixth decade, and men are affected approximately twice as often as women. Common presenting symptoms depend on the location and growth pattern of the lesions and include

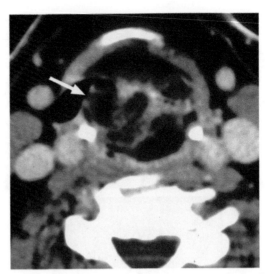

Fig. 15. Laryngeal lipoma. Axial contrast-enhanced CT image at the level of the supraglottis demonstrates a predominantly fat density (hypodense) mass centered in the right aryepiglottic fold (*arrow*). The strands of soft tissue seen in this lesion are common in benign lipomas, but their presence makes it impossible to distinguish the lesion from a low-grade liposarcoma radiographically.

hoarseness, dyspnea, voice changes, dysphagia, and cough.[51] Patients may alternatively present with a palpable or slowly enlarging neck mass, which is usually the first symptom of chondromas located in the thyroid cartilage.[53] Malignant progression to chondrosarcoma has been reported to occur in 7% of cases.[51]

Up to 80% of cartilaginous tumors of the larynx can be diagnosed reliably with CT, owing to the presence of tumoral chondroid matrix calcifications.[51,53] Chondroid calcifications typically demonstrate a fine, stippled pattern, an arclike and ringlike appearance, or a coarse popcorn-like configuration (**Fig. 16**) and, when present, allow a diagnosis of

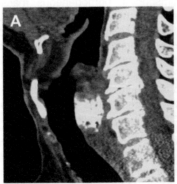
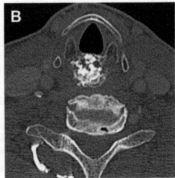

Fig. 16. Chondroma in a 67-year-old man with a 6-month history of hoarseness. Sagittal midline contrast-enhanced CT image reconstructed using a soft tissue algorithm (*A*) demonstrates a densely calcified submucosal mass deep to the posterior laryngeal wall. An axial bone algorithm CT image through the middle of the lesion (*B*) demonstrates that it appears to be arising from and expanding the posterior lamina of the cricoids cartilage. The calcifications in the tumor demonstrate a coarse popcorn-like configuration, which is typical of chondroid matrix calcification.

a cartilaginous tumor with a high degree of certainty. Unfortunately, differentiating between a chondroma and a chondrosarcoma by imaging is usually not possible, and biopsy is typically required for histologic diagnosis of the specific tumor type.[54] Chondromas tend to be smaller (usually measuring less than 3 cm in maximum diameter) than chondrosarcomas, which often exceed 3 cm (mean 3.5 cm).[53,54]

MRI provides better soft tissue contrast than CT, which may allow better characterization of tumor margins, but MRI is less well suited than CT for demonstrating fine matrix calcifications, owing to its inferior spatial resolution. The unenhanced MR signal characteristics of chondromas follow the appearance of mature hyaline cartilage— that is, predominantly low to intermediate signal intensity on T1-weighted imaging and high signal intensity on T2-weighted images.[55] When visible on MRI, chondroid matrix calcification appears as regions of low signal intensity on both T1-weighted and T2-weighted sequences. Some degree of contrast enhancement is usually present on both CT and MRI after intravenous contrast administration.

Malignant tumors

Chondrosarcoma Although rare, chondrosarcomas are the most frequently encountered nonepithelial tumors arising in the larynx.[53] Like chondromas, chondrosarcomas arise more frequently in men than in women, but they tend to occur on average a decade later in life (mean age 60–64 years) than chondromas.[54] In the larynx, they have been described after Teflon injection for treatment of vocal cord paralysis, after RT, and in association with other tumors, but it is not clear whether a true etiologic link exists or whether these associations are coincidental.[54] Most laryngeal chondrosarcomas are well-differentiated or low-grade tumors and are slow growing. Rapid growth of a cartilaginous tumor suggests the diagnosis of a dedifferentiated chondrosarcoma.[56] Metastases from laryngeal chondrosarcomas occur in 8% to 14% of patients and occur almost exclusively in patients with poorly differentiated or dedifferentiated tumors. The lung is the most common site of distant spread, and chondrosarcomas rarely metastasize to regional lymph nodes.[53]

The typical distribution and imaging characteristics of laryngeal chondrosarcomas are essentially identical to those of chondromas and most notably include the presence of chondroid matrix calcification on CT (**Fig. 17**). Larger tumor size (>3 cm), findings of nearby soft tissue invasion, and evidence of vocal cord palsy are more suggestive of malignancy, but these are neither sensitive nor specific signs.[53]

FDG-PET has been reported potentially useful for noninvasively distinguishing chondromas and chondrosarcomas. In one study examining the use of FDG-PET in non–head and neck cartilage neoplasms, FDG-PET was reported to have a sensitivity of 90.9% and a specificity of 100% for differentiating benign from malignant tumors.[57] In that report, SUVs in benign chondromas ranged from 0.8 to 1.8, whereas 10 of 11 chondrosarcomas demonstrated SUVs greater than 2.0 (range 1.4–20).

Minor salivary gland tumors Minor salivary glands (MSGs) are found throughout the submucosa of the respiratory tract. Although these glands are most numerous in the oral cavity, the typical adult larynx contains between 600 and 1600 MSGs,[58] which may give rise to neoplasms. Overall, MSG tumors make up less than 1% of laryngeal neoplasms. Like MSG tumors elsewhere in the aerodigestive tract, the majority of laryngeal MSG tumors are malignant, with adenoid cystic carcinoma accounting for most cases (40%–83%).[59,60] Most of the remaining tumors are made up of mucoepidermoid carcinoma and adenocarcinoma, with other subtypes, such as acinic cell carcinoma and myoepithelial carcinoma, less common.[59]

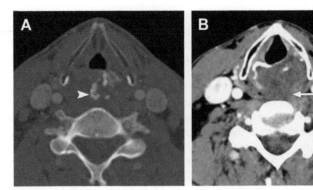

Fig. 17. Chondrosarcoma in a 44-year-old man with a 3-year history of dysphonia. Axial contrast-enhanced CT image viewed with bone windows (*A*) demonstrates a mass centered on the posterior cricoid lamina with a few scattered coarse calcifications. Note the arc-shaped calcification (*arrowhead*), which is suggestive of chondroid matrix calcification. (*B*) Axial soft tissue window CT image just caudal to (*A*) demonstrates a largely noncalcified hypodense component of the tumor which appears to be bulging through the posterior margin of the cricoid cartilage into the adjacent postcricoid hypopharynx (*arrow*). This finding is worrisome but not specific for malignancy, and chondrosarcomas are generally radiographically indistinguishable from chondromas.

Adenoid cystic carcinomas of the larynx occur primarily in middle-aged and older adults with a median age in the sixth decade and, unlike squamous cell carcinomas, are not associated with smoking.[36,59] Up to 80% of adenoid cystic carcinomas arise in the subglottis, typically at the junction with the trachea, whereas mucoepidermoid carcinoma and adenocarcinoma tend to occur in the supraglottic larynx.[6,36] Depending on the location of the tumor, patients classically present with symptoms of dysphagia (supraglottis), hoarseness (glottis), dyspnea, or stridor (subglottis). Most patients with laryngeal MSG tumors present with advanced (stage III or IV) disease, probably due in part to the predominantly subglottic location and submucosal growth pattern of these tumors, which makes early detection difficult. Approximately 20% of patients with laryngeal adenoid cystic carcinoma have regional nodal spread at the time of presentation.[59,61]

The imaging characteristics of MSG tumors in the larynx are nonspecific; however, the finding of an entirely submucosal lesion located in the subglottis or trachea should raise the suspicion for an adenoid cystic carcinoma.[36] On CT, MSG tumors classically appear as extensive soft tissue tumors with extensive submucosal spread. Subglottic tumors often demonstrate tracheal involvement and invasion of the cricoid cartilage and extralaryngeal soft tissues. Vocal cord paralysis due to invasion of the recurrent laryngeal nerve is a characteristic feature of subglottic adenoid cystic carcinomas, and its presence should alert to the possibility of perineural involvement.

MR may better depict the true extent of tumor spread in patients with MSG tumors than CT. As on CT, however, the MR signal characteristics of these tumors are nonspecific. In one small series of patients with head and neck adenoid cystic carcinomas, all the tumors demonstrated homogeneous intermediate signal intensity and diffuse contrast enhancement on T1-weighted images (**Fig. 18**). Signal intensity on T2-weighted images was much more variable, and the series found that tumors with low signal intensity on T2-weighted images were associated with higher tumor cellularity and a poorer prognosis compared with those showing high signal intensity.[62]

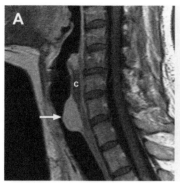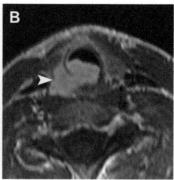

Fig. 18. Adenoid cystic carcinoma in a patient with a history of progressive shortness of breath and a posterior submucosal subglottic mass on fiberoptic laryngoscopy. Midsagittal contrast-enhanced T1-weighted MRI through the neck (*A*) demonstrates a homogeneously enhancing mass (*arrow*) involving the posterior wall of the subglottis and upper trachea. Note the oblique angle formed between the mass and the wall of the airway, suggesting the submucosal location of the lesion. An axial contrast-enhanced T1-weighted image through the mass (*B*) demonstrates that the mass has extended beyond the anatomic boundaries of the larynx into the adjacent soft tissues (*arrowhead*), which, along with tracheal involvement, makes this a T4a tumor. C, cricoid.

Non-Hodgkin lymphoma Primary non-Hodgkin lymphoma (NHL) of the larynx is rare, accounting for less than 1% of laryngeal tumors. Most (70%–85%) are of the B-cell type, with the large B-cell and mucosa-associated lymphatic tissue the most common. Mean age at presentation is in the seventh decade; however, reported patient ages range from 4 to 90 years.[63,64]

Most laryngeal lymphomas arise in the supraglottic region, presumably from either aggregates of specialized lymphoid tissue in the submucosa or from mucosa-associated lymphatic tissue located in the aryepiglottic folds and epiglottis.[63,64] In one review of 20 patients with primary laryngeal NHL, tumor involved the false cords in 85% of patients, the aryepiglottic folds in 65%, the true cords in 65%, and the epiglottis in 55%.[64] In that series, tumors involving the glottis or subglottis all had concomitant supraglottic involvement.

Symptoms and signs of primary laryngeal NHL mimic those of other laryngeal tumors and include hoarseness, cough, dysphagia, globus sensation, stridor, and systemic signs, such as weight loss and fever. Endoscopy typically reveals a submucosal swelling or a polypoid mass without ulceration.[63,64]

On CT, most laryngeal lymphomas appear as bulky homogeneous masses with submucosal involvement. Extralaryngeal extension into the hypopharynx, oropharynx, or strap muscles is common. Signal characteristics on MR are nonspecific and include intermediate signal intensity on T1-weighted images and variable signal intensities on T2-weighted images. A characteristic feature of laryngeal lymphomas is only moderate, very homogeneous contrast enhancement on both CT and MRI without calcification or necrosis (**Fig. 19**). On FDG-PET, laryngeal lymphoma consistently demonstrates FDG avidity. Associated cervical lymphadenopathy may be present in 20% to 25% of cases.[64]

Kaposi sarcoma Kaposi sarcoma (KS) is a multifocal angioproliferative disorder of vascular endothelium, which is linked to infection with human herpesvirus 8.[65,66] The lesions of KS are of intermediate (rarely metastasizing) malignant potential and most frequently affect mucocutaneous sites. Although there are 4 clinical variants described,

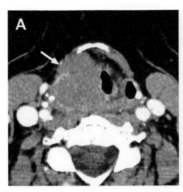
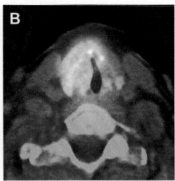

Fig. 19. NHL in a 49-year-old woman presenting with hoarseness. Axial contrast-enhanced CT image (*A*) through the supraglottis demonstrates a bulky but very homogeneous soft tissue mass centered in the right paraglottic space and potentially extending into the infrahyoid strap muscles (*arrow*). A fused axial PET/CT image through the glottis (*B*) demonstrates marked FDG uptake by the mass, suggesting it is malignant.

KS is most frequently associated with the AIDS, and it is the most common neoplasm affecting HIV-infected patients.[67] HIV-related KS is most likely to occur in the context of advanced immunosuppression and is considered an AIDS-defining illness.

Head and neck involvement by KS is not unusual, particularly in the oral cavity, but laryngeal involvement is uncommon. Presenting symptoms can include hoarseness, aphonia, dysphagia, cough, stridor, or complete airway obstruction. Physical examination findings may reveal laryngeal edema, or more commonly, one or more purple vascular lesions, which are frequently exophytic or verrucous in nature.[65,66] Diagnosis of laryngeal KS is typically established on laryngoscopy or imaging, but tissue sampling should be performed with caution, because biopsy of KS lesions in the larynx has been associated with brisk and occasionally fatal bleeding.[66]

In the appropriate clinical setting (ie, HIV-positive or immunosuppressed status), the imaging findings can be highly suggestive of the diagnosis of KS. On CT, KS lesions manifest as nodular or exophytic mucosal masses, which characteristically demonstrate avid enhancement after intravenous contrast administration (**Fig. 20**). On MRI, KS lesions demonstrate low signal intensity on T1-weighted images, high signal intensity on T2-weighted images, and strong contrast enhancement. Imaging is helpful in assessing deep involvement of the disease and to identify associated lymph node enlargement, which can be seen in approximately 13% of patients with KS.[68]

Non-neoplastic Processes

Laryngeal fractures and dislocations
Most laryngeal fractures are the result of motor vehicle accidents or sports-related injuries.[69] In the setting of acute multisystem trauma, the larynx is oftentimes imaged as part of a more extensive trauma survey that may include scans of the head, chest, and cervical spine, and approximately 50% of patients suffering acute laryngeal trauma have associated injuries, including intracranial injuries, facial fractures, cervical spine fractures, and pharyngoesophageal injuries.[14,70]

If a laryngeal injury is suspected, thin-section (2 mm or less) reformatting through the larynx using both bone and soft tissue algorithms should be performed on the acquired scan data. Although injury to ossified cartilages is usually best appreciated on dedicated bone windows, cartilage fractures in young patients, in whom the cartilages are often not

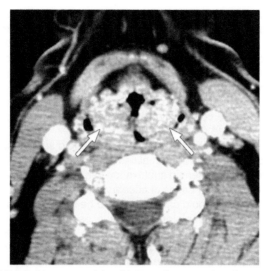

Fig. 20. KS in an HIV-positive man with a history of progressive shortness of breath. Axial contrast-enhanced CT image demonstrates nodular thickening and enhancement of both aryepiglottic folds (*arrows*), with marked contrast enhancement. In a patient with AIDS, these findings are highly suggestive of laryngeal KS.

ossified, may require close inspection using soft tissue windows, particularly in cases of nondisplaced fractures. On soft tissue windows, unossified cartilages may be only slightly hyperdense compared with nearby muscle, and any laryngeal contour deformity or soft tissue fullness should be viewed with suspicion in the setting of trauma.[4] Fortunately, laryngeal injuries are infrequent in children because their cartilages are softer, situated higher in the neck, and more protected by the mandible.[71]

The thyroid cartilage is the most frequently injured laryngeal structure, with trauma usually resulting in median or paramedian vertical fractures (**Fig. 21**).[72,73] The cricoid is

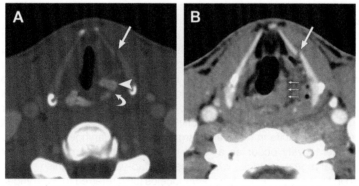

Fig. 21. Laryngeal trauma in a 31-year-old man with shortness of breath and dysphonia after being struck in the neck during a softball game. Axial bone window CT image through the level of the cricoarytenoid joints (*A*) demonstrates a displaced fracture through the left thyroid ala (*large arrow*). In addition, the left arytenoid (*arrowhead*) is anteriorly displaced and medially rotated, and there is widening of the left cricoarytenoid joint space (*curved arrow*). Slightly more cranial CT image viewed with soft tissue windows (*B*) again demonstrates the thyroid lamina fracture (*large arrow*) as well as a submucosal hematoma in the left aryepiglottic fold (*small arrows*).

next most likely to be fractured, whereas arytenoid fractures are uncommon. Fractures of the cricoid are usually bilateral due its ring-shaped structure.[4,8,72]

Laryngeal dislocations can occur at the cricoarytenoid and cricothyroid joints, with the former type more commonly reported. In published series, arytenoid dislocations have been reported due most frequently to intubation trauma (50%–87%, although some call these figures into question) and to external trauma in the minority of cases (15%–30%).[74,75] The overall trend in the literature suggests that anterior arytenoid displacement occurs more commonly than posterior displacement, but investigators differ regarding this point.[74–76]

CT can be a useful tool in the assessment of arytenoid subluxation or dislocation, because it readily demonstrates abnormalities in the orientation and positioning of the arytenoids. The findings of arytenoid subluxation can be subtle, however, and CT may appear normal in up to 36% of cases of cricoarytenoid joint injury.[74,77] Any asymmetry in the position of the arytenoid cartilage should be viewed with suspicion. In addition, a hematoma of the aryepiglottic fold is a useful indirect sign of an acute cricoarytenoid joint disruption.[4] Anterior subluxation usually results in anteromedial displacement of the arytenoid (see **Fig. 21**), and parasagittal images may demonstrate anterior tipping of the arytenoid. Furthermore, anterior arytenoid subluxation usually results in the ipsilateral vocal fold being inferiorly positioned relative to the normal side, whereas posterior subluxation results in a superiorly positioned vocal fold.[77]

Unfortunately, recurrent laryngeal nerve palsies can result in a similar malalignment of the arytenoid on CT (discussed later). Because of this, differentiating paralysis from cricoarytenoid dislocation usually requires laryngoscopy with videostroboscopy, direct palpation of the joint during direct laryngoscopy, and/or laryngeal electromyography.[77,78]

Cricothyroid joint injuries are rare but are probably under-recognized. They tend to occur in conjunction with other laryngeal fractures.[4] CT suggests cricothyroid disruption if there is asymmetric widening of the joint space, which is located between the inferior cornu of the thyroid cartilage and the lateral aspect of the cricoid.[79]

Laryngoceles and other laryngeal cysts

Laryngoceles A laryngocele is an abnormal dilatation of the laryngeal saccule, which is a pouch arising from the anterior end of the laryngeal ventricle extending superiorly between the false vocal cord and the thyroid cartilage to as high as the superior border of the thyroid cartilage.[80,81] Laryngoceles may be air-filled and freely communicate with the laryngeal lumen or may be isolated from the laryngeal lumen and fluid filled.

The etiology of laryngoceles is unclear, but it is believed that increased intralaryngeal pressure, which can be caused by activities, such as glass blowing and playing of wind instruments, results in gradual enlargement of the laryngeal saccule. Laryngoceles can alternatively occur as a result of inflammatory or neoplastic processes involving the laryngeal ventricle, which create a flap-valve mechanism causing air to be trapped in the saccule. Fluid-filled laryngoceles (also referred to as laryngeal mucoceles or saccular cysts) result from accumulation of mucus within an obstructed laryngocele.[80]

Laryngoceles are typically further classified as internal, external, or mixed based on their position relative to the thyrohyoid membrane. Internal laryngoceles, which are the most common type, are confined to the paraglottic space within the false vocal fold and are located entirely medial to the thyrohyoid membrane. External laryngoceles have a component located lateral to the thyrohyoid membrane, reflecting protrusion of the dilated saccule through the membrane into the neck; they are considered mixed if they also demonstrate an internal component.[4,80]

Dysphonia is the most common presenting complaint among patients with laryngoceles, but they can also present with symptoms of dysphagia or dyspnea or with a neck mass that may enlarge during Valsalva. On endoscopy, the internal component of a laryngocele is evident as a submucosal bulge of the false vocal fold.[81] Infected laryngoceles, referred to as laryngopyoceles, may present with an inflammatory neck mass and acute airway obstruction requiring tracheotomy and emergent drainage.

Laryngoceles can usually be diagnosed with imaging studies, and coronal or axial CT and MRI are particularly well suited for demonstrating their relationship to the thyrohyoid membrane. Laryngoceles are usually well-circumscribed lesions arising beneath the false vocal cords. Their internal characteristics depend on whether they are air-filled or cystic. Air-filled laryngoceles are easily identified due to their low CT density (approximately −1000 HU). Communication with the laryngeal airway may be seen, particularly if thin sections are used. On MR, these laryngoceles show very low signal on all pulse sequences.[80]

Fluid-filled laryngoceles can demonstrate densities ranging between those of water and soft tissue on CT. Dense mucoid or purulent contents tend to have a higher density. On MR, cystic laryngoceles show high signal intensity on T2-weighted and low signal intensity on T1-weighted images. Signal intensity on T1-weighted images may be higher than that of water if the protein content is high. After contrast administration, there should be no internal enhancement within a laryngocele, but enhancement may occasionally be seen along the periphery of the cyst, particularly in laryngopyoceles, which can arise in up to 8% of cases (**Fig. 22**).[82] Laryngopyoceles may also demonstrate air-fluid levels on imaging. Because up to 17% of laryngoceles

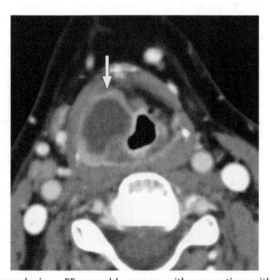

Fig. 22. Laryngopyocele in a 55-year-old woman with presenting with hoarseness and dysphagia after an upper respiratory illness. Axial contrast-enhanced image through the supraglottic larynx demonstrates a smoothly marginated cyst with a thin peripheral rim of enhancement centered in the right paraglottic space (*arrow*). Enhancement and some mild thickening of the cyst wall suggest superinfection of the cyst. The cyst did not extend lateral to the thyrohyoid membrane making this an internal laryngopyocele.

may be associated with an obstructing neoplasm, the laryngeal ventricle should be closely scrutinized for any unusual soft tissue masses.[80]

Ductal cysts are mucous retention cysts arising from obstructed submucosal glands in the larynx. They most commonly arise in infants and young children and may be congenital. They rarely arise in adults.[83,84] Ductal cysts can arise anywhere in the larynx there are submucosal glands. When they occur in the false vocal cords, they can be difficult to distinguish from an internal laryngocele or saccular cyst. Like other cysts, ductal cysts are well-demarcated, nonenhancing masses demonstrating fluid characteristics on both CT and MRI.

Thryoglossal duct cysts can bulge into the preepiglottic space between the hyoid bone and thyroid cartilage, thus mimicking a mixed laryngocele. They are generally easily distinguished from laryngoceles, however, because they are usually midline or just off midline and have an extralaryngeal component that is usually partially embedded in the strap muscles (**Fig. 23**). They may also contain thyroid remnants or ectopic thyroid tissue, which may occasionally give rise to a thyroid carcinoma.[6]

Amyloidosis

Amyloidosis is a rare disorder characterized by extracellular deposition of fibrils of amyloid in soft tissues. Amyloid refers to a family of different insoluble protein aggregates that are characteristically arranged in a highly organized β-pleated sheet configuration. Diagnosis of the condition is based on tissue biopsy demonstrating characteristic apple green birefringence under polarized light after staining with Congo red dye. Both systemic and localized forms of amyloidosis are recognized. In the systemic form, there is widespread amyloid deposition in multiple organs and tissues, whereas in the localized form of the disease, protein deposition is limited to a single organ, tissue, or site of the body.

Approximately 16% of cases of amyloidosis involve the head and neck, with the larynx accounting for 61% of these.[85,86] Amyloidosis only accounts, however, for 0.2% to 1.2% of all benign lesions of the larynx. In the majority of these cases, the disease is localized rather than associated with systemic involvement.[87,88] In most

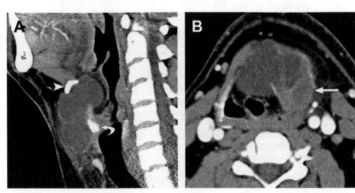

Fig. 23. Thyroglossal duct cyst/remnant in a 35-year-old man presenting with anterior neck swelling and pain. Sagittal reconstruction from a contrast-enhanced neck CT (*A*) demonstrates a cystic prelaryngeal mass, which bulges between the hyoid bone (*arrowhead*) and thyroid cartilage (*curved arrow*) into the preepiglottic space. An axial CT image just above the thyroid notch (*B*) again demonstrates the mass extending into the preepiglottic space. There is an enhancing soft tissue component along the left lateral aspect of the cyst (*arrow*) representing ectopic thyroid tissue. In these cases, papillary thyroid carcinoma arising within the ectopic thyroid tissue must be excluded.

cases of laryngeal amyloidosis, the deposited protein is immunologically identical to the variable region of the light chain fragment of immunoglobulin, but the source of the immunoglobulin protein in these cases remains unclear.[89]

Patients with laryngeal amyloidosis most commonly present in middle age with a history of progressive hoarseness. Less common complaints include dyspnea and dysphagia. The supraglottis is the most frequently affected site in the larynx, but any subsite may be involved.

On CT, the lesions of amyloid appear as well-defined, submucosal lesions demonstrating homogeneous soft tissue density with minimal, if any, contrast enhancement. One potentially distinguishing feature is calcification, which is frequently present in the lesions of amyloidosis. The calcification may range from subtle psammomatous calcification to more discrete, well-defined foci (**Fig. 24**).[86]

On MRI, amyloidosis characteristically demonstrates low signal intensity similar to that of skeletal muscle on T2-weighted images, a feature that may help to distinguish it from other submucosal lesions in the larynx, which tend to demonstrate high signal intensity.[86] On T1-weighted images, the lesions demonstrate low to intermediate signal intensity with variable contrast enhancement.[85,87,90]

Imaging Findings in Vocal Cord Paralysis

Primary innervation of the endolaryngeal muscles is via the recurrent laryngeal nerve (inferior laryngeal nerve), a branch of the vagus nerve (cranial nerve [CN] X). The nuclei of the recurrent laryngeal nerve lie within the nucleus ambiguous in the medulla, and axons exit the brainstem within CN X. The vagus nerve exits the skull base at the jugular foramen and courses into the suprahyoid neck, where it runs within the carotid space adjacent to the glossopharyngeal (CN IX), spinal accessory (CN XI), and hypoglossal nerves (CN XII). It continues inferiorly in the posterolateral aspect of the carotid sheath, and then courses in front of the subclavian arteries bilaterally. The recurrent laryngeal branches of the vagus nerve arise at the level of the aortic arch at the level of the ligamentum arteriosum on the left, and at the subclavian artery on the right, loop around the undersurfaces of these vessels, and course upward in the tracheoesophageal grooves to enter the larynx posterior

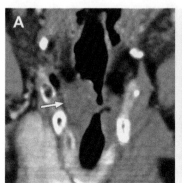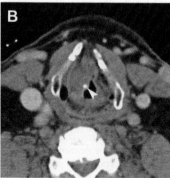

Fig. 24. Amyloidosis in a 48-year-old with a history of progressive voice changes and a supraglottic mass on fiberoptic laryngoscopy. Coronal contrast-enhanced CT image (*A*) through the midlarynx demonstrates a mass, which is homogeneously isodense to muscle spanning the right supraglottis and glottis (*arrow*). An axial CT image through the supraglottis (*B*) shows a focus of calcification in the lesion (*arrowhead*), a potentially distinguishing feature of amyloidosis.

to the cricothyroid joint. In patients with an aberrant origin of the right subclavian artery (a congenital aortic arch anomaly present in up to 2% of individuals), a nonrecurrent right laryngeal nerve is present in which the inferior laryngeal nerve branches arise directly from the cervical portion of the vagus nerve at the level of the cricoid cartilage.[91] In these cases, the anomalous subclavian artery can be seen coursing posterior to the esophagus and indenting it on the lowest cuts of a contrasted neck CT. Additional motor innervation to the larynx is through the external branch of the superior laryngeal nerve, a branch of the vagus that innervates the cricothyroid muscle and is responsible for changing vocal pitch.

The term, *vocal cord paralysis*, describes complete immobility of the cord, whereas paresis refers to partial loss of vocal cord function, both due to a neurologic injury, usually to the recurrent laryngeal or proximal vagus nerve. Most cases represent isolated recurrent laryngeal nerve palsies, with only 10% of cases due to a more central

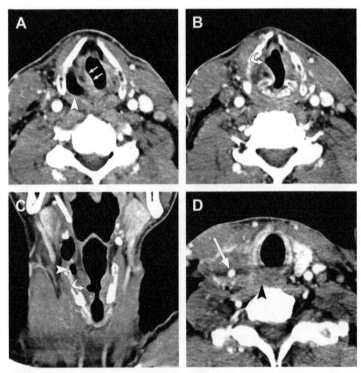

Fig. 25. 45-year-old man with right vocal cord paralysis. (*A*) Axial contrast-enhanced CT at the level of the piriform sinuses demonstrates thickening and medialization of the right aryepiglottic fold (*small arrows*) and dilation of the right piriform sinus (*arrowhead*). (*B*) Image just inferior to this demonstrates a dilated laryngeal ventricle (*curved arrow*), which gives the right false vocal fold a wavy appearance. The right arytenoid cartilage is also slightly medialized. (*C*) Corresponding coronal CT image through the larynx again demonstrates dilation of the right piriform sinus (*arrowhead*) and laryngeal ventricle (*curved arrow*). The right true vocal fold (*asterisk*) is also slightly medialized. These are characteristic findings of a unilateral right vocal cord palsy. (*D*) Axial CT image through the thyroid gland demonstrates a hypoenhancing mass of the right thyroid lobe as the likely cause of vocal cord palsy. The mass invades the tissues of the right tracheoesophageal groove (*arrowhead*) and also encases the right carotid artery (*large arrow*). This was a medullary thyroid cancer.

process.[92] Causes of vocal cord paralysis are varied and include iatrogenic or noniatrogenic trauma, tumor infiltration, or compression, Arnold-Chiari malformations, infection, drug toxicities, and neuropathies associated with neurologic disease. As many as two-thirds of cases of unilateral vocal cord paralysis may be the result of neck surgeries,[4] particularly those involving the thyroid and anterior cervical spine, for which the incidence of iatrogenic recurrent laryngeal nerve injury has been reported to be up to 13.2% and 21.6%, respectively.[91]

Diagnosis of vocal cord paralysis is usually established on clinical grounds; however, in patients in whom the glottis cannot be adequately evaluated in the office, CT imaging can be helpful to confirm the suspicion of a unilateral paralyzed fold. CT findings of a unilateral vocal cord palsy include dilatation of the ipsilateral piriform sinus, thickening and medialization of the ipsilateral aryepiglottic fold, dilatation of the ipsilateral laryngeal ventricle, anteromedial positioning of the arytenoid cartilage, fullness of the ipsilateral true vocal fold, ipsilateral subglottic fullness, and ipsilateral vallecular dilatation (**Fig. 25**). Of these imaging signs, the first 3 are the most sensitive and reliable, with each present in more than 75% of cases of unilateral cord paralysis.[92]

Imaging should also be performed to uncover potential causes of recurrent laryngeal nerve injury when an etiology is not clear on the basis of history and examination. In these cases, the entire neck and upper mediastinum should be imaged from the brainstem through the level of the left pulmonary artery (thus including the origins of both recurrent laryngeal nerves). Lesions involving the brainstem, skull base, and upper carotid space may cause additional lower cranial nerve palsies, including decreased pharyngeal tone (CN X), trapezius and sternocleidomastoid atrophy (CN XI), or tongue deviation (CN XII). Lower in the neck, identifiable causes of vocal cord palsies include tumors originating in the thyroid, hypopharynx, and cervical esophagus (see **Fig. 25**). In the chest, mediastinal and upper lobe tumors, aortic arch and right subclavian artery aneurysms, and even left atrial and pulmonary artery enlargement may cause recurrent laryngeal nerve paralysis.[4,92] In up to 85% of cases, however, a cause of paralysis may not be seen on imaging.

REFERENCES

1. Henrot P, Blum A, Toussaint B, et al. Dynamic maneuvers in local staging of head and neck malignancies with current imaging techniques: principles and clinical applications. Radiographics 2003;23(5):1201–13.
2. Kim BS, Ahn KJ, Park YH, et al. Usefulness of laryngeal phonation CT in the diagnosis of vocal cord paralysis. AJR Am J Roentgenol 2008;190(5):1376–9.
3. Becker M, Zbaren P, Laeng H, et al. Neoplastic invasion of the laryngeal cartilage: comparison of MR imaging and CT with histopathologic correlation. Radiology 1995;194(3):661–9.
4. Glastonbury CM. Non-oncologic imaging of the larynx. Otolaryngol Clin North Am 2008;41(1):139–56, vi.
5. Pameijer FA, Hermans R. Imaging techniques, radiologic anatomy, and normal variants. In: Hermans R, editor. Imaging of the larynx. Berlin, Heidelberg: Springer; 2001. p. 9–21.
6. Curtin HD. The larynx. In: Som PM, Curtin HD, editors. Head and neck imaging, vol. 2. St Louis (MO): Mosby; 2003. p. 1595–699.
7. Garvin HM. Ossification of laryngeal structures as indicators of age. J Forensic Sci 2008;53(5):1023–7.

8. Becker M, Burkhardt K, Dulguerov P, et al. Imaging of the larynx and hypopharynx. Eur J Radiol 2008;66(3):460–79.

9. Blitz AM, Aygun N. Radiologic evaluation of larynx cancer. Otolaryngol Clin North Am 2008;41(4):697–713, vi.

10. Kallmes DF, Phillips CD. The normal anterior commissure of the glottis. AJR Am J Roentgenol 1997;168(5):1317–9.

11. Curtin HD. Imaging of the larynx: current concepts. Radiology 1989;173(1):1–11.

12. Schwartz SR, Cohen SM, Dailey SH, et al. Clinical practice guideline: hoarseness (dysphonia). Otolaryngol Head Neck Surg 2009;141(3 Suppl 2):S1–31.

13. Lee WT, Eliashar R, Eliachar I. Acute external laryngotracheal trauma: diagnosis and management. Ear Nose Throat J 2006;85(3):179–84.

14. Bhojani RA, Rosenbaum DH, Dikmen E, et al. Contemporary assessment of laryngotracheal trauma. J Thorac Cardiovasc Surg 2005;130(2):426–32.

15. Schaefer SD. The acute management of external laryngeal trauma. A 27-year experience. Arch Otolaryngol Head Neck Surg 1992;118(6):598–604.

16. Eliachar I, Lewin JS. Imaging evaluation of laryngotracheal stenosis. J Otolaryngol 1993;22(4):265–77.

17. Parida PK, Gupta AK. Role of spiral computed tomography with 3-dimensional reconstruction in cases with laryngeal stenosis–a radioclinical correlation. Am J Otolaryngol 2008;29(5):305–11.

18. American Cancer Society. Cancer facts & figures 2011. Atlanta (GA): American Cancer Society; 2011.

19. American Joint Committee on Cancer. Larynx. In: Edge SB, Byrd DR, Compton CC, et al, editors. AJCC cancer staging manual. 7th edition. New York: Springer; 2010. p. 57–67.

20. Silver CE, Beitler JJ, Shaha AR, et al. Current trends in initial management of laryngeal cancer: the declining use of open surgery. Eur Arch Otorhinolaryngol 2009;266(9):1333–52.

21. Loevner LA, Yousem DM, Montone KT, et al. Can radiologists accurately predict preepiglottic space invasion with MR imaging? AJR Am J Roentgenol 1997; 169(6):1681–7.

22. Dursun G, Keser R, Akturk T, et al. The significance of pre-epiglottic space invasion in supraglottic laryngeal carcinomas. Eur Arch Otorhinolaryngol 1997; 254(Suppl 1):S110–2.

23. Murakami R, Nishimura R, Baba Y, et al. Prognostic factors of glottic carcinomas treated with radiation therapy: value of the adjacent sign on radiological examinations in the sixth edition of the UICC TNM staging system. Int J Radiat Oncol Biol Phys 2005;61(2):471–5.

24. Ferreiro-Arguelles C, Jimenez-Juan L, Martinez-Salazar JM, et al. CT findings after laryngectomy. Radiographics 2008;28(3):869–82 [quiz: 914].

25. Chawla S, Carney AS. Organ preservation surgery for laryngeal cancer. Head Neck Oncol 2009;1:12.

26. Patel UA, Howell LK. Local response to chemoradiation in T4 larynx cancer with cartilage invasion. Laryngoscope 2011;121(1):106–10.

27. Becker M, Zbaren P, Delavelle J, et al. Neoplastic invasion of the laryngeal cartilage: reassessment of criteria for diagnosis at CT. Radiology 1997;203(2):521–32.

28. Yousem DM, Hatabu H, Hurst RW, et al. Carotid artery invasion by head and neck masses: prediction with MR imaging. Radiology 1995;195(3):715–20.

29. Hsu WC, Loevner LA, Karpati R, et al. Accuracy of magnetic resonance imaging in predicting absence of fixation of head and neck cancer to the prevertebral space. Head Neck 2005;27(2):95–100.

30. Som PM, Brandwein MS. Lymph nodes. In: Som PM, Curtin HD, editors. Head and neck imaging, vol. 2. St Louis (MO): Mosby; 2003. p. 1865–934.

31. Mukherji SK, Armao D, Joshi VM. Cervical nodal metastases in squamous cell carcinoma of the head and neck: what to expect. Head Neck 2001;23(11): 995–1005.

32. Chu MM, Kositwattanarerk A, Lee DJ, et al. FDG PET with contrast-enhanced CT: a critical imaging tool for laryngeal carcinoma. Radiographics 2010;30(5):1353–72.

33. Schwartz DL, Rajendran J, Yueh B, et al. FDG-PET prediction of head and neck squamous cell cancer outcomes. Arch Otolaryngol Head Neck Surg 2004; 130(12):1361–7.

34. Mukherji SK, Weadock WJ. Imaging of the post-treatment larynx. Eur J Radiol 2002;44(2):108–19.

35. Glastonbury CM, Parker EE, Hoang JK. The postradiation neck: evaluating response to treatment and recognizing complications. AJR Am J Roentgenol 2010;195(2):W164–71.

36. Becker M, Moulin G, Kurt AM, et al. Non-squamous cell neoplasms of the larynx: radiologic-pathologic correlation. Radiographics 1998;18(5):1189–209.

37. Brouwer J, Hooft L, Hoekstra OS, et al. Systematic review: accuracy of imaging tests in the diagnosis of recurrent laryngeal carcinoma after radiotherapy. Head Neck 2008;30(7):889–97.

38. Horiuchi C, Taguchi T, Yoshida T, et al. Early assessment of clinical response to concurrent chemoradiotherapy in head and neck carcinoma using fluoro-2-deoxy-d-glucose positron emission tomography. Auris Nasus Larynx 2008; 35(1):103–8.

39. Zbaren P, Caversaccio M, Thoeny HC, et al. Radionecrosis or tumor recurrence after radiation of laryngeal and hypopharyngeal carcinomas. Otolaryngol Head Neck Surg 2006;135(6):838–43.

40. Hunter SE, Scher RL. Clinical implications of radionecrosis to the head and neck surgeon. Curr Opin Otolaryngol Head Neck Surg 2003;11(2):103–6.

41. Hermans R, Pameijer FA, Mancuso AA, et al. CT findings in chondroradionecrosis of the larynx. AJNR Am J Neuroradiol 1998;19(4):711–8.

42. Furuta Y, Homma A, Oridate N, et al. Surgical complications of salvage total laryngectomy following concurrent chemoradiotherapy. Int J Clin Oncol 2008;13(6):521–7.

43. Ganly I, Patel S, Matsuo J, et al. Postoperative complications of salvage total laryngectomy. Cancer 2005;103(10):2073–81.

44. van la Parra RF, Kon M, Schellekens PP, et al. The prognostic value of abnormal findings on radiographic swallowing studies after total laryngectomy. Cancer Imaging 2007;7:119–25.

45. O-Lee TJ, Messner A. Subglottic hemangioma. Otolaryngol Clin North Am 2008; 41(5):903–11, viii–ix.

46. Perkins JA, Duke W, Chen E, et al. Emerging concepts in airway infantile hemangioma assessment and management. Otolaryngol Head Neck Surg 2009;141(2): 207–12.

47. Nozawa K, Aihara T, Takano H. MR imaging of a subglottic hemangioma. Pediatr Radiol 1995;25(3):235–6.

48. Yilmaz MD, Aktepe F, Altuntas A. Cavernous hemangioma of the left vocal cord. Eur Arch Otorhinolaryngol 2004;261(6):310–1.

49. Jungehulsing M, Fischbach R, Pototschnig C, et al. Rare benign tumors: laryngeal and hypopharyngeal lipomata. Ann Otol Rhinol Laryngol 2000;109(3):301–5.

50. Powitzky R, Powitzky ES, Garcia R. Liposarcoma of the larynx. Ann Otol Rhinol Laryngol 2007;116(6):418–24.

51. Chiu LD, Rasgon BM. Laryngeal chondroma: a benign process with long-term clinical implications. Ear Nose Throat J 1996;75(8):540–2, 544–9.
52. Hyams VJ, Rabuzzi DD. Cartilaginous tumors of the larynx. Laryngoscope 1970; 80(5):755–67.
53. Baatenburg de Jong RJ, van Lent S, Hogendoorn PC. Chondroma and chondrosarcoma of the larynx. Curr Opin Otolaryngol Head Neck Surg 2004;12(2): 98–105.
54. Thompson LD, Gannon FH. Chondrosarcoma of the larynx: a clinicopathologic study of 111 cases with a review of the literature. Am J Surg Pathol 2002;26(7):836–51.
55. Stiglbauer R, Steurer M, Schimmerl S, et al. MRI of cartilaginous tumours of the larynx. Clin Radiol 1992;46(1):23–7.
56. Sakai O, Curtin HD, Faquin WC, et al. Dedifferentiated chondrosarcoma of the larynx. AJNR Am J Neuroradiol 2000;21(3):584–6.
57. Feldman F, Van Heertum R, Saxena C, et al. 18FDG-PET applications for cartilage neoplasms. Skeletal Radiol 2005;34(7):367–74.
58. Bak-Pedersen K, Nielsen KO. Subepithelial mucous glands in the adult human larynx. Studies on number, distribution and density. Acta Otolaryngol 1986; 102(3–4):341–52.
59. Ganly I, Patel SG, Coleman M, et al. Malignant minor salivary gland tumors of the larynx. Arch Otolaryngol Head Neck Surg 2006;132(7):767–70.
60. Mahlstedt K, Ussmuller J, Donath K. Malignant sialogenic tumours of the larynx. J Laryngol Otol 2002;116(2):119–22.
61. Batsakis JG, Luna MA, el-Naggar AK. Nonsquamous carcinomas of the larynx. Ann Otol Rhinol Laryngol 1992;101(12):1024–6.
62. Sigal R, Monnet O, de Baere T, et al. Adenoid cystic carcinoma of the head and neck: evaluation with MR imaging and clinical-pathologic correlation in 27 patients. Radiology 1992;184(1):95–101.
63. Markou K, Goudakos J, Constantinidis J, et al. Primary laryngeal lymphoma: report of 3 cases and review of the literature. Head Neck 2010;32(4):541–9.
64. Siddiqui NA, Branstetter BF, Hamilton BE, et al. Imaging characteristics of primary laryngeal lymphoma. AJNR Am J Neuroradiol 2010;31(7):1261–5.
65. Fatahzadeh M. Kaposi sarcoma: review and medical management update. Oral Surg Oral Med Oral Pathol Oral Radiol Endod 2012;113(1):2–16.
66. Pantanowitz L, Dezube BJ. Kaposi sarcoma in unusual locations. BMC Cancer 2008;8:190.
67. Cheung MC, Pantanowitz L, Dezube BJ. AIDS-related malignancies: emerging challenges in the era of highly active antiretroviral therapy. Oncologist 2005; 10(6):412–26.
68. Restrepo CS, Martinez S, Lemos JA, et al. Imaging manifestations of Kaposi sarcoma. Radiographics 2006;26(4):1169–85.
69. Bell RB, Verschueren DS, Dierks EJ. Management of laryngeal trauma. Oral Maxillofac Surg Clin North Am 2008;20(3):415–30.
70. Jewett BS, Shockley WW, Rutledge R. External laryngeal trauma analysis of 392 patients. Arch Otolaryngol Head Neck Surg 1999;125(8):877–80.
71. Shires CB, Preston T, Thompson J. Pediatric laryngeal trauma: a case series at a tertiary children's hospital. Int J Pediatr Otorhinolaryngol 2011;75(3):401–8.
72. Robinson S, Juutilainen M, Suomalainen A, et al. Multidetector row computed tomography of the injured larynx after trauma. Semin Ultrasound CT MR 2009; 30(3):188–94.
73. Shockley WW, Ball SS. Laryngeal trauma. Curr Opin Otolaryngol Head Neck Surg 2000;8:497–502.

74. Rubin AD, Hawkshaw MJ, Moyer CA, et al. Arytenoid cartilage dislocation: a 20-year experience. J Voice 2005;19(4):687–701.
75. Sataloff RT, Bough ID Jr, Spiegel JR. Arytenoid dislocation: diagnosis and treatment. Laryngoscope 1994;104(11 Pt 1):1353–61.
76. Stack BC Jr, Ridley MB. Arytenoid subluxation from blunt laryngeal trauma. Am J Otolaryngol 1994;15(1):68–73.
77. Alexander AE Jr, Lyons GD, Fazekas-May MA, et al. Utility of helical computed tomography in the study of arytenoid dislocation and arytenoid subluxation. Ann Otol Rhinol Laryngol 1997;106(12):1020–3.
78. Norris BK, Schweinfurth JM. Arytenoid dislocation: an analysis of the contemporary literature. Laryngoscope 2011;121(1):142–6.
79. Sataloff RT, Rao VM, Hawkshaw M, et al. Cricothyroid joint injury. J Voice 1998; 12(1):112–6.
80. Alvi A, Weissman J, Myssiorek D, et al. Computed tomographic and magnetic resonance imaging characteristics of laryngocele and its variants. Am J Otolaryngol 1998;19(4):251–6.
81. Dursun G, Ozgursoy OB, Beton S, et al. Current diagnosis and treatment of laryngocele in adults. Otolaryngol Head Neck Surg 2007;136(2):211–5.
82. Weissler MC, Fried MP, Kelly JH. Laryngopyocele as a cause of airway obstruction. Laryngoscope 1985;95(11):1348–51.
83. Aubry K, Kapella M, Ketterer S, et al. A case of laryngeal ductal cyst: antenatal diagnosis and peripartum management. Int J Pediatr Otorhinolaryngol 2007; 71(10):1639–42.
84. Ozgursoy OB, Batikhan H, Beton S, et al. Sudden-onset life-threatening stridor in an adult caused by a laryngeal ductal cyst. Ear Nose Throat J 2009;88(3):828–30.
85. Chin SC, Fatterpeckar G, Kao CH, et al. Amyloidosis concurrently involving the sinonasal cavities and larynx. AJNR Am J Neuroradiol 2004;25(4):636–8.
86. Gean-Marton AD, Kirsch CF, Vezina LG, et al. Focal amyloidosis of the head and neck: evaluation with CT and MR imaging. Radiology 1991;181(2):521–5.
87. Arslan A, Ceylan N, Cetin A, et al. Laryngeal amyloidosis with laryngocele: MRI and CT. Neuroradiology 1998;40(6):401–3.
88. Bartels H, Dikkers FG, van der Wal JE, et al. Laryngeal amyloidosis: localized versus systemic disease and update on diagnosis and therapy. Ann Otol Rhinol Laryngol 2004;113(9):741–8.
89. Thompson LD, Derringer GA, Wenig BM. Amyloidosis of the larynx: a clinicopathologic study of 11 cases. Mod Pathol 2000;13(5):528–35.
90. Gilad R, Milillo P, Som PM. Severe diffuse systemic amyloidosis with involvement of the pharynx, larynx, and trachea: CT and MR findings. AJNR Am J Neuroradiol 2007;28(8):1557–8.
91. Rubin AD, Sataloff RT. Vocal fold paresis and paralysis. Otolaryngol Clin North Am 2007;40(5):1109–31, viii–ix.
92. Chin SC, Edelstein S, Chen CY, et al. Using CT to localize side and level of vocal cord paralysis. AJR Am J Roentgenol 2003;180(4):1165–70.

Cervical Lymph Node Evaluation and Diagnosis

Thomas C. Bryson, MD, Gaurang V. Shah, MD*,
Ashok Srinivasan, MBBS, MD, Suresh K. Mukherji, MD

KEYWORDS

• Lymphadenopathy • Lymph node • Head and neck cancer • CT • MRI

KEY POINTS

• In many cases of cervical lymphadenopathy, the clinical history, physical examination, and routine laboratory investigations can establish a presumptive diagnosis of reactively enlarged nodes related to viral or bacterial infection. Imaging these patients is generally unnecessary, unless atypical symptoms or findings concerning for aggressive infection are noted.

• Imaging, particularly computed tomography (CT), is valuable in cases concerning for suppurative lymphadenitis or deep neck infection by identifying abscesses requiring surgical drainage.

• Imaging findings such as stranding of adjacent fat on CT may help distinguish suppurative nodes from metastatic disease; however, common imaging findings such as nodal enlargement, enhancement, and hypodensity seen in the setting of lymphadenitis caused by typical or atypical pathogens can also be seen with nodal metastasis.

• In asymptomatic patients and patients with nonspecific symptoms, imaging may be indicated to assist in evaluating a palpable neck mass.

INTRODUCTION

Cervical lymphadenopathy is a common clinical finding, which can be related to reactive nodal hypertrophy, granulomatous processes, lymphoma and head and neck cancers or mimicked by nonnodal neck masses. Cross-sectional imaging has the ability to quickly assess the extent of cervical lymphadenopathy with greater accuracy than the physical examination and provide information regarding the relationship with

Dr Mukherji is a consultant with Phillips Medical Systems. The other authors have nothing to disclose.
Department of Radiology, University of Michigan Hospital and Health Systems, 1500 East Medical Center Drive, Ann Arbor, MI 48109-5030, USA
* Corresponding author. Department of Radiology UH-B2-A209, University of Michigan Health Systems, 1500 East Medical Center Drive, Ann Arbor, MI 48109-5030, USA.
E-mail address: gvshah@med.umich.edu

Otolaryngol Clin N Am 45 (2012) 1363–1383
http://dx.doi.org/10.1016/j.otc.2012.08.007

oto.theclinics.com

adjacent vital structures. This information can have significant management implications in cases of acute infection, but is perhaps most important when applied to staging of head and neck malignancies. Head and neck squamous cell carcinomas (HNSCC) are the most common malignancy of the upper aerodigestive tract, and lymphatic spread is the most important mechanism of metastasis in these patients. Accurately staging nodal disease in HNSCC has both important prognostic and management implications. This article discusses the rationale for imaging cervical lymph nodes and reviews nodal anatomy and common drainage patters, imaging features of pathologic lymph nodes, and the advantages of various imaging modalities available.

RATIONALE FOR IMAGING

In many cases of cervical lymphadenopathy, the clinical history, physical examination, and routine laboratory investigations can establish a presumptive diagnosis of reactively enlarged nodes related to viral or bacterial infection. Imaging these patients is generally unnecessary, unless atypical symptoms or findings concerning for aggressive infection are noted. Imaging, particularly computed tomography (CT), has proved valuable in cases concerning for suppurative lymphadenitis or deep neck infection by identifying abscesses requiring surgical drainage.[1,2] Imaging findings such as stranding of adjacent fat on CT may help distinguish suppurative nodes from metastatic disease; however, common imaging findings such as nodal enlargement, enhancement, and hypodensity seen in the setting of lymphadenitis caused by typical or atypical (eg, mycobacterial or bacillary) pathogens can also be seen with nodal metastasis (Fig. 1).[3]

In asymptomatic patients and patients with nonspecific symptoms, imaging may be indicated to assist in evaluating a palpable neck mass. In the case of a solitary

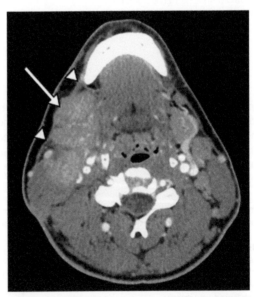

Fig. 1. Contrast-enhanced CT shows a conglomerate of enlarged, heterogeneously enhancing right level I and II lymph nodes (*arrow*) in an immunosuppressed patient with fungal lymphadenitis. Note the adjacent inflammatory stranding and thickening of the platysma muscle (*arrowheads*).

palpable neck mass, imaging with ultrasonography (US), CT, or magnetic resonance imaging (MRI) may identify congenital cysts such as thyroglossal and branchial cleft cysts. Imaging findings in many of these patients are nonspecific, and recent studies have questioned the ability of US to make a confident preoperative diagnosis.[4] However, imaging in these types of patients should be able to differentiate between nodal disease and nonnodal neoplasms in most cases. Nonnodal findings on imaging can also affect the differential diagnosis. For example, multiple cystic lesions within the parotid glands seen in combination with cervical lymphadenopathy can suggest the diagnosis of human immunodeficiency virus infection.

The prognostic value of accurate staging in the case of head and neck malignancies has produced a well-defined role for the use of imaging. Squamous cell carcinomas (SCC), which make up 80% to 90% of all upper aerodigestive tract malignancies, have shown a high predilection for metastasis to regional lymph nodes, with nodal metastases present in 20% to 30% of patients at the time of diagnosis depending on the site.[5,6] The presence or absence of lymph node metastasis in these patients at the time of diagnosis has a profound impact on 5-year disease-specific survival rates. In 1 series evaluating HNSCC from multiple sites, the 5-year survival was reduced from 67.9% to 39.9% based solely on the presence of nodal metastases. Nodal stage in this series also affected survival, with advanced N2 or N3 patients, according to the American Joint Committee on Cancer (AJCC) staging system,[7] showing significantly worse outcomes.[8] Staging examinations by palpation alone have shown limited sensitivity of approximately 64%, specificity of 85%, and overall accuracy of approximately 75%.[9] Also, clinical examination has proved inaccurate at evaluating size of cervical nodes regardless of clinical experience.[10] The ability of imaging studies to evaluate nodal groups occult to palpation (such as retropharyngeal nodes) and provide accurate nodal measurements can increase sensitivity and specificity up to 81% and 96%, respectively,[9] with imaging identifying palpably occult nodal metastases in up to 27% of patients.[11]

Patients who are deemed N0 by clinical staging typically undergo elective treatment of cervical lymph nodes such as neck dissection if there is a 20% risk of occult metastases.[12] Imaging studies may increase sensitivity and specificity over palpation; however, identification of micrometastases (metastatic deposits less than 3 mm in size) remains a significant challenge for imaging. Up to 25% of neck dissection specimens may harbor only micrometastases[13] and use of highly sensitive molecular pathology techniques can show evidence for micrometastases in even more cases than traditional light microscopy.[14,15] Treatment of these N0 patients remains controversial, and some investigators have suggested that the rate of occult metastases in patients undergoing thorough staging examinations including CT or MRI is low (less than 10%), making observation a viable option with equivalent outcomes to elective neck dissection.[8] Other investigators have advocated reducing the number of staging evaluations used in patients with small primary tumors[16]; however, they continue to advocate the use of cross-sectional imaging as an accurate and expedient way to evaluate both the primary tumor and potential nodal metastases.

NODAL CLASSIFICATION

The complex anatomy of cervical lymph nodes has led to numerous attempts at organization. The most widely used schemes historically have been those, such as that of Rouvière,[17] describing nodal groups based on proximity to adjacent structures. This type of organization resulted in the familiar large groupings of cervical nodes such as the jugular or spinal accessory chains, which were then subdivided into superficial or deep, upper or lower, and medial or lateral subgroups. With the development of more advanced surgical approaches to head and neck cancer, including techniques such as selective neck dissections, a less cumbersome scheme was needed that could accurately reflect patterns of lymphatic drainage and standardize communication between clinicians. Building on the work of earlier investigators such as Lindberg[18] and Shah and colleagues,[19] the American Head and Neck Society (AHNS) and American Academy of Otolaryngology–Head and Neck Surgery developed a 6-level system of nodal classification.[20–22] Some of the surgical boundaries initially defined proved difficult to define by imaging; therefore, surrogate landmarks were identified and an imaging-based classification of cervical lymph nodes was developed.[23] The most recent AHNS consensus statement on nodal classification has been updated to reflect this system and the role of imaging in evaluating cervical lymph nodes in the setting of head and neck cancer.[24] The result has been a widely accepted division of cervical lymph nodes into 7 numbered nodal levels with well-defined anatomic boundaries that can be easily identified by both surgeons and radiologists (**Fig. 2**).

On cross-sectional imaging, level I lymph nodes are found inferior to the myelohyoid muscle, anterior to a line drawn at the posterior margin of the submandibular glands and within the boundaries of the mandible. This region can be subdivided into levels IA and IB by the anterior bellies of the digastric muscles, with level IA lymph nodes medial and level IB nodes lateral to the anterior belly of the digastric muscle.

Level II lymph nodes are found posterior to the line drawn at the posterior margin of the submandibular glands, anterior to the posterior margin of the sternocleidomastoid muscle and between the lower margin of the hyoid bone and the skull base (**Fig. 3**). Level II nodes can also be subdivided into levels IIA and IIB, with level IIA nodes along the internal jugular vein and level IIB nodes posterior to the internal jugular vein and separated by a fat plane.

Level III lymph nodes are found lateral to the carotid arteries, anterior to the posterior margin of the sternocleidomastoid muscle and between the lower margin of the hyoid bone and lower margin of the cricoid cartilage (see **Fig. 3**).

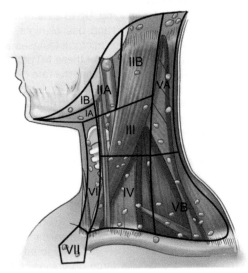

Fig. 2. Cervical lymph nodes divided into 7 levels, with subdivision of levels I, II, and V.

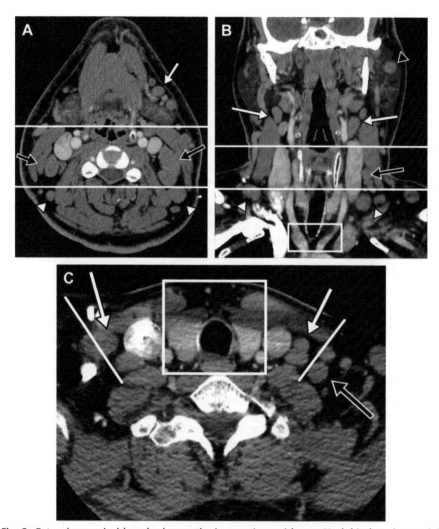

Fig. 3. Extensive cervical lymphadenopathy in a patient with non-Hodgkin lymphoma. (*A*) Axial CT image with horizontal lines demarcating the posterior margins of the submandibular glands and sternocleidomastoid (SCM) muscles. These lines separate lymph nodes within levels I (*white arrow*), II (*black arrow*), and V (*white arrowhead*). (*B*) Coronal CT image with horizontal lines demarcating the levels of the hyoid bone and cricoid cartilage. These lines separate lymph nodes within levels II (*white arrows*), III (*black arrow*), and IV (*white arrowheads*). An intraparotid node is also seen (*black arrowhead*). The white rectangle demarcates where level VII nodes would be seen. (*C*) Axial CT image with oblique lines demarcating the plane between the posterior margins of the SCM and anterior scalene muscles. These lines separate lymph nodes within levels IV (*white arrows*) and V (*black arrow*). The white rectangle demarcates where level VI nodes would be seen.

Level IV lymph nodes are found lateral to the carotid arteries, anterior to the line connecting the posterior margins of the sternocleidomastoid and anterior scalene muscles and between the lower margin of the cricoid cartilage and the clavicle (see **Fig. 3**).

Level V lymph nodes are found posterior to the posterior margin of the sternocleido-mastoid muscle from the skull base to the clavicle. Level V nodes can be subdivided in to levels VA and VB, with level VA nodes located between the skull base and lower margin of the cricoid cartilage and level VB nodes located between the lower margin of the cricoid and the clavicle anterior to the anterior margin of the trapezius muscle (see **Fig. 3**).

Levels VI and VII are outside the traditional boundaries of the radical neck dissection and, although they have been defined in the literature, may be less widely applied in clinical practice. Level VI lymph nodes encompass those found in the anterior central or visceral compartment medial to the carotid arteries and between the lower margin of the hyoid bone and the upper margin of the manubrium. Level VII lymph nodes encompass those found in a paratracheal location medial to the carotid arteries within the superior mediastinum between the upper margin of the manubrium and the innominate artery (see **Fig. 3**).

Some nodal sites, such as the nodal groups of the superior pericervical region including intraparotid, buccinator, suboccipital, and retroauricular lymph nodes, lie outside these defined levels and retain their traditional anatomic descriptors. Nodes found medial to the carotid arteries superior to the hyoid bone are referred to as retropharyngeal nodes (Rouvière), a similar example of an anatomically named nodal distribution.

PATTERNS OF NODAL DRAINAGE

The 7-level nodal classification system was designed to reflect common patterns of lymphatic drainage, and most malignancies of the head and neck have a predictable pattern of metastasis along these routes. Although the detailed anatomy of the lymphatic system of the head and neck and upper aerodigestive tract is beyond the scope of this review, recent works have mapped lymphatic drainage patterns[25] and these anatomic pathways have been found to mirror clinical experience in patterns of metastatic disease in a variety of head and neck malignancies.[26–28] The presence of predictable drainage patterns, particularly in the case of HNSCC, have led to the clinical practice of selective neck dissection involving nodal groups at highest risk rather than more comprehensive, and morbid, radical neck dissection. Therefore, a basic understanding of these patterns is essential when evaluating cervical lymph nodes in the setting of malignancy either clinically or by imaging. However, these patterns are not immutable, and skip metastasis to more distal nodal groups without involvement of usual proximal drainage pathways can occur in up to 15% of cases.[29]

Oral Cavity Lymphatic Drainage

Lymphatic drainage of the oral cavity may extend from level I to level IV, depending on the location of the primary tumor. Anterior regions including the anterior floor of mouth, anterior mandibular gingival, and medial lower lip drain preferentially to level IA nodes, with the upper lip, lateral lower lip, buccal mucosal, and contiguous mucosa of the anterior palate draining preferentially to level IB nodes. The posterior portions of the oral cavity drain preferentially to level II.

Tongue Lymphatic Drainage

Drainage of the tongue is complex, with the ventral tongue following drainage patterns of the floor of mouth to level IA anteromedially and IB laterally (**Fig. 4**). The dorsal oral tongue may drain either to level I nodes medially or level II nodes laterally. The tongue base shows drainage patterns more akin to pharyngeal drainage, primarily involving levels II and III (**Fig. 5**). Level IV nodes may be involved in advanced disease, or via alternative drainage pathways. Midline lesions may have bilateral drainage patterns.

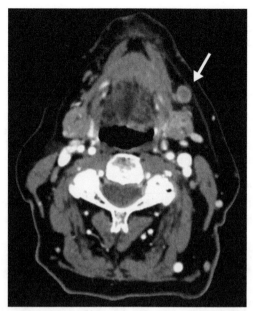

Fig. 4. Abnormal level Ib lymph node (*white arrow*) in a patient with SCC of the anterior lateral floor of mouth involving the oral tongue. This node is borderline by size criteria, but abnormally rounded and centrally nonenhancing.

Nasopharynx Lymphatic Drainage

The nasopharynx is richly supplied with lymphatics and shows one of the highest rates of nodal metastasis when involved with SCC.[30] The nasopharynx also serves as the catchment basin for lymphatic drainage of most of the nasal cavity and paranasal sinuses. The predominant lymphatic drainage pattern for these regions is to lateral

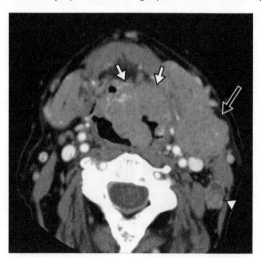

Fig. 5. Abnormal level IIa and level IIb lymph nodes (*black arrows* and *white arrowhead*, respectively) in a patient with a large tongue base SCC extending into the vallecula (*white arrows*). These nodes are abnormally enlarged and heterogeneously enhancing. Borderline enlarged right level II lymph nodes were also seen in this patient, whose tumor crossed midline.

retropharyngeal nodes and level II nodes, with drainage to more distal level III and IV nodal groups in more advanced disease and through alternative drainage patterns (**Fig. 6**). Unlike other areas of the pharyngeal mucosa, nasopharyngeal lesions may drain posteriorly to level V. Midline lesions of the nasopharynx may result in bilateral drainage patterns.

Oropharyngeal Lymphatic Drainage

Oropharyngeal structures, including the soft palate, palatine and lingual tonsils, and posterior pharyngeal wall show a similar drainage pattern to that previously described for the tongue base. Drainage is primarily to level II and III nodal groups, with less common involvement of retropharyngeal and level IV nodes.

Hypopharynx Lymphatic Drainage

The hypopharynx is surpassed only by the nasopharynx in density of lymphatic drainage, with particularly dense confluence of lymphatic drainage in the piriform

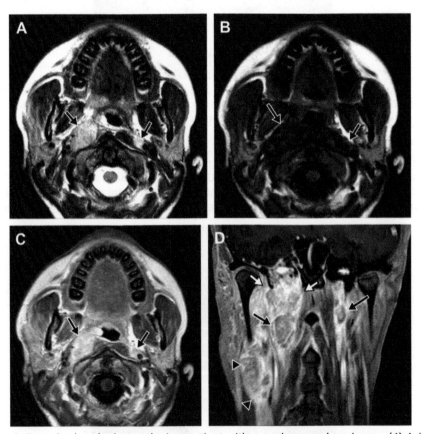

Fig. 6. Extensive lymphadenopathy in a patient with nasopharyngeal carcinoma. (*A*) Axial T2-weighted MRI shows bilateral retropharyngeal lymph node enlargement (*black arrows*). (*B*) Axial unenhanced T1-weighed MRI and (*C*) axial T1-weighted postgadolinium MRI show abnormal enhancement of these retropharyngeal nodes (*black arrows*). (*D*) Coronal postgadolinium fat-suppressed T1-weighted image shows bilateral retropharyngeal lymph nodes (*black arrows*), extensive right level II and III lymph nodes (*black arrowheads*), and the primary nasopharyngeal carcinoma (*white arrows*).

sinuses. Drainage of the hypopharynx is similar to that of the oropharynx, with predominant involvement of levels II to IV and occasional drainage to retropharyngeal nodes from the posterior hypopharyngeal wall. Anterior hypopharyngeal lymphatic drainage channels may directly communicate with laryngeal lymphatics, with eventual involvement of level VI nodes.

Laryngeal Lymphatic Drainage

Laryngeal drainage patterns can be divided into supraglottic, glottic, and subglottic patterns. Supraglottic structures, including the epiglottis and aryepiglottic folds, drain primarily to level III, with occasional drainage cephalad to level II. Prominent horizontal drainage patterns lead to an increased risk for bilateral metastasis. Glottic structures such as the true vocal fold and vocal ligaments have poor lymphatic drainage, making nodal metastasis from small glottic lesions less likely. More advanced glottic lesions, with involvement of the muscles of phonation, may have involvement of nodal levels II to IV and VI (**Fig. 7**). Subglottic processes have primarily lateral drainage to levels III and IV.

Paratracheal Lymphatic Drainage

Processes involving the cervical esophagus, thyroid and parathyroid glands, and some subglottic locations show primarily paratracheal drainage to levels VI and VII. Other less common processes, including malignant melanoma and other cutaneous malignancies, have less predictable patterns of metastases. Melanoma may initially involve superficial nodes such as postauricular or suboccipital nodal groups, with additional involvement of posterior level V nodes depending on the location of the primary lesion.[31,32]

IMAGING CHARACTERISTICS OF PATHOLOGIC LYMPH NODES
Size

Size criteria are widely used in evaluating lymph nodes on cross-sectional imaging and are integral to the AJCC nodal staging system. Criteria for nodal enlargement have been studied by multiple groups advocating different techniques and cutoff values, with variability in the resulting sensitivity and specificity for detecting

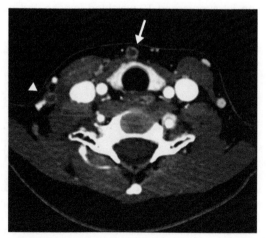

Fig. 7. Peripherally enhancing anterior level VI (Delphian, *arrow*) and right level IV/V lymph nodes (*arrow head*) in a patient with laryngeal carcinoma.

malignancy.[13,33–35] Nodes may be measured in either greatest diameter (long axis) or minimal diameter (short axis). Nodes measuring greater than 1.5 cm in greatest diameter in levels I or II and greater than 1.0 cm in all other levels are considered abnormal and harbor metastatic disease in approximately 80% of cases.[36] Other investigators claim minimal diameter measurements are more accurate and reproducible on both CT and US, with diameters exceeding 11 mm in levels I and II or 10 mm elsewhere considered abnormal.[37] Nodes meeting these minimal diameter criteria harbor metastatic disease in approximately 75% of cases.[13] Retropharyngeal nodes have been considered separately by some investigators, with those exceeding 6 to 8 mm in greatest diameter concerning for metastasis, particularly in the setting of nasopharyngeal tumors.[38,39] Some investigators have suggested alternative measurement criteria for sonography, considering minimum diameter measurements greater than 6 to 7 mm in levels I and II or 5 mm in levels III and IV abnormal.[40]

Shape

Size criteria alone may misinterpret reactive nodes as malignant and overlook small metastases. Therefore, additional morphologic criteria have been proposed. Normal lymph nodes tend to be flat or kidney-bean–shaped, with a fat-containing hilum. Malignant nodes typically show a rounded shape, with loss of the normal fatty hilum or focal cortical expansion (**Fig. 8**).[41,42] It has been suggested that a maximal diameter/minimal diameter ratio greater than 2 favors benign nodes and a ratio less than 2 favors malignancy.[36,43] Nodal grouping can also help identify pathologic nodes. Grouping refers to 3 or more nodes in continuity with each other, each measuring at least 8 to 10 mm in diameter. Although not individually enlarged by these criteria, groupings of nodes such as this along the expected drainage pathway for a known malignancy are concerning and increase sensitivity for metastases.[13]

Density

Nodal necrosis, with its focal central hypodensity on CT and thick rind of surrounding enhancing tissue, is an important diagnostic criterion considered virtually pathognomonic for metastatic disease in patients with HNSCC. Similar imaging findings can be seen on MRI, including a focal defect in enhancement centrally on gadolinium-enhanced T1-weighted imaging. This nonenhancing central region is typically hyperintense on fat-suppressed T2-weighted images, but may show variable

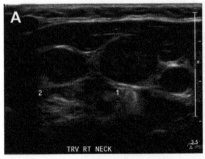 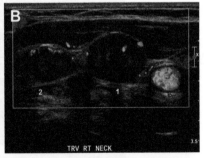

Fig. 8. Abnormal level III lymph nodes in a patient with metastatic papillary thyroid carcinoma. (*A*) Gray-scale sonographic image showing the rounded shape of 2 lymph nodes with abnormal maximal diameter/minimal diameter ratio. (*B*) Color Doppler sonographic image showing loss of the normal fatty hilum and normal hilar vasculature. Peripheral blood flow is seen.

signal characteristics depending on the makeup of the necrotic tissue (**Fig. 9**). Although it is difficult to apply these characteristics to small foci of necrosis less than 3 mm in size, they are generally accurate in detecting necrotic nodes, with sensitivities of 91% and 93% and specificities of 93% and 89% for CT and MRI, respectively.[44] Although some studies have suggested that CT is superior to MRI in detection of central nodal necrosis, both have been shown to be more sensitive than US.[44,45] Central nodal necrosis is more common in larger nodes, occurring in 56% to 63% of metastatic nodes larger than 1.5 cm and 10% to 33% of nodes smaller than 1 cm; however, as many as 35% of all necrotic nodes are less than 1 cm in size.[33,34,46] Rarely, metastatic lymph nodes may appear cystic, with central fluid characteristics and a thin rim of tissue. This situation occurs more commonly in papillary thyroid carcinoma, but can occur in HNSCC. These cystic nodes can be misinterpreted as branchial cleft cysts, and care should be taken to evaluate for possible primary malignancy when cystic lesions are seen in adults.[47]

Extracapsular Spread

Extracapsular spread of malignancy and invasion of adjacent structures are of key clinical importance in determining a patient's prognosis and surgical options. Extracapsular spread is a histologic diagnosis in many cases, with imaging features such as blurring of nodal margins and soft tissue infiltration of adjacent fat or muscle producing sensitivities and specificities of only 63% to 81% and 60% to 72% for CT and up to 77% and 72% for MRI, respectively (**Fig. 10**).[48–50] Other studies reported an accuracy of 90% for CT and 78% for MRI in detecting extracapsular spread.[45] When present, findings of macroscopic extracapsular spread identifiable by imaging increase the rate of local recurrence by a factor of 3.5 compared with those without evidence of extracapsular nodal disease.[51] In addition, if 2 or more nodes show extracapsular spread, the risk of local recurrence is 58.3%, rate of distant metastases is 33.3%, and median survival is less than 1 year.[52] Larger nodes are more likely to show extracapsular spread of disease, with up to 75% of nodes greater than 3 cm in size showing evidence either by imaging or microscopically.

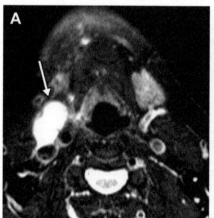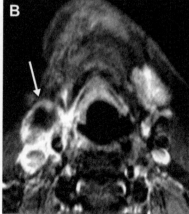

Fig. 9. Abnormal right level II lymph node in a patient with SCC of the right tonsil. (*A*) Axial T2-weighted MRI image shows increased signal within this necrotic lymph node (*white arrow*). (*B*) Axial postgadolinium fat-suppressed T1-weighted image shows thick irregular peripheral enhancement of this node consistent with nodal necrosis (*white arrow*).

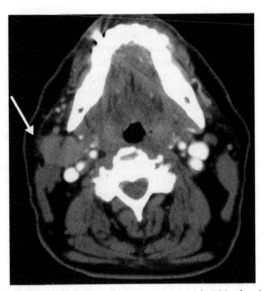

Fig. 10. Enlarged right level II lymph node in a patient with SCC of unknown primary site (*arrow*). Poor definition of the lateral node margin and stranding of adjacent fat are consistent with extracapsular spread of neoplasm.

Invasion of Adjacent Structures

When nodal disease is advanced, confluent masses of cervical adenopathy may invade adjacent structures such as the carotid artery or jugular vein. Carotid invasion in most cases renders the mass unresectable, and further preoperative testing, such as balloon occlusion testing, may be required if carotid sacrifice is to be considered. Fat planes separating an infiltrating mass from the vessels should be evaluated to determine the degree of circumferential involvement. If less than 180° of the vessel circumference is involved, then direct vascular invasion is unlikely. However, if greater than 270° of circumferential encasement is present by cross-sectional imaging, arterial wall invasion can be presumed with a relatively high degree of sensitivity and specificity (**Fig. 11**).[53] Maneuvers on real-time sonography to determine mobility of a mass relative to vessels can also be useful to determine if vessel invasion has occurred.[54]

ADVANCED IMAGING TECHNIQUES
Contrast-Enhanced CT

Traditionally, cross-sectional anatomic imaging with CT, MRI, or US has formed the cornerstone of head and neck imaging, with the choice of initial imaging modality depending on the individual center and clinical indication. Contrast-enhanced CT is widely used because of its short examination times, ubiquitous availability, high inherent contrast between lymph nodes and cervical fat, and relatively high spatial resolution with modern multidetector scanners. The short examination times and relatively wider gantry bore are better tolerated by claustrophobic patients compared with MRI and CT images are typically less affected by motion artifacts. MRI, with its high-contrast resolution and multiplanar imaging capabilities, can also readily detect abnormal lymph nodes, and modern turbospin echo sequences have shortened

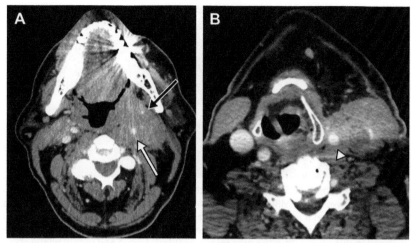

Fig. 11. Confluent lymphadenopathy causing vascular encasement in a patient with unresectable oropharyngeal SCC. (*A*) Confluent level II adenopathy with encasement of the left internal carotid (*white arrow*) and external carotid (*black arrow*) arteries. (*B*) Additional confluent level III adenopathy with resultant encasement of the left common carotid artery (*white arrowhead*).

examination times. MRI has added value in evaluating a primary neoplastic process, with improved detection of bone marrow involvement and perineural spread of disease.[55] Overall, most studies comparing the accuracy of CT and MRI in evaluating the important clinically negative (N0) neck have found no significant difference between the 2 modalities, with imaging detecting approximately 40% to 60% of occult metastases and micrometastases going largely undetected.[56–59]

US

US, particularly in combination with ultrasound-guided fine-needle aspiration, has gained popularity in Europe. In general, US is superior to palpation in detection of nodal metastases and may outperform CT and MRI.[59–61] Doppler techniques evaluating patterns of hilar and peripheral blood flow have been found to offer added value in identifying nodal metastases.[62–64] Ultrasound-guided fine-needle aspiration cytology has been shown to be superior to CT and MRI, with specificity for nodal metastases approaching 100%.[65] These techniques are highly operator dependent and labor intensive to achieve this degree of accuracy.

Diffusion-Weighted MRI

Recently, techniques such as diffusion-weighted MRI (DWI) and perfusion have added new tools to the imaging armamentarium. HNSCC can show areas of restricted diffusion and corresponding decreased signal on apparent diffusion coefficient maps, likely because of their highly cellular nature.[66] Several studies have now shown that DWI can aid in differentiation of benign reactive lymphadenopathy from metastatic malignancy and may be particularly helpful in evaluating the posttreatment neck (**Fig. 12**).[67–69] These studies have shown sensitivities of 84% to 89%, specificities of 94% to 97%, and accuracy of 91% to 94% for detection of metastatic lymph nodes by DWI, significantly outperforming conventional turbospin echo imaging in each

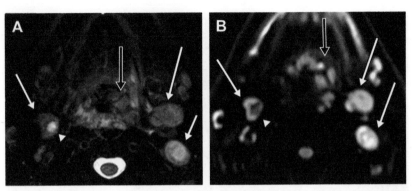

Fig. 12. Metastatic lymph nodes in a patient with tongue base SCC on T2 and DWI. (*A*) Axial fat-suppressed T2-weighted MRI shows irregular left tongue base mass (*black arrow*) and bilateral abnormal level II lymph nodes (*white arrows*). A small focus of increased T2 signal is seen within one of the nodes (*white arrowhead*) (*B*) Axial DWI at a corresponding level shows impeded diffusion within the primary tumor (*black arrow*) and within bilateral metastatic lymph nodes (*white arrows*). Note the small focus of necrosis within the right-sided node does not impede diffusion (*white arrowhead*).

case. As with other modalities, DWI sensitivity for metastatic disease decreases to 76% in subcentimeter nodal metastases. This technique is still not standardized, and these values are dependent on the apparent diffusion coefficient cutoff values chosen. Also, magnetic field inhomogeneity or improper coil placement can negatively affect image quality and limit diagnostic usefulness.[70]

Contrast-Enhanced CT and MRI

The role of contrast-enhanced imaging in CT and MRI is well established. Iodinated contrast enables evaluation of nodal architecture by CT and is required for identification of nodal necrosis in most cases. Gadolinium contrast media may be less integral to the evaluation of cervical lymph nodes by MRI, but add value in evaluating for nodal necrosis and in evaluating characteristics of the primary lesion, such as perineural spread of malignancy.[71] Newer contrast-enhanced techniques, such as perfusion imaging, are now being used to provide functional evaluations of cervical lymph nodes. Perfusion techniques evaluate dynamic microscopic blood flow changes by documenting changes in signal intensity (MRI) or attenuation (CT) in a given region of interest after bolus administration of contrast material. These techniques, like DWI, are noninvasive and can be obtained without adding significant additional time to imaging protocols.[72] CT perfusion characteristics of neoplastic tissue have been shown to be different from adjacent normal tissue, with SCC of the upper aerodigestive tract showing increased blood volume and blood flow, with corresponding decreases in mean transit time (**Fig. 13**).[73] Perfusion characteristics may be able to direct therapy, with some studies linking increased blood volume/flow with increased chemosensitivity.[74] Although some studies have suggested that CT perfusion was not useful when applied to lymph nodes,[75] more recent studies have shown that these perfusion techniques can be applied to help differentiate metastatic nodes from reactive benign lymph nodes.[76] Similarly, recent studies of dynamic susceptibility-weighted perfusion MRI have shown promise in differentiating metastases from benign lymph nodes and may be able to differentiate between metastases and lymphoma.[77]

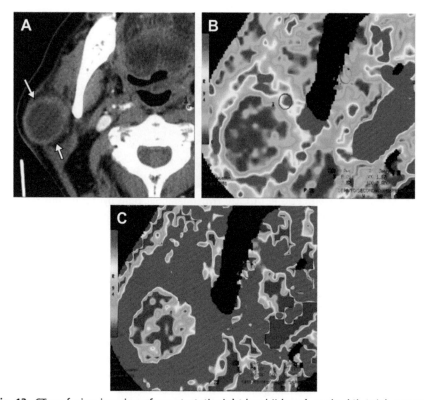

Fig. 13. CT perfusion imaging of a metastatic right level II lymph node. (*A*) Axial contrast-enhanced CT image obtained during perfusion imaging shows peripheral enhancement of this abnormal lymph node (*white arrows*). Corresponding increases (*red on the color scale*) in blood volume (*B*) and blood flow (*C*) are seen on perfusion maps at the periphery of this node.

POSITRON EMISSION TOMOGRAPHY AND [^{18}F]FLUORODEOXYGLUCOSE POSITRON EMISSION TOMOGRAPHY

Positron emission tomography (PET) with [^{18}F]fluorodeoxyglucose (FDG), and modern fused PET/CT, are powerful tools that are able to evaluate glucose metabolism within cervical lymph nodes. This ability to provide metabolic information, and now fuse it with anatomic imaging, has proved powerful, with FDG-PET and PET/CT routinely out-performing conventional CT and MRI in the detection of nodal disease in patients who have head and neck cancer.[78–81] PET imaging in these studies has shown sensitivity for nodal metastases of up to 90% and specificity approaching 100%. Although the technical resolution of PET imaging is 4 to 5 mm and micrometastases remain a significant challenge, FDG-PET is capable of detecting metastases within lymph nodes of 4 to 6 mm, which would be overlooked by anatomic imaging alone.[78,82,83] Current practice does not use PET/CT routinely for initial staging; however, it has the capability to alter therapy through detection of previously occult nodal and distant metastases and can provide functional information about the primary lesion (**Fig. 14**). Primary tumors, but not metastatic lymph nodes, with higher objective measures of metabolic activity (higher standardized uptake values) have been shown to have higher rates of locoregional recurrence and may benefit from more aggressive therapy.[84] Some investigators

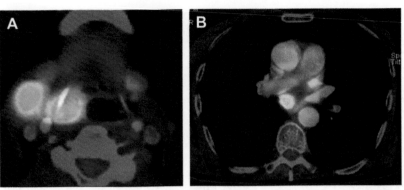

Fig. 14. Staging study with FDG-PET/CT. (*A*) Hypermetabolic right pyriform sinus SCC with regional right level III nodal metastasis. (*B*) Whole-body PET/CT imaging can detect distant metastases, as in this case of hypermetabolic mediastinal lymph nodes concerning for distant metastases.

have suggested that a negative PET examination can decrease the risk of occult metastases in clinically N0 patients with T1 to T3 primary tumors to 15% or less, a rate at which elective nodal treatments may be deferred.[80] In the posttherapy neck, PET has proved superior to CT or MRI in detecting residual nodal metastases.[85]

SUMMARY AND RECOMMENDATIONS

Cross-sectional imaging, particularly CT and MRI, is a valuable tool in the armamentarium of the head and neck surgeon for evaluation of cervical lymph nodes, particularly in the setting of head and neck malignancies. The evaluation of nodal size, morphology, and enhancement characteristics is the primary means of identifying abnormal lymph nodes on cross-sectional imaging, and understanding the nodal classification scheme is required to effectively communicate the location of abnormal nodes to other physicians. Imaging techniques outperform the clinical examination in detection of metastatic lymph nodes and can detect 40% to 60% of occult metastatic disease, but continue to be insensitive for detection of micrometastases. Newer techniques such as DWI, perfusion imaging, and FDG-PET/CT may improve the imaging evaluation of the N0 neck.

REFERENCES

1. Lazor JB, et al. Comparison of computed tomography and surgical findings in deep neck infections. Otolaryngol Head Neck Surg 1994;111(6):746–50.
2. Smith JL 2nd, Hsu JM, Chang J. Predicting deep neck space abscess using computed tomography. Am J Otolaryngol 2006;27(4):244–7.
3. McKellop JA, Bou-Assaly W, Mukherji SK. Emergency head & neck imaging: infections and inflammatory processes. Neuroimaging Clin North Am 2010; 20(4):651–61.
4. Sidell DR, Shapiro NL. Diagnostic accuracy of ultrasonography for midline neck masses in children. Otolaryngol Head Neck Surg 2011;144(3):431–4.
5. Byers RM, Wolf PF, Ballantyne AJ. Rationale for elective modified neck dissection. Head Neck Surg 1988;10(3):160–7.
6. Giacomarra V, et al. Predictive factors of nodal metastases in oral cavity and oropharynx carcinomas. Laryngoscope 1999;109(5):795–9.

7. Edge SB. American Joint Committee on Cancer and American Cancer Society. AJCC cancer staging handbook from the AJCC cancer staging manual. New York: Springer; 2010. p. 1 online resource (xix, 718 p).
8. Layland MK, Sessions DG, Lenox J. The influence of lymph node metastasis in the treatment of squamous cell carcinoma of the oral cavity, oropharynx, larynx, and hypopharynx: N0 versus N+. Laryngoscope 2005;115(4):629–39.
9. Haberal I, et al. Which is important in the evaluation of metastatic lymph nodes in head and neck cancer: palpation, ultrasonography, or computed tomography? Otolaryngol Head Neck Surg 2004;130(2):197–201.
10. Alderson DJ, et al. Observer error in the assessment of nodal disease in head and neck cancer. Head Neck 2001;23(9):739–43.
11. Atula TS, et al. Assessment of cervical lymph node status in head and neck cancer patients: palpation, computed tomography and low field magnetic resonance imaging compared with ultrasound-guided fine-needle aspiration cytology. Eur J Radiol 1997;25(2):152–61.
12. Weiss MH, Harrison LB, Isaacs RS. Use of decision analysis in planning a management strategy for the stage N0 neck. Arch Otolaryngol Head Neck Surg 1994;120(7):699–702.
13. van den Brekel MW, et al. Cervical lymph node metastasis: assessment of radiologic criteria. Radiology 1990;177(2):379–84.
14. Brennan JA, et al. Molecular assessment of histopathological staging in squamous-cell carcinoma of the head and neck. N Engl J Med 1995;332(7): 429–35.
15. Hamakawa H, et al. Keratin mRNA for detecting micrometastasis in cervical lymph nodes of oral cancer. Cancer Lett 2000;160(1):115–23.
16. Braunius WW, et al. Observing stage-shifts in head and neck squamous cell carcinoma from initial clinical outpatient staging to definite clinical tumour board staging using radiological and endoscopical investigations: will less do? Clin Otolaryngol 2011;36(4):352–60.
17. Rouvière H, Tobias MJ. Anatomy of the human lymphatic system. Ann Arbor (MI): Edwards brothers, inc; 1938. ix, p. 318.
18. Lindberg R. Distribution of cervical lymph node metastases from squamous cell carcinoma of the upper respiratory and digestive tracts. Cancer 1972;29(6): 1446–9.
19. Shah JP, et al. Surgical grand rounds. Neck dissection: current status and future possibilities. Clin Bull 1981;11(1):25–33.
20. Robbins KT, et al. Standardizing neck dissection terminology. Official report of the Academy's Committee for Head and Neck Surgery and Oncology. Arch Otolaryngol Head Neck Surg 1991;117(6):601–5.
21. Robbins KT. Classification of neck dissection: current concepts and future considerations. Otolaryngol Clin North Am 1998;31(4):639–55.
22. Robbins KT, et al. Neck dissection classification update: revisions proposed by the American Head and Neck Society and the American Academy of Otolaryngology-Head and Neck Surgery. Arch Otolaryngol Head Neck Surg 2002;128(7):751–8.
23. Som PM, Curtin HD, Mancuso AA. An imaging-based classification for the cervical nodes designed as an adjunct to recent clinically based nodal classifications. Arch Otolaryngol Head Neck Surg 1999;125(4):388–96.
24. Robbins KT, et al. Consensus statement on the classification and terminology of neck dissection. Arch Otolaryngol Head Neck Surg 2008;134(5): 536–8.

25. Werner JA, Dunne AA, Myers JN. Functional anatomy of the lymphatic drainage system of the upper aerodigestive tract and its role in metastasis of squamous cell carcinoma. Head Neck 2003;25(4):322–32.

26. de Wilt JH, et al. Correlation between preoperative lymphoscintigraphy and metastatic nodal disease sites in 362 patients with cutaneous melanomas of the head and neck. Ann Surg 2004;239(4):544–52.

27. King AD, et al. Neck node metastases from nasopharyngeal carcinoma: MR imaging of patterns of disease. Head Neck 2000;22(3):275–81.

28. Shah JP. Patterns of cervical lymph node metastasis from squamous carcinomas of the upper aerodigestive tract. Am J Surg 1990;160(4):405–9.

29. Byers RM, et al. Frequency and therapeutic implications of "skip metastases" in the neck from squamous carcinoma of the oral tongue. Head Neck 1997;19(1):14–9.

30. Wang Y, Ow TJ, Myers JN. Pathways for cervical metastasis in malignant neoplasms of the head and neck region. Clin Anat 2012;25(1):54–71.

31. Pathak I, et al. Do nodal metastases from cutaneous melanoma of the head and neck follow a clinically predictable pattern? Head Neck 2001;23(9):785–90.

32. Wagner JD, et al. Cervical sentinel lymph node biopsy for melanomas of the head and neck and upper thorax. Arch Otolaryngol Head Neck Surg 2000;126(3): 313–21.

33. Don DM, et al. Evaluation of cervical lymph node metastases in squamous cell carcinoma of the head and neck. Laryngoscope 1995;105(7 Pt 1):669–74.

34. Friedman M, et al. Nodal size of metastatic squamous cell carcinoma of the neck. Laryngoscope 1993;103(8):854–6.

35. van den Brekel MW, Castelijns JA, Snow GB. The size of lymph nodes in the neck on sonograms as a radiologic criterion for metastasis: how reliable is it? AJNR Am J Neuroradiol 1998;19(4):695–700.

36. Som PM. Detection of metastasis in cervical lymph nodes: CT and MR criteria and differential diagnosis. AJR Am J Roentgenol 1992;158(5):961–9.

37. Sumi M, Ohki M, Nakamura T. Comparison of sonography and CT for differentiating benign from malignant cervical lymph nodes in patients with squamous cell carcinoma of the head and neck. AJR Am J Roentgenol 2001;176(4): 1019–24.

38. Mancuso AA, et al. Computed tomography of cervical and retropharyngeal lymph nodes: normal anatomy, variants of normal, and applications in staging head and neck cancer. Part II: pathology. Radiology 1983;148(3):715–23.

39. Mancuso AA, et al. Computed tomography of cervical and retropharyngeal lymph nodes: normal anatomy, variants of normal, and applications in staging head and neck cancer. Part I: normal anatomy. Radiology 1983;148(3):709–14.

40. Yonetsu K, et al. Contribution of doppler sonography blood flow information to the diagnosis of metastatic cervical nodes in patients with head and neck cancer: assessment in relation to anatomic levels of the neck. AJNR Am J Neuroradiol 2001;22(1):163–9.

41. Rubaltelli L, et al. Sonography of abnormal lymph nodes in vitro: correlation of sonographic and histologic findings. AJR Am J Roentgenol 1990;155(6):1241–4.

42. Vassallo P, et al. Differentiation of benign from malignant superficial lymphadenopathy: the role of high-resolution US. Radiology 1992;183(1):215–20.

43. Bruneton JN, et al. Very high frequency (13 MHz) ultrasonographic examination of the normal neck: detection of normal lymph nodes and thyroid nodules. J Ultrasound Med 1994;13(2):87–90.

44. King AD, et al. Necrosis in metastatic neck nodes: diagnostic accuracy of CT, MR imaging, and US. Radiology 2004;230(3):720–6.

45. Yousem DM, et al. Central nodal necrosis and extracapsular neoplastic spread in cervical lymph nodes: MR imaging versus CT. Radiology 1992;182(3):753–9.
46. Eida S, et al. Combination of helical CT and Doppler sonography in the follow-up of patients with clinical N0 stage neck disease and oral cancer. AJNR Am J Neuroradiol 2003;24(3):312–8.
47. Gor DM, Langer JE, Loevner LA. Imaging of cervical lymph nodes in head and neck cancer: the basics. Radiol Clin North Am 2006;44(1):101–10, viii.
48. Carvalho P, et al. Accuracy of CT in detecting squamous carcinoma metastases in cervical lymph nodes. Clin Radiol 1991;44(2):79–81.
49. Steinkamp HJ, et al. Extracapsular spread of cervical lymph node metastases: Diagnostic value of magnetic resonance imaging. Rofo 2002;174(1): 50–5 [in German].
50. Steinkamp HJ, et al. The extracapsular spread of cervical lymph node metastases: the diagnostic value of computed tomography. Rofo 1999;170(5): 457–62 [in German].
51. Brasilino de Carvalho M. Quantitative analysis of the extent of extracapsular invasion and its prognostic significance: a prospective study of 170 cases of carcinoma of the larynx and hypopharynx. Head Neck 1998;20(1):16–21.
52. Greenberg JS, et al. Extent of extracapsular spread: a critical prognosticator in oral tongue cancer. Cancer 2003;97(6):1464–70.
53. Yousem DM, et al. Carotid artery invasion by head and neck masses: prediction with MR imaging. Radiology 1995;195(3):715–20.
54. Gritzmann N, et al. Invasion of the carotid artery and jugular vein by lymph node metastases: detection with sonography. AJR Am J Roentgenol 1990;154(2): 411–4.
55. Weber AL, Romo L, Hashmi S. Malignant tumors of the oral cavity and oropharynx: clinical, pathologic, and radiologic evaluation. Neuroimaging Clin North Am 2003;13(3):443–64.
56. Curtin HD, et al. Comparison of CT and MR imaging in staging of neck metastases. Radiology 1998;207(1):123–30.
57. Hillsamer PJ, et al. Improving diagnostic accuracy of cervical metastases with computed tomography and magnetic resonance imaging. Arch Otolaryngol Head Neck Surg 1990;116(11):1297–301.
58. Lenz M, Kersting-Sommerhoff B, Gross M. Diagnosis and treatment of the N0 neck in carcinomas of the upper aerodigestive tract: current status of diagnostic procedures. Eur Arch Otorhinolaryngol 1993;250(8):432–8.
59. van den Brekel MW, et al. Modern imaging techniques and ultrasound-guided aspiration cytology for the assessment of neck node metastases: a prospective comparative study. Eur Arch Otorhinolaryngol 1993;250(1):11–7.
60. Prayer L, et al. Sonography versus palpation in the detection of regional lymph-node metastases in patients with malignant melanoma. Eur J Cancer 1990;26(7): 827–30.
61. Vassallo P, et al. In-vitro high-resolution ultrasonography of benign and malignant lymph nodes. A sonographic-pathologic correlation. Invest Radiol 1993;28(8): 698–705.
62. Ahuja AT, Ying M. Sonographic evaluation of cervical lymph nodes. AJR Am J Roentgenol 2005;184(5):1691–9.
63. Ariji Y, et al. Power Doppler sonography of cervical lymph nodes in patients with head and neck cancer. AJNR Am J Neuroradiol 1998;19(2):303–7.
64. Tschammler A, et al. Vascular patterns in reactive and malignant lymphadenopathy. Eur Radiol 1996;6(4):473–80.

65. van den Brekel MW, et al. Occult metastatic neck disease: detection with US and US-guided fine-needle aspiration cytology. Radiology 1991;180(2): 457–61.

66. Wang J, et al. Head and neck lesions: characterization with diffusion-weighted echo-planar MR imaging. Radiology 2001;220(3):621–30.

67. Dirix P, et al. Diffusion-weighted MRI for nodal staging of head and neck squamous cell carcinoma: impact on radiotherapy planning. Int J Radiat Oncol Biol Phys 2010;76(3):761–6.

68. Holzapfel K, et al. Value of diffusion-weighted MR imaging in the differentiation between benign and malignant cervical lymph nodes. Eur J Radiol 2009;72(3): 381–7.

69. Vandecaveye V, et al. Head and neck squamous cell carcinoma: value of diffusion-weighted MR imaging for nodal staging. Radiology 2009;251(1): 134–46.

70. Hermans R, Vandecaveye V. Diffusion-weighted MRI in head and neck cancer. Cancer Imaging 2007;7:126–7.

71. Hudgins PA. Contrast enhancement in head and neck imaging. Neuroimaging Clin North Am 1994;4(1):101–15.

72. Shah GV, et al. New directions in head and neck imaging. J Surg Oncol 2008; 97(8):644–8.

73. Gandhi D, et al. Computed tomography perfusion of squamous cell carcinoma of the upper aerodigestive tract. Initial results. J Comput Assist Tomogr 2003;27(5): 687–93.

74. Zima A, et al. Can pretreatment CT perfusion predict response of advanced squamous cell carcinoma of the upper aerodigestive tract treated with induction chemotherapy? AJNR Am J Neuroradiol 2007;28(2):328–34.

75. Bisdas S, et al. Quantitative measurements of perfusion and permeability of oropharyngeal and oral cavity cancer, recurrent disease, and associated lymph nodes using first-pass contrast-enhanced computed tomography studies. Invest Radiol 2007;42(3):172–9.

76. Trojanowska A, et al. Squamous cell cancer of hypopharynx and larynx–evaluation of metastatic nodal disease based on computed tomography perfusion studies. Eur J Radiol 2011.

77. Abdel Razek AA, Gaballa G. Role of perfusion magnetic resonance imaging in cervical lymphadenopathy. J Comput Assist Tomogr 2011;35(1):21–5.

78. Adams S, et al. Prospective comparison of 18F-FDG PET with conventional imaging modalities (CT, MRI, US) in lymph node staging of head and neck cancer. Eur J Nucl Med 1998;25(9):1255–60.

79. Hannah A, et al. Evaluation of 18 F-fluorodeoxyglucose positron emission tomography and computed tomography with histopathologic correlation in the initial staging of head and neck cancer. Ann Surg 2002;236(2):208–17.

80. Ng SH, et al. Prospective study of [18F]fluorodeoxyglucose positron emission tomography and computed tomography and magnetic resonance imaging in oral cavity squamous cell carcinoma with palpably negative neck. J Clin Oncol 2006;24(27):4371–6.

81. Roh JL, et al. Utility of 2-[18F] fluoro-2-deoxy-D-glucose positron emission tomography and positron emission tomography/computed tomography imaging in the preoperative staging of head and neck squamous cell carcinoma. Oral Oncol 2007;43(9):887–93.

82. Benchaou M, et al. The role of FDG-PET in the preoperative assessment of N-staging in head and neck cancer. Acta Otolaryngol 1996;116(2):332–5.

83. Jabour BA, et al. Extracranial head and neck: PET imaging with 2-[F-18]fluoro-2-deoxy-D-glucose and MR imaging correlation. Radiology 1993;186(1): 27–35.
84. Schwartz DL, et al. FDG-PET prediction of head and neck squamous cell cancer outcomes. Arch Otolaryngol Head Neck Surg 2004;130(12):1361–7.
85. Kim SY, et al. Evaluation of 18F-FDG PET/CT and CT/MRI with histopathologic correlation in patients undergoing salvage surgery for head and neck squamous cell carcinoma. Ann Surg Oncol 2011;18(9):2579–84.

Lesions of the Skull Base
Imaging for Diagnosis and Treatment

Asim F. Choudhri, MD[a,b,c,]*, Hemant A. Parmar, MD[d],
Robert E. Morales, MD[e], Dheeraj Gandhi, MD[e,f]

KEYWORDS

• Skull base • Tumor • Temporal bone • Head and neck

KEY POINTS

• A specific diagnosis is not always possible based on imaging alone; however, a systematic approach to the imaging of skull base lesions can allow the rapid formation of a concise and logical differential diagnosis.
• CT of the skull base provides excellent anatomic detail of osseous structures.
• MRI provides excellent soft tissue detail, although no single "routine" MRI protocol exists that will work for all skull base pathology.
• Positron emission tomography (PET)/CT is an important tool for the diagnosis and follow-up of head and neck malignancies.

INTRODUCTION

Lesions of the skull base can be challenging to diagnose and treat because of the complex anatomy, proximity to cranial nerves and important vasculature, and wide variety of pathology that may be infrequently encountered. Modern imaging techniques can help characterize skull base lesions, determine a diagnosis, and formulate a plan for tissue diagnosis and/or subsequent treatment.

Disclosures: No disclosures.
[a] Department of Radiology, University of Tennessee Health Science Center, 50 North Dunlap – G216, Memphis, TN 38103, USA; [b] Department of Neurosurgery, University of Tennessee Health Science Center, 50 North Dunlap – G216, Memphis, TN 38103, USA; [c] Department of Radiology, Le Bonheur Neuroscience Institute, Le Bonheur Children's Hospital, 50 North Dunlap – G216, Memphis, TN 38103, USA; [d] Department of Radiology, University of Michigan, 1500 E. Medical Center Drive, TC- 132-A, Ann Arbor, MI 48109, USA; [e] Department of Radiology, Division of Neuroradiology, University of Maryland, 22 South Greene Street G2K14, Baltimore, MD 21201, USA; [f] Departments of Neurology and Neurosurgery, University of Maryland, 22 South Greene Street G2K14, Baltimore, MD 21201, USA
* Corresponding author. Department of Radiology, Le Bonheur Children's Hospital, 50 North Dunlap – G216, Memphis, TN 38103.
E-mail address: achoudhri@uthsc.edu

Otolaryngol Clin N Am 45 (2012) 1385–1404
http://dx.doi.org/10.1016/j.otc.2012.08.008
0030-6665/12/$ – see front matter © 2012 Elsevier Inc. All rights reserved.
oto.theclinics.com

IMAGING CONSIDERATIONS FOR SKULL BASE

CT

CT of the skull base provides excellent anatomic detail of osseous structures. CT is a widely available technique that can be performed quickly. When using a helical acquisition technique, the raw data can be processed within the scanner to provide reconstructions in any imaging plane from a single acquisition. Although orthogonal axes are most commonly used (axial, sagittal, and coronal), oblique planes can be used to correct for head tilt or provide optimal visualization of a specific structure (eg, simulated Stenvers or Pöschl views).

CT source data can be rendered into images of varying thicknesses, with thinner sections providing higher anatomic detail at the expense of more image noise. CT source data can also be subjected to sharpening algorithms to enhance osseous detail. Soft tissue–optimized images ("soft tissue algorithm") can be adjusted to show osseous detail ("bone window"), however, with less osseous resolution than the dedicated bone algorithm images.

When tumor, infection, or a vascular lesion is suspected, intravenous iodinated contrast may be a helpful adjunct. If the CT images are obtained during the initial arterial phase after administering contrast, the study provides excellent vascular detail (ie, CT angiography). CT images performed 1 to 3 minutes after contrast administration provide less angiographic detail; however, tumors with capillary/venous pooling and hyperemic tissue associated with an infectious process will become more conspicuous. When evaluating cerebrospinal fluid (CSF) leaks, intrathecal iodinated contrast can be administered via lumbar puncture and then used to diagnose and localize a leak.[1]

Given the ionizing radiation required for CT examinations, carefully identifying the diagnostic question before the scan helps maximize utility of the study while minimizing excess radiation. Efforts to reduce radiation dose, possibly through use of alternative imaging modalities, may be especially important in children.[2]

MRI

MRI provides excellent soft tissue detail; however, no single "routine" MRI protocol exists that will work for all skull base abnormalities. The imaging protocol required will be based on the suspected abnormality, the available imaging equipment, and local imaging expertise.

T1- and T2-weighted sequences are the 2 basic MR pulse sequences that can be performed in different planes and with different slice thicknesses. Typically, fat, proteinaceous material, and some blood products (particularly methemoglobin) have a hyperintense (or "bright") appearance on T1-weighted imaging. Fat and water tend to be hyperintense on T2-weighted imaging. Note that subtle variations between sequences on different protocols, at different field strengths, and using equipment from different manufacturers can significantly vary the appearance of structures, and thus familiarity with locally used protocols is important for proper interpretation of images.

Intravenous administration of gadolinium chelates serves a similar contrast-enhancement role for MR that iodinated contrast does for CT. Enhancing lesions will be hyperintense, or "bright," on postcontrast T1-weighted sequences; however, 2 pitfalls can occur if one is not careful. A finding that has intrinsic hyperintense signal on T1-weighted images (T1 hyperintense appearance) will be hyperintense on postcontrast sequences even in the absence of enhancement, and therefore comparison with precontrast T1-weighted imaging is important. As fat has a hyperintense appearance on T1-weighted images, a small enhancing lesion surrounded by fat can be difficult to detect. For this reason, special MR sequences in which the signal of fat is nulled (fat suppression) can improve conspicuity of lesions surrounded by fat. Often, however, using non–fat-suppressed imaging at the skull base is preferred because of the image degradation and artifacts that can occur with fat suppression techniques. Moreover, because of its intrinsic bright signal, fat provides excellent contrast with low-intensity structures, such as nerves and vessels. Diffusion-weighted imaging is a technique commonly used in the brain to detect stroke; however, it has recently become recognized for its ability to characterize abscesses and head and neck tumors, and to differentiate cholesteatoma from granulation tissue.[3]

High-resolution fluid-sensitive balanced steady state free precession sequences, often referred to by manufacturers proprietary acronyms, such as CISS (constructive interference in the steady state; Siemens AG, Munich, Germany) or FIESTA (fast imaging employing steady state acquisition; GE, Fairfield, CT) can provide submillimeter resolution and are excellent for detecting cranial nerve abnormalities and finding fluid communications in suspected meningoceles/encephaloceles.

Intrathecal gadolinium to detect skull base CSF leaks has been described in several reports, although this technique is not currently approved by the U.S. Food and Drug Administration and therefore is not discussed in this report. However, this technique may emerge as an important problem-solving tool in the future.[4]

Angiography

Angiography remains an important tool for confirming the diagnosis of vascular lesions of the skull base,[5] and can serve as a therapeutic option in many cases, either on its own or for presurgical embolization.

Nuclear Medicine

Although PET/CT is an important tool for the diagnosis and follow-up of head and neck malignancies[6,7] and metastases, it is not significantly discussed in this article. Radionuclide cisternography can be helpful for confirming a CSF leak, but it has less spatial resolution than either CT or MR cisternography.[1,4] Nuclear medicine studies can also help confirm whether a tumor has a neuroendocrine origin, such as in glomus tumors/paragangliomas.[8,9]

ANTERIOR SKULL BASE
Anatomy

The anterior skull base includes the pterygopalatine fossa, cribriform plate, and planum sphenoidale, and thus abnormalities can have an intracranial, neurovascular, or sinonasal origin (**Table 1**). Traumatic and congenital abnormalities are also commonly encountered.

The pterygopalatine fossa is a crossroads of nerves and vessels that communicates with the intracranial contents via foramen rotundum posteriorly (**Fig. 1**C, G, J), the central skull base/carotid canal via the vidian canal posteriorly (**Fig. 1**D, G), the orbit via the infraorbital foramen superiorly (**Fig. 1**J), the paranasal sinuses via the sphenopalatine foramen medially (**Fig. 1**C), the masticator space via the pterygomaxillary fissure laterally (**Fig. 1**C, D), and the hard palate via the greater and lesser palatine foramina inferiorly. Therefore, the pterygopalatine fossa is often involved in perineural spread of head and neck neoplasms and should be especially scrutinized in patients with head and neck, orbital, and sinonasal abnormalities.

Congenital Lesions

Congenital anomalies of the anterior skull base often present in infancy, and their complexity is rich enough for a dedicated article.[10–13] Because occasionally patients

Table 1 Anterior skull base lesions	
Neoplasms	Sinonasal carcinoma Metastatic lesions Sinonasal undifferentiated carcinoma Juvenile nasal angiofibroma Sinonasal melanoma Hemangiopericytoma Non-Hodgkin's lymphoma, sinonasal Nerve sheath tumor Esthesioneuroblastoma Meningioma
Congenital	Sincipital encephalocele
Infection/other	Empyema of sinonasal origin Mucocele Fibrous dysplasia Sinonasal osteoma

may present later in childhood or adulthood, it is important to be aware of and exclude these entities before biopsy or excision of an anterior skull base lesion. Sincipital encephaloceles can be subdivided by location into frontonasal, frontoethmoidal, and sphenoid encephaloceles. Embryologic rests of tissue can also result in masses such as a nasal glioma and a nasal dermoid. High-resolution fluid-sensitive sequences (eg, CISS/FIESTA) can help identify CSF/dural extension through the skull base, thereby helping to characterize these lesions.

Tumors

Many types of neoplastic processes may involve the anterior skull base, including juvenile nasal angiofibroma (JNA), esthesioneuroblastoma, sinonasal malignancies, and meningioma. When the mass is large, the center of the mass may become difficult to accurately localize, and the precise diagnosis may similarly become difficult to determine.

JNA

JNA is a vascular tumor that arises in the sphenopalatine foramen and extends into the posterior nasal cavity.[14] The classic presentation is that of an adolescent boy with recurrent unilateral epistaxis. Because it arises from the medial recess of the pterygopalatine fossa, it is not unexpected that the arterial supply is predominantly from the internal maxillary artery. CT typically shows an intensely enhancing mass that causes expansion of the sphenopalatine foramen, an imaging hallmark for this neoplasm. MR often shows heterogeneous signal on T1- and T2-weighted imaging and avid contrast enhancement, with internal flow voids confirming the internal vascularity. Larger masses characteristically produce posterior scalloping and mass effect on the posterior wall of the maxillary sinus. Angiography and embolization are often required as preoperative adjuncts.

Esthesioneuroblastoma

Esthesioneuroblastoma, or olfactory neuroblastoma, is a neural tumor arising from branches of the olfactory nerve and is therefore typically centered at the cribriform plate.[15] Differentiation from other abnormalities involving the cribriform plate can be difficult, but esthesioneuroblastoma will often demonstrate peripheral cystic components along the superior (intracranial) margin (**Fig. 2**).

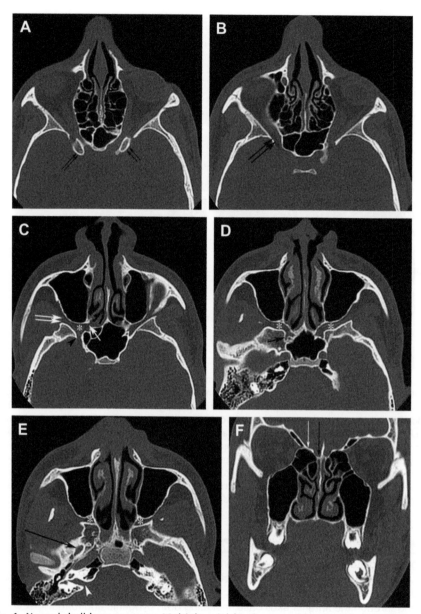

Fig. 1. Normal skull base anatomy. Multiple axial (*A–E*), coronal (*F–H*), mid-sagittal (*I*), and parasagittal (*J*) bone algorithm CT images of the skull base. Axial images in a cranial-to-caudal direction, and the coronal images are anterior to posterior. The following structures can be seen: foramen rotundum (*black arrowheads*); vidian canal (*short black arrows*); foramen ovale (*long black arrows*); pterygopalatine fossa (*white asterisks*); internal auditory canal (*white arrowhead*); sphenopalatine foramen (*short white arrows*); pterygomaxillary fissure (*double white arrows*); inferior orbital fissure (*long white arrows*); superior orbital fissure (*double black arrows*); cribriform plate (*thin black arrows*); fovea ethmoidalis (*thin white arrows*); anterior clinoid processes (*double thin black arrow*); and tegmen tympani (*double black arrowheads*).

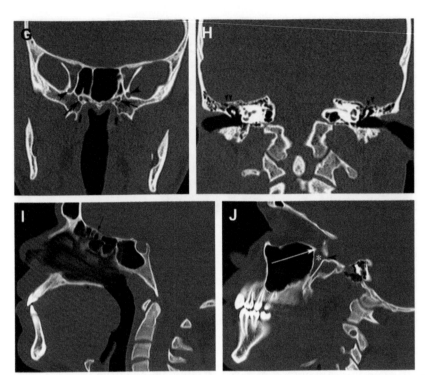

Fig. 1. (continued). Normal skull base anatomy. Multiple axial (*A–E*), coronal (*F–H*), mid-sagittal (*I*), and parasagittal (*J*) bone algorithm CT images of the skull base. Axial images in a cranial-to-caudal direction, and the coronal images are anterior to posterior. The following structures can be seen: foramen rotundum (*black arrowheads*); vidian canal (*short black arrows*); foramen ovale (*long black arrows*); pterygopalatine fossa (*white asterisks*); internal auditory canal (*white arrowhead*); sphenopalatine foramen (*short white arrows*); pterygomaxillary fissure (*double white arrows*); inferior orbital fissure (*long white arrows*); superior orbital fissure (*double black arrows*); cribriform plate (*thin black arrows*); fovea ethmoidalis (*thin white arrows*); anterior clinoid processes (*double thin black arrow*); and tegmen tympani (*double black arrowheads*).

Nonesthesioneuroblastoma Cribriform Plate Invasion

Cribriform plate invasion can occur from nearly any sinonasal primary malignancy, including sinonasal undifferentiated carcinoma, squamous cell carcinoma, adenocarcinoma, inverted papilloma, melanoma, and metastases.[16] Sinonasal infections can extend through the anterior skull base, including both pyogenic and fungal infections. Pyogenic infections can often be identified through a rim of peripheral enhancement surrounding a fluid collection on CT and MR, and diffusion restriction within the central purulent contents on diffusion-weighted MR imaging. Pyogenic infections may have ill-defined margins, and often induce edema in the adjacent brain parenchyma. In contrast, fungal infections tend to have circumscribed margins and may demonstrate solid enhancement pattern. A high density on unenhanced CT and internal foci of very low signal on T2-weighted MR sequence from high mineral content may be identified in fungal infections and can serve as an important imaging clue.[17,18]

Intracranial masses, particularly extradural lesions such as a meningioma (**Fig. 3**), can extend through the cribriform plate. A cribriform plate meningioma will typically

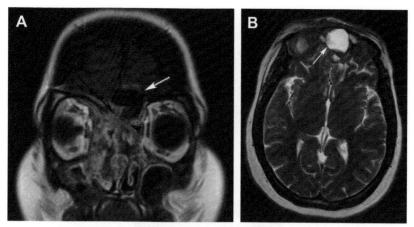

Fig. 2. Esthesioneuroblastoma. Coronal T1-weighted MR image of the anterior skull base performed after the administration of intravenous gadolinium (*A*) and an axial T2-weighted MR image (*B*) shows a predominantly solid enhancing mass filling the ethmoid air cells (*black arrow*) and extending through the cribriform plate (*black arrowhead*). Small cystic areas (*white arrow*) along the interface of the solid lesion and the brain are a characteristic feature of esthesioneuroblastoma.

have imaging features commonly seen in meningiomas, such as a dural tail (suggesting an extra-axial origin), and the center of the mass will typically be above the cribriform plate.

Trauma/CSF leak

Fractures of the anterior skull base, in particular the lamina papyracea and fovea ethmoidalis, may incompletely heal and can result in CSF leak. CT can show high-resolution osseous detail, but it may be difficult to determine the site of leakage without the help of intrathecal contrast injection (CT cisternogram).

If CSF leak is confirmed with either beta-2-transferrin or nuclear medicine cisternogram, CT cisternography can help localize the leak to allow targeted repair/patching.[1] Intrathecal gadolinium-enhanced MR cisternography may have a greater role in the future,[4] but the safety profile of intrathecal gadolinium has not yet been established.

Perineural spread

Head and neck tumors can often have perineural spread that involves the pterygopalatine fossa,[19–21] most commonly squamous cell, adenoid cystic, and mucoepidermoid carcinomas. Tumors of the sinonasal cavity, palate, oral cavity, parapharyngeal space, and masticator space can spread via the perineural route to the pterygopalatine fossa and then gain access intracranially or into the orbit.

CENTRAL SKULL BASE
Anatomy

The primary structure of the central skull base is the sphenoid bone and clivus (**Table 2**). The clivus (**Fig. 1I**) is composed of the basisphenoid and basiocciput, separated by the sphenooccipital synchondrosis in childhood. The sella turcica is an intracranial "saddle-shaped" concavity along the superior surface of the basisphenoid (**Fig. 1I**). The central skull base also includes the sphenoid wings, which is the location

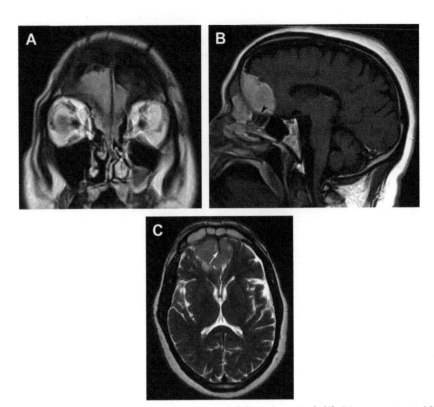

Fig. 3. Cribriform plate meningioma. Coronal (*A*) and sagittal (*B*) T1 postcontrast MR imaging of the anterior skull base shows an enhancing mass along the inferior aspect of the bilateral anterior cranial fossae that extends through the cribriform plate (*black arrowhead*) to involve the frontal sinuses and anterior ethmoid air cells. Axial T2-weighted image of the brain (*C*) shows the mass is predominantly hypointense, reflective of low water content. The mass also preserves the anterior aspect of the falx cerebri (*white arrow*), which would be atypical of an aggressive sinonasal neoplasm or an esthesioneuroblastoma.

of the carotid canal (**Fig. 1**D, E), and the major skull base foramina, including the foramen rotundum (**Fig. 1**C, G, J), ovale, spinosum, and lacerum (**Fig. 1**E). The internal carotid artery traverses the cavernous sinus, which is lateral to the basisphenoid. Inferolateral to the cavernous sinus is Meckel cave, an extradural compartment containing the gasserian ganglion.

Several different processes can manifest in the central skull base, including masses arising from the pituitary fossa, cavernous sinuses, nerves, meninges, and bone. On occasion, giant aneurysms may be encountered arising from the petrous or cavernous segments of the carotid artery. The pituitary masses and meningiomas commonly occur in the middle cranial fossa but are not discussed here.

Nerve Sheath Tumors

Nerve sheath tumors can occur along any cranial nerves, particularly in the setting of neurofibromatosis type II. Nerve sheath tumors may present as lesions of the cavernous sinus or Meckel cave, or result in expansion of foramen rotundum and ovale. Perineural spread of head and neck carcinomas often traverse the central skull

Table 2 Central skull base lesions	
Neoplasms	Chordoma Chondrosarcoma Ecchordosis physaliphora Pituitary macroadenomas Craniopharyngioma Schwannoma Meningioma Skull base metastasis Hemangiopericytoma Multiple myeloma Non-Hodgkin's lymphoma
Congenital	Sphenoid dysplasia (neurofibromatosis type I) Transsphenoidal cephalocele
Infection/other	Fibrous dysplasia Osteomyelitis Tolosa-hunt syndrome Arachnoid granulation Paget disease Fibrous dysplasia

base, particularly when arising from the maxillary (V2) and mandibular (V3) nerves spreading through the foramen rotundum and foramen ovale, respectively.[19–21] The foramen ovale has been referred to as the "chimney of the masticator space" for its propensity to serve as a conduit for perineural spread.

Cavernous Sinus Lesions

The cavernous sinus masses can be neoplastic or nonneoplastic.[22,23] Neoplastic entities of the cavernous sinus include meningiomas, nerve sheath tumors, rhabdomyosarcoma, lymphoma, and metastases, and direct invasion of other skull base neoplasms, such as chordoma, chondrosarcoma, and pituitary primary neoplasms. Nonneoplastic entities can present as cavernous sinus masses, including noninfectious inflammation in Tolosa-Hunt syndrome, sarcoidosis, and Langerhans cell histiocytosis. Vascular abnormalities can present as mass-like lesions, including aneurysms of the cavernous carotid artery, cavernous sinus thrombosis, and a carotid-cavernous sinus arteriovenous fistula.

Differentiating these lesions requires close evaluation of adjacent structures, such as the clivus and pituitary gland, to ensure they are not involved. Vascular evaluation with MR angiography, CT angiography, or conventional angiography may be needed. In particular, a high index of suspicion for aneurysm is required, and excluding an aneurysm as a cause for a lesion is critical before biopsy or resection is attempted.

Osseous Lesions

Osseous lesions of the clivus include primary and secondary lesions.[24,25] Secondary neoplastic involvement of the clivus can be related to direct invasion of nasopharyngeal carcinoma, invasive pituitary lesions, sinonasal carcinoma, or hematogenous spread. Osteomyelitis of the clivus can also occur from direct sinonasal extension or from hematogenous spread.

Chordoma and chondrosarcoma are primary neoplastic lesions of the clivus that can be difficult to differentiate on imaging (**Fig. 4**).[24,25] Chordomas arise from primitive

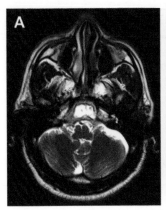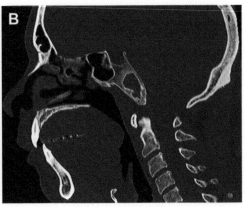

Fig. 4. Chordoma of the clivus. Axial T2-weighted MR image (*A*) shows a hyperintense lesion within the clivus. Sagittal bone algorithm CT image (*B*) shows a centrally lytic lesion with a thin peripheral rim of sclerosis, and also that the clivus is slightly expanded. A chondrosarcoma could have a similar appearance.

notochordal remnants at the sphenooccipital synchondrosis, whereas chondrosarcomas originate from primitive mesenchymal cells or from embryonic rest of the cartilaginous matrix of the cranium. Arising from notochordal remnants, chordomas are generally midline in location, whereas chondrosarcomas are located laterally and involve the petrous bone. However, when relatively large in size, the distinction between these lesions is more difficult. Both lesions tend to enhance and be hyperintense on T2-weighted imaging. Arc-like calcifications are more likely to be seen in chondrosarcoma, but are not always present. Furthermore, chordomas tend to calcify to some degree, and the distinction can be difficult. In addition to chordoma, a cystic clivus lesion in a child raises the possibility of an intraosseous craniopharyngioma.

Although MRI provides excellent soft tissue detail and should be performed on all indeterminate osseous lesions, bony detail is best depicted on CT. A classic example of the utility of CT is that of fibrous dysplasia, a common central skull base osseous lesion that can have varied appearances on MR but typically has a characteristic ground-glass matrix on CT (**Fig. 5**).[26] CT of fibrous dysplasia also commonly shows osseous expansion with preservation of the cortex. Although fibrous dysplasia can have internal cystic areas, the appearance is more circumscribed than a lytic "punched-out" lesion in an osseous metastasis.

Ecchordosis physaliphora is an additional clival lesion to consider. It is a benign notochordal remnant seen in approximately 2% of autopsy specimens, but is less commonly seen on imaging because it is generally small and below imaging resolution.[27-29] Ecchordosis physaliphora is embryologically related to a chordoma but will not enhance on postcontrast sequences. Follow-up imaging may be required to document stability if distinction from more sinister lesions such as chordoma or chondrosarcoma is necessary.

Mucoceles

Mucoceles have marked expansile potential and may extend intracranially, particularly those of the frontal and sphenoid sinuses.[30,31] The imaging diagnosis is generally straightforward given the location and expansion of the involved sinus. Before surgical treatment of sphenoid sinus mucoceles, the osseous integrity of the margins must be scrutinized because thinning/dehiscence of the osseous plate separating the

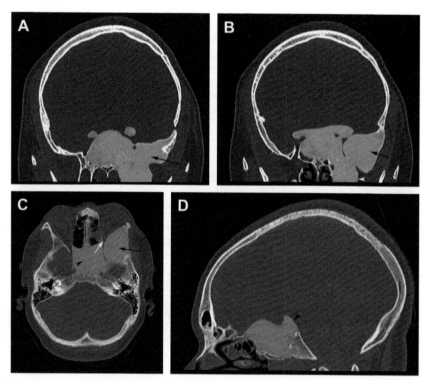

Fig. 5. Fibrous dysplasia of the central skull base. Coronal (*A, B*), axial (*C*), and sagittal (*D*) bone algorithm CT images show an expansile osseous abnormality involving the basisphenoid (*black arrow head*), the left pterygoid process (*white arrowhead*) and pterygoid plates, and the left sphenoid wing (*black arrow*). The lesion has a fairly homogeneous ground-glass matrix without focal lytic or sclerotic areas. The margins appear expanded but smooth, with a narrow zone of transition between involved and uninvolved bone, suggesting a nonaggressive process. This patient presented with symptoms from impingement of the left optic nerve at the orbital apex (*white arrow*).

sphenoid sinus from the cavernous sinus and internal carotid artery may be present. A mucocele with intracranial extension must also be differentiated from an encephalocele or pseudomeningocele.[32]

POSTERIOR SKULL BASE AND TEMPORAL BONES
Anatomy

The posterior skull base is composed predominantly of the temporal and occipital bones (**Table 3**). The petrous temporal bone includes the middle and inner ear structures (**Fig. 1**D, E, H), and medially the triangular temporal bone is directed anterior and superiorly to form the petrous apex (**Fig. 1**D, H). Several important canals and foramina are located in the posterior fossa, including the jugular foramina, hypoglossal canals, internal auditory canals, foramen magnum, and mastoid foramina.

Paragangliomas

Paragangliomas are vascular lesions that can occur along the course of the internal jugular vein (glomus jugulare) or along the cochlear promontory (glomus tympanicum),

Table 3 Posterior skull base lesions	
Neoplasms	Schwannoma (jugular foramen, hypoglossal nerve) Endolymphatic sac tumor Meningioma–jugular foramen Skull base metastasis Arachnoid granulation (dural sinus) Glomus jugulare paraganglioma Chordoma/chondrosarcoma Plasmacytoma Giant cell tumor
Congenital	Epidermoid/cholesteatoma
Infection/other	Petrous apicitis Cholesterol granuloma Bell palsy Facial nerve venous malformation (facial nerve hemangioma) Dural sinus thrombosis, skull base Dural arteriovenous fistula Fibrous dysplasia

or can be trans-spatial (glomus jugulotympanicum). Although paragangliomas are typically hyperintense on T2-weighted imaging, as they get larger internal "flow voids" they will typically be seen related to the macroscopic vascular prominence. Flow voids are focal areas of hypointense signal caused by medium- and large-sized blood vessels, and thus typically will be round or tubular, depending on the orientation of the vessel with respect to the imaging plane. Because of their vascular nature, paragangliomas enhance avidly on CT and MRI, and show rapid early arterial filling on angiography.[5,8,9]

A glomus tympanicum should be differentiated from other lesions that may be located along the cochlear promontory, such as schwannoma, hemangioma, meningioma, choristoma, and adenoma. Other lesions in this location to be distinguished include pars tensa cholesteatoma (which would restrict diffusion and would not enhance) and an aberrant vascular structure, such as a persistent stapedial artery or aberrant internal carotid artery.

The leading differential considerations for a glomus jugulare are a jugular foramen schwannoma (originating from cranial nerve IX, X, or XI), a jugular foramen meningioma, and hypervascular metastases.[33–35] MRI flow artifacts can result in a "jugular-bulb pseudomass," and a high index of suspicion is warranted to prevent incorrect diagnosis.

Internal Auditory Canal and Inner Ear

Vestibular schwannomas are common tumors of the internal auditory canal, which can extend through the porus acousticus into the cerebellopontine angle cistern as they enlarge. Bilateral vestibular schwannomas are pathognomonic for neurofibromatosis type II, and unilateral vestibular schwannomas are often sporadic (**Fig. 6**). When extending to the cerebellopontine angle, the leading differential consideration of an enhancing lesion is a meningioma, and nonenhancing lesions are most commonly arachnoid cysts and epidermoids; however, other entities can occur in this location.[36] Statistically, the primary differential consideration on imaging for a small intracanicular schwannoma is an infectious/inflammatory lesion, such as seen in Bell palsy and Ramsey Hunt syndrome[37]; however, these entities can be differentiated based on clinical

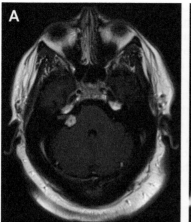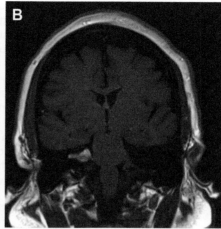

Fig. 6. Vestibular schwannoma. Axial (*A*) and coronal (*B*) postcontrast T1-weighted MR images show an enhancing lesion filling the right internal auditory canal. The mass expands the porus acousticus (*B*) and is larger and round in shape in the cerebellopontine angle cistern (*A*) creating an "ice-cream cone" appearance. The contralateral cerebellopontine angle and internal auditory canal were normal.

presentation, the mass-like appearance of schwannomas, and appearance on follow-up imaging. Schwannomas can occur in the facial nerve, anywhere along its course.[38]

The endolymph and perilymph within the inner ear is considered by MRI to be nearly pure water, given that electrolytes do not significantly alter the T1 and T2 properties of water. Accordingly, the inner ear structures should suppress on fluid-attenuated inversion recovery (FLAIR) imaging, which nulls the signal of pure water. Proteinaceous material may be present within the vestibule and semicircular canals in cases of vestibular schwannoma because of microextension of the tumor into the labyrinth.

Incomplete FLAIR suppression can also be seen secondary to viral labyrinthitis, trauma/hemorrhage, and pyogenic infections.[39] Hemolabyrinth will often have hyperintense signal on T1-weighed imaging because of methemoglobin.

Facial Nerve Hemangioma

The facial nerve hemangioma is not a true hemangioma, but rather a venous malformation of the facial nerve typically centered at the geniculate ganglion.[38,40,41] The lesions may have a salt-and-pepper osseous pattern and typically enhance on postcontrast T1-weighted imaging. Differentiation from an intrinsic facial nerve tumor, such as a facial schwannoma or perineural spread along the facial nerve, may not always be possible; however, a facial nerve hemangioma typically is centered at the geniculate ganglion and does not longitudinally expand the nerve as commonly occurs with neoplasms.

Lesions of the Petrous Apex

Lesions of the petrous apex can be difficult to diagnose and characterize in the absence of a systematic approach and understanding of the anatomy and pathophysiology of processes in this location. Even with a well-thought-out analysis, a specific diagnosis can be difficult.

A cholesterol granuloma is one of the most common lesions encountered in the skull base, most commonly at the petrous apex (**Fig. 7**). Although the mechanism of origin remains theoretical, chronic hemorrhage/giant cell reactions secondary to negative pressure from middle ear dysfunction seems to be one of the most plausible explanations to which experts subscribe. Still another possible explanation is hyperpneumatization of the petrous apex and secondary bone marrow exposure, which leads to cholesterol granuloma development.[42] In either case, chronic blood products composed of methemoglobin produce T1 shortening. Cholesterol granulomas should not restrict diffusion nor display areas of solid enhancement.

A cholesteatoma/epidermoid of the petrous apex is a circumscribed lesion, histologically similar to a middle ear cholesteatoma and an intracranial epidermoid. Accordingly, this lesion will show characteristic diffusion restriction[42] related to the densely packed keratin that limits the free movement of water molecules.

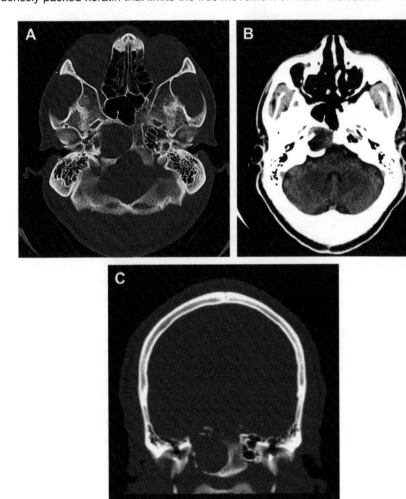

Fig. 7. Petrous apex cholesterol granuloma. Axial CT images in bone (*A*) and soft tissue algorithm (*B*), and a coronal bone algorithm CT image (*C*) show an expansile lesion in the right petrous apex that has circumscribed nonaggressive appearing margins (*A, C*) and a low-density appearance centrally (*B*).

Secondary neoplastic involvement of the petrous apex can occur from hematogenous metastatic disease or through direct extension of sinonasal carcinoma (**Fig. 8**). Extension of a chordoma, chondrosarcoma, intraosseous schwannoma, or intraosseous craniopharyngioma can also be present.

Pneumatization of the petrous apex is a normal variant that can be unilateral or bilateral. Unilateral pneumatization of the petrous apex can result in a "pseudolesion" in the nonaerated side on MRI, because the marrow will be hyperintense on T1-weighted imaging and can be mistaken for an enhancing lesion. Reviewing precontrast T1-weighted imaging to see that the hyperintense signal is intrinsic and not related to enhancement can help confirm that this normal variant does not represent a mass. If further confirmation is needed, imaging both with and without fat-saturation techniques can help, because the hyperintense signal of fat within bone marrow in a nonaerated petrous apex on T1-weighted images will suppress using fat saturation, whereas an enhancing lesion will not. Additionally, performing a CT scan (or reviewing a scan that has already been performed) can make understanding the pseudolesion easier (**Fig. 9**).

A pneumatized petrous apex has the potential to be filled with fluid (effusion) and may get infected (petrous apicitis). This condition can result in retroorbital pain from irritation of the ophthalmic branch of the trigeminal nerve, ipsilateral abducens nerve palsy from irritation of the abducens nerve within the adjacent Dorello canal, otalgia, facial pain, and otitis media, a constellation of findings referred to as *Gradenigo syndrome*.[42]

Mastoid Disease and Lesions

The most commonly encountered abnormality of the mastoid air cells is infection, which can result in demineralization of the osseous septae in the process called

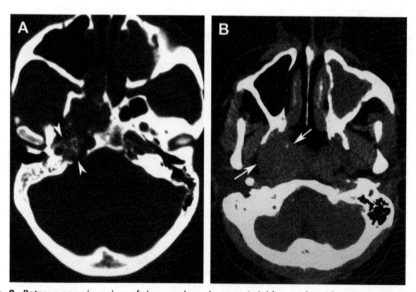

Fig. 8. Petrous apex invasion of sinonasal carcinoma. Axial bone algorithm CT image of the petrous apices (*A*) shows a lytic process in the right petrous apex with poorly defined margins and an irregular border (*white arrowheads*), suggesting an aggressive process. Axial soft tissue CT image of the nasopharynx (*B*) shows a soft tissue mass effacing the right fossa of Rosenmüller (*white arrow*), which had eroded into the petrous apex. (*Courtesy of* Matthew T. Whitehead, MD, University of Tennessee Health Science Center, Memphis, Tennessee).

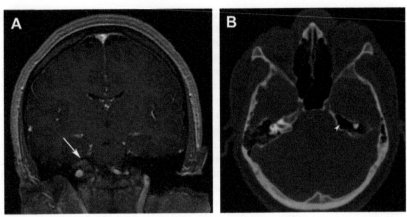

Fig. 9. Petrous apex pseudolesion. Coronal postcontrast T1-weighted MRI imaging of the petrous apices (*A*) shows asymmetric hyperintense signal in the right petrous apex (*white arrow*), which was initially mistaken for an enhancing lesion. Evaluation of precontrast images (not shown) shows that the hyperintense signal was present before contrast, indicating that there is likely not a discrete lesion. Axial bone algorithm CT (*B*) shows asymmetric pneumatization of the left petrous apex (*white arrowhead*), which is a normal variant. As a result, T1-weighted MR images will show hyperintense signal from fat within the bone marrow in the nonpneumatized petrous apex.

coalescent mastoiditis. Mastoiditis can then extend through the outer table of the skull into the postauricular soft tissues or can have posteromedial extension thorough the sigmoid plate or cephalad extension through the tegmen mastoideum. Erosion through the outer table can result in a soft tissue abscess/fluid collection; if extension to the sternocleidomastoid muscle occurs, it can lead to a Bezold abscess. Extension through the sigmoid plate carries the risk of both an epidural empyema and sigmoid sinus thrombosis, and CT or MR venography may be warranted for further evaluation. Extension through the tegmen tympani and tegmen mastoideum can result in an epidural empyema along the floor of the middle cranial fossa, with possible direct involvement of the inferior temporal lobe (inferior temporal gyrus, occipitotemporal gyrus, parahippocampal gyrus).

Langerhans Cell Histiocytosis

An inflammatory process of the mastoid air cells does not necessarily represent neoplasm. Langerhans cell histiocytosis (LCH) is a noninfectious inflammatory process that can mimic coalescent mastoiditis.[43] Differentiation between these processes may require postcontrast MRI showing solid mass-like enhancement in LCH, but ultimately biopsy may be needed to confirm the diagnosis and exclude neoplastic causes.

Endolymphatic Sac Tumor

Papillary cystadenoma of the endolymphatic sac is a tumor resulting in cystic dilation of the vestibular aqueduct and the endolymphatic sac along the petrous ridge.[44,45] This slow-growing lesion may be visible on CT because of osseous remodeling, but it is most readily evident on MRI (**Fig. 10**). Beyond its specific location of origin, spontaneous hyperintensity on T1-weighted images and calcifications are characteristic clues suggesting the diagnosis. Although this tumor can occur sporadically, it is strongly associated with von Hippel-Lindau disease, and further workup of these

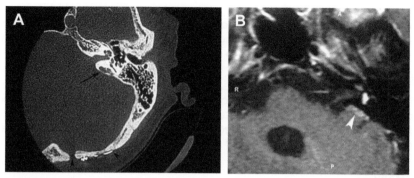

Fig. 10. Endolymphatic sac tumor. Axial bone algorithm CT of the left temporal bone (*A*) shows a focally lytic process subjacent to the left petrous ridge (*black arrow*) in the expected location of the vestibular aqueduct. Axial T1-weighted postcontrast image (*B*) shows focal enhancement in the area of the osseous abnormality (*white arrowhead*). Note that the CT image (*A*) shows evidence of prior posterior fossa surgery (*black arrowheads*) for a hemangioblastoma in this patient with von Hippel-Lindau disease.

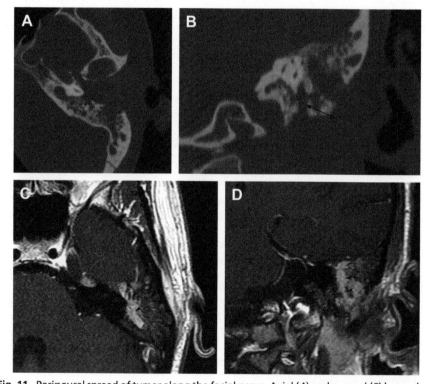

Fig. 11. Perineural spread of tumor along the facial nerve. Axial (*A*) and coronal (*B*) bone algorithm CT of the left temporal bone show a destructive process throughout the opacified middle ear cavity and mastoid air cells. Postcontrast T1-weighted axial (*C*) and coronal (*D*) MRI shows that the opacification is largely related to a soft tissue mass, and not simply infected fluid. There is expansion of the canal for the mastoid segment of the left facial nerve (*black arrow*), extending superiorly from the stylomastoid foramen (*B*), with linear enhancement seen along the expected course of the tympanic (*C*) and mastoid (*D*) segments of the facial nerve (*black arrowheads*). Biopsy of the middle ear portion of the mass showed adenoid-cystic carcinoma, which had spread along the facial nerve from the parotid gland. (*Courtesy of* C. Bruce Macdonald, MD, University of Tennessee Health Science Center, Memphis, Tennessee).

patients, including fundoscopic examination, may be beneficial.[45–47] If the results are positive, contrast-enhanced MR imaging of the entire neural axis and imaging of the kidneys and pancreas are warranted to look for other associated tumors.

Perineural Spread

Perineural tumor spread can extend to the posterior skull base, particularly when parotid (or parotid region) tumors extend along the facial nerve (**Fig. 11**).[19–21,37] Recognizing the pattern of tumor spread is the key to diagnosing perineural spread, which may be the initial presentation of a tumor in a distant location.

SUMMARY

Through understanding skull base anatomy and common and uncommon pathologic entities, expected pathways of extension (eg, perineural spread) can be predicted, narrowing the differential diagnoses and helping to accurately stage tumors. With knowledge of appropriate imaging studies, skull base lesions do not have to remain confusing or intimidating. Although ultimately one must understand that a specific diagnosis will not always be possible based on imaging alone, a systematic approach to the imaging of skull base lesions can allow the rapid formation of a concise and logical differential diagnosis.

REFERENCES

1. La Fata V, McLean N, Wise S, et al. CSF leaks: correlation of high-resolution CT and multiplanar reformations with intraoperative endoscopic findings. AJNR Am J Neuroradiol 2008;29(3):536–41.
2. Goske MJ, Applegate KE, Bullas D, et al. Image Gently: progress and challenges in CT education and advocacy. Pediatr Radiol 2011;41(Suppl 2):461–6.
3. Dremmen MH, Hofman PA, Hof JR, et al. The diagnostic accuracy of non-echo-planar diffusion-weighted imaging in the detection of residual and/or recurrent cholesteatoma of the temporal bone. AJNR Am J Neuroradiol 2012;33(3):439–44.
4. Selcuk H, Albayram S, Ozer H, et al. Intrathecal gadolinium-enhanced MR cisternography in the evaluation of CSF leakage. AJNR Am J Neuroradiol 2010;31(1):71–5.
5. Carmody RF, Seeger JF, Horsley WW, et al. Digital subtraction angiography of glomus tympanicum and jugulare tumors. AJNR Am J Neuroradiol 1983;4:263–5.
6. Hain SF. Positron emission tomography in cancer of the head and neck. Br J Oral Maxillofac Surg 2005;43:1–6.
7. Harvey RJ, Pitzer G, Nissman DB. PET/CT in the assessment of previously treated skull base malignancies. Head Neck 2010;32(1):76–84.
8. Whiteman ML, Serafini AN, Telischi FF, et al. 111In octreotide scintigraphy in the evaluation of head and neck lesions. AJNR Am J Neuroradiol 1997;18:1073–80.
9. Bustillo A, Telischi F, Weed D, et al. Octreotide scintigraphy in the head and neck. Laryngoscope 2004;114(3):434–40.
10. Nunez S, Mantilla MT, Burmudez S. Midline congenital malformations of the brain and skull. Neuroimaging Clin N Am 2011;21(3):429–82.
11. Kathuria S, Chen J, Gregg L, et al. congenital arterial and venous anomalies of the brain and skull base. Neuroimaging Clin N Am 2011;21(3):545–62.
12. Arshad AR, Selvapragasam T. Frontoethmoidal encephalocele: treatment and outcome. J Craniofac Surg 2008;19(1):175–83.
13. Lowe LH, Booth TN, Joglar JM, et al. Midface anomalies in children1. Radiographics 2000;20(4):907–22.

14. Lio Z, Wang D, Sun X, et al. The site of origin and expansive routes of juvenile naso-pharyngeal angiofibroma (JNA). Int J Pediatr Otorhinolaryngol 2011;75(9):1088–92.
15. Thompson LD. Olfactory neuroblastoma. Head Neck Pathol 2009;3(3):252–9.
16. Hanna E, DeMonte F, Ibrahim S, et al. Endoscopic resection of sinonasal cancers with and without craniotomy: oncologic results. Arch Otolaryngol Head Neck Surg 2009;135(12):1219.
17. Zinreich SJ. Imaging of the nasal cavity and paranasal sinuses. Curr Opin Radiol 1992;4(1):112–6.
18. Som PM, Curtin HD. Chronic inflammatory sinonasal diseases including fungal infections. The role of imaging. Radiol Clin North Am 1993;31(1):33–44.
19. Maroldi R, Farina D, Borghesi A, et al. Perineural tumor spread. Neuroimaging Clin N Am 2008;18:413–29.
20. Nemec ST, Herneth AM, Czerny C. Perineural tumor spread in malignant head and neck tumors. Top Magn Reson Imaging 2007;18:467–71.
21. Warden KF, Parmar H, Trobe JD. Perineural spread of cancer along the three trigeminal divisions. J Neuroophthalmol 2009;29:300–7.
22. Razek AA, Castillo M. Imaging lesions of the cavernous sinus. AJNR Am J Neuro-radiol 2009;30(3):444–52.
23. Yousem DM, Atlas SW, Grossman RI, et al. MR imaging of Tolosa-Hunt syndrome. AJNR 1989;10:1181–4.
24. Kimura F, Kim KS, Friedman H, et al. MR imaging of the normal and abnormal clivus. AJNR 1990;11:1015–21.
25. Erdem E, Angtuaco EC, Van Hemert R, et al. Comprehensive review of intracra-nial chordoma. Radiographics 2003;23(4):995–1009.
26. Schreiber A, Villaret AB, Maroldi R, et al. Fibrous dysplasia of the sinonasal tract and adjacent skull base. Curr Opin Otolaryngol Head Neck Surg 2012;20(1):45–52.
27. Mehnert F, Beschorner R, Küker W, et al. Retroclival ecchordosis physaliphora: MR imaging and review of the literature. AJNR Am J Neuroradiol 2004;25(10):1851–5.
28. Ling SS, Sader C, Robbins P, et al. A case of giant ecchordosis physaliphora: a case report and literature review. Otol Neurotol 2007;28(7):931–3.
29. Macdonald RL, Deck JH. Immunohistochemistry of ecchordosis physaliphora and chordoma. Can J Neurol Sci 1990;17(4):420–3.
30. Ichimura K, Ohta Y, Maeda YI, et al. Mucoceles of the paranasal sinuses with intracranial extension-postoperative course. Am J Rhinol 2001;15(4):243–7.
31. Soon SR, Lim CM, Singh H, et al. Sphenoid sinus mucocele: 10 cases and liter-ature review. J Laryngol Otol 2010;124(1):44–7.
32. Vaezi A, Snyderman CH, Saleh HA, et al. Pseudomeningoceles of the sphenoid sinus masquerading as sinus pathology. Laryngoscope 2011;121(12):2507–13.
33. Eldevik OP, Gabrielsen TO, Jacobsen EA. Imaging findings in schwannomas of the jugular foramen. AJNR Am J Neuroradiol 2000;21:1139–44.
34. Davagnanam I, Chavda SV. Identification of the normal jugular foramen and lower cranial nerve anatomy: contrast-enhanced 3D fast imaging employing steady-state acquisition MR imaging. AJNR Am J Neuroradiol 2008;29(3):574–6.
35. Linn J, Peters F, Moriggl B, et al. The jugular foramen: imaging strategy and detailed anatomy at 3T. AJNR Am J Neuroradiol 2009;30(1):34–41.
36. Bonneville F, Sarrazin JL, Marsot-Dupuch K, et al. Unusual lesions of the cerebel-lopontine angle: a segmental approach. Radiographics 2001;21(2):419–38.
37. Tien R, Dillon WP, Jackler RK. Contrast-enhanced MR imaging of the facial nerve in 11 patients with Bell's palsy. AJNR Am J Neuroradiol 1990;11:735–41.

38. Wiggins RH, Harnsberger HR, Salzman KL, et al. The many faces of facial nerve schwannoma. AJNR Am J Neuroradiol 2006;27(3):694–9.

39. Seltzer S, Mark AS. Contrast enhancement of the labyrinth on MR scans in patients with sudden hearing loss and vertigo: evidence of labyrinthine disease. AJNR Am J Neuroradiol 1991;12:13–6.

40. Friedman O, Neff BA, Willcox TO, et al. Temporal bone hemangiomas involving the facial nerve. Otol Neurotol 2002;23(5):760–6.

41. Balkany T, Fradis M, Jafek BW, et al. Hemangioma of the facial nerve: role of the geniculate capillary plexus. Skull Base Surg 1991;1(1):59–63.

42. Razek AA, Huang BY. Lesions of the petrous apex: classification and findings at CT and MR Imaging. Radiographics 2012;32(1):151–73.

43. D'Ambrosio N, Soohoo S, Warshall C, et al. Craniofacial and intracranial manifestations of Langerhans cell histiocytosis: report of findings in 100 patients. Am J Roentgenol 2008;191(2):589–97.

44. Michaels L. Origin of endolymphatic sac tumor. Head Neck Pathol 2007;1(2): 104–11.

45. Leung RS, Biswas SV, Duncan M, et al. Imaging features of von Hippel-Lindau disease. Radiographics 2008;28(1):65–79 [Quiz: 323].

46. Butman JA, Kim HJ, Baggenstos M, et al. Mechanisms of morbid hearing loss associated with tumors of the endolymphatic sac in von Hippel-Lindau disease. JAMA 2007;298(1):41–8.

47. Lonser RR, Kim HJ, Butman JA, et al. Tumors of the endolymphatic sac in von Hippel-Lindau disease. N Engl J Med 2004;350(24):2481.

Postoperative and Postradiation Changes on Imaging

Philip Lobert, MD[a], Ashok Srinivasan, MBBS, MD[b],*,
Gaurang V. Shah, MD[a], Suresh K. Mukherji, MD[a]

KEYWORDS

• Neck dissection • Post radiation neck • Diffusion neck • Perfusion neck

KEY POINTS

• Assessment of the posttherapy neck creates compound challenges because of alterations in normal anatomy that usually provide a framework for interpretation for the radiologist.
• Interpreting imaging in the immediate postoperative period is often complicated by a variety of normal trauma-related changes involving the soft tissue in and around the operative bed: subcutaneous emphysema, edema, hemorrhage, cellulitis, and lymph or suppurative fluid collections.
• The imaging appearance of flap reconstruction depends on the specific surgery performed. In general, the nerve supply to myocutaneous flaps is interrupted, which in combination with disuse leads to muscular fatty atrophy.
• Changes from radiation therapy are visible on posttreatment CT and MRI, most pronounced in the first month or two after irradiation, and may include thickening of the skin and platysma muscle, retropharyngeal edema, postradiation sialadenitis, lymphatic tissue atrophy, and thickening and increased enhancement of the pharyngeal walls and of the laryngeal structures.

INTRODUCTION

Imaging has always played an important role in pretherapy assessment of head and neck cancer providing crucial information on the anatomic extent of primary tumors, lymph nodal metastases, and involvement of critical adjacent structures that can preclude surgical resection. Although assessment of the pretherapy neck has its

Dr Mukherji is a consultant with Philips Medical Systems. The other authors have nothing to disclose.
[a] Department of Radiology, University of Michigan Health Systems, 1500 E Medical center drive, Ann Arbor, MI 48109, USA; [b] Division of Neuroradiology, Department of Radiology, University of Michigan Health System, B1-132 TC, Ann Arbor, MI 48109, USA
* Corresponding author.
E-mail address: ashoks@med.umich.edu

own challenges (eg, poor contrast enhancement in tumors causing difficulty in margin delineation), these are only compounded in the posttherapy neck because of alterations in normal anatomy that usually provide a framework for interpretation for the radiologist. This article discusses the normal appearance of the posttherapy neck after common surgical procedures and chemoradiation therapy. The recognition of complications and disease recurrence is emphasized with illustrated examples.

THE POSTSURGICAL NECK
Types of Neck Dissection

Although there are a variety of classification schemes for the surgical management of neck disease in head and neck cancer, the nomenclature most widely used is the one developed by the Committee for Head and Neck Surgery and Oncology of the American Academy of Otolaryngology/Head and Neck Surgery.[1] It is based on the concept that a full radical neck dissection (RND) is the standard for treating nodal cervical disease in patients with head and neck cancer, and all other procedures involve one or more modifications of the RND. There are five limited surgeries that involve the preservation of one or more nonnodal structures or nodal groups[1]: (1) modified RND (MND), (2) supraomohyoid selective neck dissection (SND), (3) lateral SND, (4) posterolateral SND, (5) anterior compartment SND.

The option to perform a more extensive operation than the full RND also exists, and is referred to as an extended RND. On occasion surgeries do not precisely fit into this classification scheme because certain nodal levels were or were not resected, and should be described accordingly. If MND is performed for limited disease in an N1 or N2 neck, the nonnodal structures spared should be specifically mentioned in the report.

RND

The imaging-based numerical cervical lymph node classification scheme devised by Som and colleagues[2] as a radiologic adjunct to the widely accepted clinically based scheme devised by the American Joint Committee on Cancer and the American Academy of Otolaryngology-Head and Neck Surgery[1,2] is used in this article. In the setting of extensive neck disease, with or without extracapsular nodal spread, RND is the operation of choice and is often followed by radiation therapy (RT) (the effects of radiation as it pertains to imaging are described later). Traditionally, this applies to patients with disease surrounding the spinal accessory nerve (SAN) or the internal jugular vein (IJV). The procedure includes en bloc resection of all ipsilateral cervical lymph nodes extending from the body of the mandible superiorly to the clavicle inferiorly, and from the lateral border of the sternohyoid muscle, hyoid bone, and contralateral anterior belly of the digastric muscle anteriorly to the anterior border of the trapezius muscle posteriorly.[1] Included along with the levels I through V lymph node groups are the ipsilateral SAN, IJV, submandibular gland (SMG), and sternocleidomastoid muscle (**Fig. 1**).

MND

MND is performed in patients with limited nodal disease not fixed to or directly infiltrating the aforementioned nonlymphatic structures. The MND involves en bloc resection of lymph node groups I through V, but spares one or more of the ipsilateral nonlymphatic structures removed during RND: the SAN, IJV, SMG, and SCM (**Fig. 2**). As such, it is important to specifically mention what structures were preserved

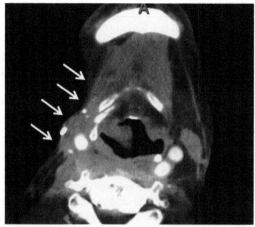

Fig. 1. Typical postoperative appearance of the neck after a radical neck dissection. Contrast-enhanced axial computed tomography (CT) image of the neck in a patient with head and neck cancer after radical neck dissection demonstrating surgical absence of the right sternocleidomastoid muscle, right submandibular gland, and right internal jugular vein (*arrows*).

when describing an MND, either surgically or for imaging follow-up. The major advantage of an MND is related to morbidity encountered when the SAN is removed. Morbidity related to SCM or IJV resection is more relevant when bilateral neck dissections are required.

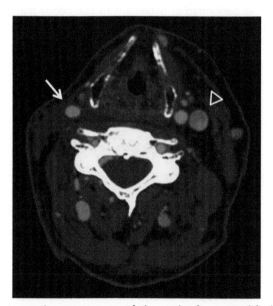

Fig. 2. Typical postoperative appearance of the neck after a modified neck dissection. Contrast-enhanced axial CT image of the neck in a patient with head and neck cancer after a modified neck dissection demonstrating surgical absence of the right internal jugular vein (*arrow*) compared with the normal left side (*arrowhead*). The right sternocleidomastoid is preserved.

SND

SND is performed in N0 patients at risk for lymphatic spread of disease. The rationale for SND is based on anatomic studies performed by Rouviere[3] and Fisch and Sigel[4] and clinicopathologic studies performed by Lindberg,[5] Skolnik and coworkers,[6] and Shah,[7] demonstrating that lymphatic drainage of the mucosal surfaces in the head and neck follow relatively predictable routes, and therefore removal of selective high-risk lymph node groups based on the location of the primary lesion can be performed to better preserve functionality and cosmesis. The four types are described next according to the nodal groups resected.

Supraomohyoid SND

Supraomohyoid SND is performed in patients with oral cavity cancer and N0 necks. It involves en bloc resection of level I, II, and III lymph nodes; and whenever level I lymph nodes are resected, the ipsilateral SMG is also removed to control spread of disease (**Fig. 3**).[8] For tongue carcinoma, the dissection is extended to the level IV lymph nodes, referred to as an extended supraomohyoid SND. Contralateral neck dissection is indicated for cancers in the floor or the mouth, ventral tongue, or midline tongue involvement when postoperative RT is not planned.[1]

Lateral SND

Lateral SND is performed in patients with oropharynx, hypopharynx, and supraglottic larynx carcinomas with N0 necks. It involves en bloc resection of the level II, III, and IV lymph nodes, and is typically performed on both sides because visceral midline neck structures have bilateral lymphatic drainage (**Fig. 4**).[1]

Posterolateral SND

Posterolateral SND is performed in patients with cutaneous malignancies and soft tissue sarcomas of the posterior scalp, nuchal ridge, occiput, or posterior upper

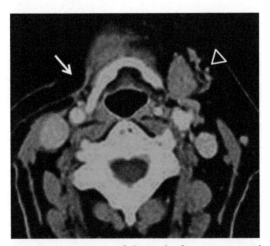

Fig. 3. Typical postoperative appearance of the neck after a supraomohyoid selective neck dissection. Contrast-enhanced axial CT image of the neck in a patient with head and neck cancer after a right supraomohyoid selective neck dissection demonstrating surgical absence of the right submandibular gland (*arrow*), which is easily identifiable when compared with the normal contralateral submandibular gland (*arrowhead*), and preservation of the right internal jugular vein and right sternocleidomastoid muscle.

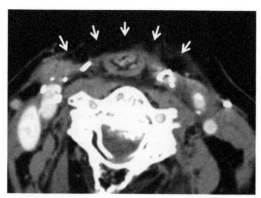

Fig. 4. Typical postoperative appearance of a lateral selective neck dissection. Contrast-enhanced axial CT image of the neck in a patient with laryngeal cancer after total laryngectomy and a bilateral lateral selective neck dissection demonstrating surgical absence of the larynx and bilateral level III lymph nodes with preservation of the internal jugular veins and sternocleidomastoid muscles (*arrows*).

neck. The dissection consists of en bloc removal of levels II through V and the suboccipital and postauricular nodes. Perifacial and external jugular nodes may also be resected.[8] The intervening subcutaneous fat and fascia between lymph node groups and the primary disease are removed to eliminate small nests of tumor cells.[1]

Anterior compartment SND

Anterior compartment SND is performed in patients with cancers of the thyroid gland, hypopharynx, cervical trachea or esophagus, and subglottic larynx. The dissection consists of en bloc removal of the level VI lymph nodes, extending from the hyoid bone superiorly, the carotid sheaths laterally, and the suprasternal notch inferiorly. If there is known disease near the suprasternal notch, level VII nodes are also resected. Occasionally, this can be performed as a unilateral procedure, eliminating the need for parathyroid reimplantation.[1]

Extended RND

Extended RND refers to removal of one or more lymph node groups or nonlymphatic structures not included in a routine RND. This may include retropharyngeal, superior mediastinal (VII), perifacial, and paratracheal (VI) nodes. Examples of nonlymphatic structures that may be included in an extended RND are carotid artery, hypoglossal nerve, vagus nerve, and paraspinal muscles. Special mention of retropharyngeal nodes should be made, either as a pertinent positive or negative finding, with pretreatment imaging of primary pharyngeal carcinomas, and tongue base, tonsillar, soft palate, and retromolar trigone cancers that have spread to the lateral or posterior oropharyngeal walls.[8]

ROUTINE POSTOPERATIVE IMAGING CHANGES

Interpreting imaging in the immediate postoperative period (before 4–6 weeks) is often complicated by a variety of normal trauma-related changes involving the soft tissue in and around the operative bed: subcutaneous emphysema, edema, hemorrhage, cellulitis, and lymph or suppurative fluid collections. In most cases these changes minimize by 4 to 6 weeks with return to a near normal postsurgical appearance of the neck.

However, in some cases the edematous changes, skin thickening, and fluid collections can persist for months or even years after surgery. This tends to occur more commonly in patients who have received postoperative RT or have diminished healing capacity from any cause.

On CT, the primary findings within the subcutaneous fat include reticular soft tissue stranding related to obstructed venules and lymphatic capillaries and a generalized increase in the fat attenuation secondary to increased interstitial fluid. The latter is typically not appreciated with MRI. These treatment-related changes typically resolve within the first month after surgery. However, the onset of reticular fat stranding may be delayed in patients that receive postoperative RT. Hematomas, serosanguinous, and chylous fluid collections are not uncommon in the immediate postoperative period and should recede over time. Maturational changes of blood products may be appreciated early on, including relatively high attenuation hematomas in the first couple of weeks (60–90 Hounsfield units), which gradually contract and become near water attenuation (0 Hounsfield units) with ongoing hemolysis and release of methemoglobin into solution.

Vertical skin incisions are typically seen as a small infolding of the skin using axial imaging techniques. Although recurrence could potentially look like this, the diagnosis should be clinically evident. Horizontal incisions are typically not well seen with axial image acquisition. Identifying a SND with imaging can be difficult. The best clue is often reduced subcutaneous fat volume in the region of surgery. MND and RND should be easily identifiable by imaging with flattening of the ipsilateral neck contour, nonvisualization of ipsilateral lymph nodes, and absence of all or some of the ipsilateral SCM, SMG, and IJV. Although the SAN cannot be directly visualized with imaging, the effects of SAN denervation are often present, and include shoulder drooping, atrophy of the ipsilateral upper trapezius muscle, and compensatory hypertrophy of the ipsilateral levator scapulae muscle.

SURGERY WITH RECONSTRUCTION

There are two broad categories of surgery for head and neck cancer: primary disease resection with an appropriate nodal dissection that does not require reconstruction, and those that require surgical reconstruction to close or repair the surgical defect for improved cosmesis or function.

A wide spectrum of pedicle or free flap techniques, grafts, and prosthesis are currently available for surgical reconstruction. Knowledge in this regard is important, because flap reconstructions do add a dimension of complexity to the imaging appearance of the postoperative neck. Recognition of normal changes over time related to the myocutaneous flap reconstruction is crucial so as not to confuse normal postoperative change within the surgical bed, and in the myocutaneous flap, with disease recurrence.

Pedicle Flaps

These consist of rotated regional skin and its underlying muscle with a preserved vascular pedicle and primary feeding nutrient vessels. The named vascular pedicle with which the flap is rotated is typically identifiable on surveillance imaging, helping to distinguish it from free flap techniques (**Fig. 5**). Common donor sites for pedicle flap reconstruction include the ipsilateral chest wall (ie, pectoralis major, trapezius, latissimus dorsi) and the head and neck musculature (ie, temporalis, sternocleidomastoid, and levator scapulae). Because the vascular supply to pedicle myocutaneous flap is excellent, they are typically preferred for closing defects in irradiated necks.

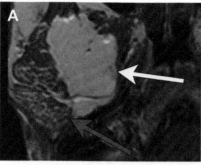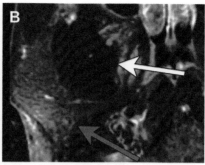

Fig. 5. Typical MRI appearance of a myocutaneous graft reconstruction. (*A*) Unenhanced axial T1-weighted MRI and (*B*) axial T2-weighted MRI with fat saturation demonstrate the normal homogenous appearance of fat (*white arrow*) and muscle (*gray arrow*) after myocutaneous free flap reconstruction in a patient with right parotid mucoepidermoid carcinoma.

Free Flaps

These can consist of skin, soft tissue, muscle, and sometimes bone, and are transferred from distant sites to the surgical field for reconstruction, where they are anastomosed to local vessels using microvascular techniques. In these cases there is no identifiable vascular pedicle with imaging. Examples of free flap reconstructions include cutaneous flaps for oral cavity defects; osseous flaps for mandibular reconstruction; and neopharynx creation using myocutaneous flaps (most commonly pectoralis major pedicle flaps) or jejunal interposition after laryngopharyngectomy.

The imaging appearance of flap reconstruction depends on the specific surgery performed. In general, the nerve supply to myocutaneous flaps is interrupted, which in combination with disuse leads to muscular fatty atrophy. This takes time, and early surveillance imaging may demonstrate relative preservation of muscle bulk in the transposed graft. Curvilinear soft tissue densities within myocutaneous flaps years after surgery are characteristic of atrophic muscle, which needs to be recognized to avoid potential false positivity. Mild overlying skin thickening of surgical flaps is a common finding. Neopharyngeal reconstruction using a pectoralis major myocutaneous flap has a characteristic appearance in which the flap has a rolled or tubular appearance resulting in a reversal of tissue planes, with the skin forming the inner pseudomucosal layer of the neopharynx.[9]

RT

Depending on the clinical scenario, RT (with or without chemotherapy) is not only used as an adjunct to surgery, but also as an effective primary treatment approach in certain cases.[10] The doses delivered, radiation ports, and timing of radiation administration are tailored to the patient and the status of their primary and secondary cervical disease. Changes from RT are visible on posttreatment CT (**Fig. 6**) and MRI, and may include the following[11]:

- Thickening of the skin and platysma muscle
- Reticular soft tissue thickening within subcutaneous and deep fat planes
- Retropharyngeal edema
- Postradiation sialadenitis: increased enhancement of major salivary glands followed by relative glandular atrophy
- Lymphatic tissue atrophy of lymph nodes and Waldeyer tonsillar ring

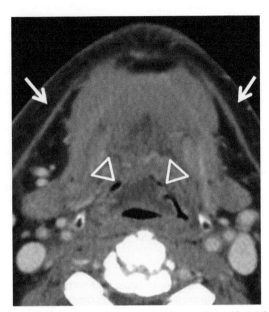

Fig. 6. Typical postradiation therapy changes. Contrast-enhanced axial CT images of the neck in a patient with supraglottic laryngeal squamous cell carcinoma after radiation therapy demonstrates symmetric reticular superficial and deep compartment fat stranding and platysmal muscle thickening (*arrows*) along with supraglottic visceral space mucosal edema (*arrowheads*).

- Thickening and increased enhancement of the pharyngeal walls
- Thickening of the laryngeal structures
- Fatty marrow replacement in vertebrae contained within the radiation portal

These changes are most pronounced in the first month or two after irradiation, and gradually resolve with time. Changes from RT may persist for years, and prolong healing and imaging changes to surgery. Although changes related to RT are commonly bilateral, they can appear asymmetric depending on the radiation portal used.[11]

IMAGING DETECTION OF POSTTHERAPEUTIC COMPLICATIONS
Vascular Complications

Thrombosis of the IJV is not uncommon after therapy and is typically clinically silent. The incidence of IJV thrombosis has been shown to occur in less than half of patients after MND or RT alone, to nearly 80% of patients after MND and RT in combination.[12] Many cases of posttherapy IJV thrombosis have also been shown to recanalize outside of the immediate postoperative week.[13] Carotid artery thrombosis can also occur, either from direct ligation or other surgery-related trauma. Radiation-induced carotid arteritis, a potentially serious complication of therapy, is occasionally identified during surveillance imaging as smooth long segment arterial wall thickening and enhancement with luminal narrowing. Irradiated patient can also develop accelerated atherosclerosis.[14–17]

Mandibular Osteoradionecrosis

A rare but feared complication of radiation is mandibular osteoradionecrosis, commonly appearing after trauma or surgical/dental manipulation in which the surrounding irradiated tissues cannot meet the increased demands for healing.[18] This complication can occur in native mandibles and in osteomyocutaneous free flap reconstructions. CT findings of osteonecrosis include cortical disruption; rarefaction; sequestration; pathologic fracture; thickened surrounding soft tissue (sometimes gas containing); and fistula formation (**Fig. 7**). These finding may be indistinguishable from infection and tumor recurrence. If they occur at a site distant from the primary tumor, osteoradionecrosis is most likely. Biopsy is often necessary to distinguish among radionecrosis, infection, and recurrence.

Persistent severe edema and radionecrosis is an uncommon complication occurring in approximately 1% to 5% of treated patients.[19] Its peak incidence is temporaneous with tumor recurrence during the first 12 months posttreatment. Although cartilage is relatively radioresistant, when the perichondrium is broached by trauma or tumor, the exposed irradiated cartilage becomes vulnerable to airway microorganisms, which leads to perichondritis, necrosis, and eventual collapse.[11] Patients with laryngeal necrosis are typically symptomatic, and on CT thickening of the surrounding soft tissue with a small amount of adjacent fluid is often all that is seen.[20] Cartilaginous abnormalities (eg, sclerosis, fragmentation, chondrolysis, collapse, and arytenoid dislocation [potentially sloughing into the airway]), are often not apparent until later.

Chylous Fistula

Occurring in 1% to 2% of patients with neck dissection, these typically present after level IV nodal dissections where there is potential for injury to the thoracic duct. With CT and MRI these are typically identified as persistent cystic masses or fluid collections in the lower neck near the carotid sheath in the expected location of the thoracic duct.[8]

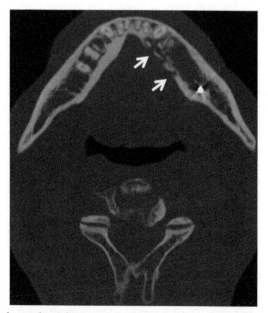

Fig. 7. Contrast-enhanced axial CT image of the neck in a patient status postradiation therapy for a left tongue base squamous cell carcinoma demonstrates cortical disruption, rarefaction, and sequestered bone fragments along the lingual surface of the left mandible (*arrows*), typical of osteoradionecrosis.

Posttraumatic Neuroma

Posttraumatic neuroma is a rare complication after neck surgery, and is not a true neoplasm. It occurs at the proximal margin of a transected peripheral nerve and is related to a normal proliferative reparative-type response to injury in which the nerve ends cannot meet and the axonal growth pattern become haphazard and overly exuberant. Posttraumatic neuromas are typically less than 2 cm in diameter and most commonly occur along the dorsal margin of the neck incision, involving the cutaneous nerves of the cervical plexus.[21–29] They cannot be readily differentiated from recurrence and scar by imaging alone.

Dermal Metastasis

Development of skin metastasis is a rare complication of therapy typically occurring within the first 6 posttherapeutic months. Extensive nodal disease with extracapsular spread and immunocompromise are risk factors for the development of skin metastasis. This diagnosis carries a very poor prognosis.[30]

Other Long-Term Complications of RT

Other long-term complications of radiotherapy include soft tissue fibrosis, delayed central nervous system reaction, radiation myelopathy, cranial nerve palsy, and secondary tumors.

ROUTINE SURVEILLANCE IMAGING

In most patients with head and neck cancer, CT is adequate for evaluating the posttherapeutic neck. MRI is preferred in cases of nasopharyngeal, sinonasal, and skull base tumors. The time frame in which to acquire the sentinel posttherapeutic imaging study is a balance between resolving therapeutic changes and the risk of disease recurrence, which could be misidentified as normal on the initial imaging examination, if baseline imaging is acquired too late. There are a host of factors that determine the risk of disease recurrence (ie, host resistance, the presence of tumor-free margins at the time of surgery, biologic aggressiveness of the primary tumor), and obtaining CT or MRI is recommended after surgery, radiation, or combined therapy for head and neck cancers with a high-risk profiles.[31,32] Although there is no consensus on the best time to perform baseline posttherapeutic imaging, it has been suggested that it be obtained 3 to 6 months after therapy completion,[11] although these recommendation are evolving and probably best done on a case-by-case basis. The primary added value of surveillance imaging is early detection of complications or disease recurrence before clinical manifestations. Baseline CT and MRI may also carry some predictive information regarding eventual outcomes in primarily irradiated laryngeal and hypopharyngeal cancers[31] and in advanced head and neck cancer treated with chemoradiation therapy,[33] although there are newer advanced biologic imaging modalities that may be more useful in this regard.

IMAGING OF DISEASE RECURRENCE

Comparing with prior studies is critical for the accurate interpretation of all posttherapy imaging in the head and neck. The fundamental tenets of detecting disease recurrence are twofold: a new or enlarging neck mass must be considered recurrence until proved otherwise, and the most likely location for tumor recurrence is either in the operative bed or along the surgical margins.

The primary imaging characteristics of recurrent tumors are progressively enlarging neck mass, neck lymph nodes, or appearance of new abnormal lymph node.[34,35] Tumor typically attenuates similar to muscle on CT, but can contain areas of central fluid attenuation suggestive of cavitation and necrosis (**Fig. 8**). Recurrent tumors can appear as discrete masses with well-defined margins, spiculated masses, or as a very infiltrative process, such that it would exceedingly difficult to accurately trace its true extent. Recurrent tumors can demonstrate a variety of enhancement patterns, and just like primary lesions can erode bone, encase vital structure, and spread along nerves.

The posttherapy changes, particularly in multimodality treatment regimens with or without surgical reconstruction, can make detection of tumor recurrence very difficult because of anatomic distortion in the surgical bed, the most likely location for recurrence. In general, CT has a high sensitivity (63%–100%) and moderate specificity (24%–80%) for differentiating recurrent tumor from posttreatment changes.[36–40] The accuracy of CT is improved in this regard when evaluating early stage primary tumor response to nonsurgical therapy. Complete resolution is indicative of cure, 50% to 75% reduction in tumor volume is an indeterminate response requiring close follow-up, and less than 50% reduction in size is considered treatment failure.[41]

The MRI criteria for recurrence is an enlarging enhancing mass that is of intermediate to high signal intensity on T2-weighted sequences. Dense scar and vascularized granulation tissue can enhance and appear irregular and infiltrative, just like recurrent tumor. However, one potential advantage of MRI over CT is its superior soft tissue contrast resolution, illustrated by several studies that have suggested that decreased T2-weighted signal in an abnormal mass in the operative bed is strongly suggestive of dense scar or fibrotic tissue as opposed to recurrent tumor.[34,35,40,42,43] There is good evidence that MRI should be performed as the primary surveillance imaging modality in cases of nasopharyngeal, sinonasal, and skull base tumors at risk of perineural or intracranial invasion. The diagnostic accuracy of MRI to detect recurrent head and neck squamous cell carcinoma in the other mucosal spaces of the head and neck

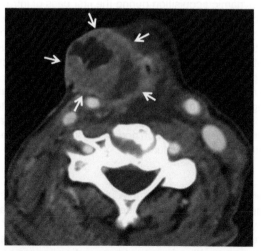

Fig. 8. CT appearance of recurrent neoplasm after therapy. Contrast-enhanced axial CT image in a patient with total laryngectomy, bilateral lateral SND, and radiation therapy for laryngeal squamous cell carcinoma demonstrates an enhancing mass in the surgical bed with necrotic contents (*arrows*) suggestive of tumor recurrence.

is not as well established, but seems to be dependent on the experience of the individual interpreting the study.[44] Current MRI techniques of the neck are still limited by suboptimal signal-to-noise ratios and patient motion artifact related to relatively slow acquisition times compared with CT.

ROLE OF ADVANCED IMAGING TECHNIQUES

There are several promising advanced neuroimaging techniques that may help evaluate the posttherapeutic neck by alleviating uncertainty regarding tumor response to therapy and potential recurrence. In this regard, the current status and applications of MR spectroscopy, CT perfusion (CTP), diffusion weighted imaging (DWI), perfusion-weighted MRI, and ^{18}F-fluorodeoxyglucose (FDG) positron emission tomography (PET) are discussed next.

Proton MR Spectroscopy

MR spectroscopy has the unique ability to detect concentrations of certain metabolites within tissue. Although obtaining adequate quality spectra in the head and neck is more technically challenging than in the brain, studies have demonstrated higher quantities of certain metabolites in different head and neck pathologies.[45–50] Because choline (Cho) is a marker of cell membrane turnover, residual and recurrent cancer after treatment can be expected to demonstrate this metabolite in excess on MR spectroscopy. This has been shown in a study of posttreatment masses in which elevated concentrations of Cho in an indeterminate mass correlated significantly with residual or recurrent cancer. Although the absences of Cho had a lesser negative predictive value (81%), the presence of excess Cho in a posttreatment mass had a positive predictive value of 100%.[51]

CTP

The fundamental principle of acquiring CTP is continuous recording of attenuation over a fixed area of interest during passage of iodinated contrast medium through a region. This is a dynamic acquisition during the first pass of intravascular iodinated contrast through a regional vascular bed.[52,53] Time-attenuation curves are created allowing for generation of perfusion parameters, such as blood volume, blood flow (BF), mean transit time, and capillary permeability, which allow evaluation of the hemodynamic status of a particular lesion. Because recurrent head and neck cancers develop neoangiogenesis similar to primary malignancies, CTP is a promising means of evaluating this neovascularity. In a study comparing tumor recurrence with posttherapeutic changes, recurrent tumors tended to demonstrate increased BF compared with posttherapy masses (**Fig. 9**). However, perfusion parameters did not differentiate benign and malignant lymph nodes and there was no correlation between perfusion parameters and tumor volume.[54]

DWI

DWI has the potential to reflect water molecular motion in the tissue microenvironment. The fundamental premise is that tissue that is more compact at the cellular level (eg, high cellularity) tends to show a reduction in water molecular motion, which is expressed by lower apparent diffusion coefficient (ADC) values. Identifying recurrent tumor in the posttherapy setting from posttherapeutic changes can be challenging, but potentially lessened to some extent with DWI. Recurrent tumor shows decreased ADC compared with radionecrosis, presumably because of increased free water in necrosis and increased cellularity in recurrent tumors (**Fig. 10**).[55–57] Although this

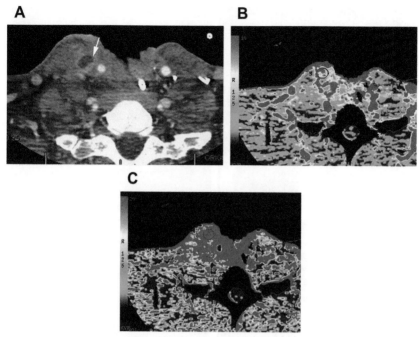

Fig. 9. Posttherapy disease recurrence on CT and CT perfusion. (*A*) Contrast-enhanced CT of the neck in a patient with laryngeal squamous cell carcinoma status post total laryngectomy, bilateral lateral SND, and radiation therapy demonstrates asymmetric soft tissue fullness surrounding a thrombosed right internal jugular vein (*arrow*). On the corresponding CT perfusion blood volume (*B*) and blood flow (*C*) color maps, significantly increased blood volume and flow is seen in this region (*black circles*) suggestive of residual tumor.

has been shown in multiple studies, there is still no threshold ADC that can be used clinically for this distinction. However, it suffices to say that DWI can be a useful tool in addition to conventional imaging to help in making management decisions (eg, when the ADC values are significantly decreased in an conventionally indeterminate posttherapy mass, it increases the suspicion of neoplastic recurrence and thus guides early intervention).

Perfusion-Weighted MRI

Similar to CTP, perfusion-weighted MRI measures BF dynamics at the microcirculatory level and is able to generate perfusion parameters, such as blood volume, BF, and mean transit time. The most widely available technique for performing perfusion-weighted MRI is T2*-weighted dynamic contrast-enhanced imaging, requiring the bolus injection of paramagnetic contrast medium and rapid acquisition of images during first-pass intravascular perfusion of the capillary bed.[58] Other techniques, such as dynamic T1-weighted contrast imaging (providing assessment of tumor permeability) and arterial spin-labeling (intra-arterial water is used as an endogenous tracer) are currently only used at a few centers.[59] Perfusion-weighted MRI has shown some promise in evaluation of early tumor response to chemoradiation therapy and assessment of posttreatment masses. One study showed a transient increase in tumor blood volume within 2 weeks of starting chemoradiation in patients who responded well to therapy compared with patients who had early locoregional failure.[60]

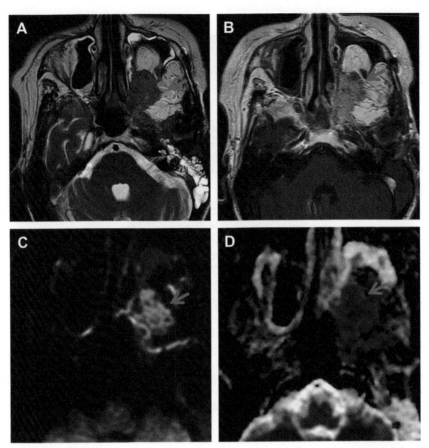

Fig. 10. MRI appearance of recurrent neoplasm after graft reconstruction. (*A*) Axial T2-weighted and (*B*) T1-weighted postcontrast MRIs in a patient status post partial maxillectomy with myocutaneous graft reconstruction for a minor salivary gland tumor demonstrate a suspicious soft tissue mass at the free edge of the fat graft (*arrow*). Review of the (*C*) diffusion weighted images (DWI) and (*D*) ADC maps from this MRI shows impeded diffusion within the mass as seen by bright signal on the DWI image with corresponding low ADC map signal (*arrows*). Reduced ADC values in posttherapy masses have been shown to be more suggestive of recurrent tumor than granulation tissue in multiple studies.

FDG-PET

FDG-PET imaging relies on the transport of FDG into cells, thereby allowing a direct way of visualizing groups of abnormal cells. This modality is already being used extensively to diagnosis, stage, and follow-up head and neck cancers. Although FDG is not a specific radiotracer (inflammatory lesions also accumulate FDG), FDG-PET is still one of the most accurate modalities available for differentiating posttreatment change from residual or recurrent disease.[61,62] Although false-positive (brown fat, muscular activity, inflammation) and false-negative (small tumor, low glycolytic activity) results can occur, the specificity and sensitivity of FDG-PET has been consistently high (89% and 97%, respectively) for the detection of residual neck disease in patients with head and neck cancer treated with concurrent chemoradiation (**Fig. 11**).[63] Meta-analysis has shown that the pooled sensitivity, specificity, and positive and

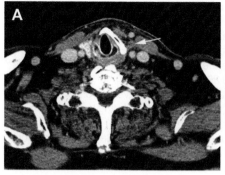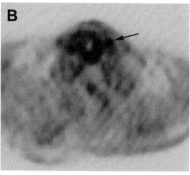

Fig. 11. (A) Axial contrast-enhanced CT of the neck demonstrates asymmetric soft tissue medial to the left sternocleidomastoid muscle (*arrow*) that demonstrates (*B*) intense FDG avidity on the corresponding PET scan (*arrow*) in a patient with laryngeal carcinoma treated with radiation therapy. This is suggestive of tumor recurrence.

negative predictive values of FDG-PET for detecting residual and recurrent head and neck cancer is 94%, 82%, 75%, and 95%, respectively.[64]

SUMMARY

Although interpretation of the posttreatment neck is challenging even for the expert, this article provides an overview of expected postsurgery and postradiation changes on imaging, and introduces the concept of advanced neck imaging that may become the mainstay of posttherapy evaluation in the future.

REFERENCES

1. Robbins KT. Classification of neck dissection: current concepts and future considerations. Otolaryngol Clin North Am 1998;31:639–55.
2. Som PM, Curtin HD, Mancuso AA. Imaging-based nodal classification for evaluation of neck metastatic adenopathy. Am J Roentgenol 2000;174:837–44.
3. Rouviere H. Anatomy of the human lymphatic system. Ann Arbor (MI): Edwards Bros. Inc; 1938.
4. Fisch UP, Sigel ME. Cervical lymphatic system as visualized by lymphography. Ann Otol Rhinol Laryngol 1964;73:870–82.
5. Lindberg R. Distribution of cervical lymph node metastases from squamous cell carcinoma of the upper respiratory and digestive tracts. Cancer 1972;29:1446–9.
6. Skolnik EM, Yee KF, Friedman M, et al. The posterior triangle in radical neck surgery. Arch Otolaryngol 1976;102:1–4.
7. Shah JP. Patterns of cervical lymph node metastasis from squamous carcinomas of the upper aerodigestive tract. Am J Surg 1990;160:405–9.
8. Som PM, Lawson W, Urken ML. The posttreatment neck: clinical and imaging considerations. Head and neck imaging. 5th edition. St Louis (MO): Mosby; 2003. p. 2239–72.
9. Wester DJ, Whiteman ML, Singer S, et al. Imaging of the postoperative neck with emphasis on surgical flaps and their complications. Am J Roentgenol 1995;164: 989–93.
10. Zelefsky M. Nonsurgical and combined therapy for squamous cell cancer of the neck. In: Harrison LB, Sessions RS, Hong WK, editors. Head and neck cancer: a multidisciplinary approach. Philadelphia: Lippincott-Raven; 1999. p. 379–89.

11. Hermans R. Posttreatment imaging in head and neck cancer. Eur J Radiol 2008; 66:501–11.
12. Medina J, Houck J, O'Malley B. Management of cervical lymph nodes in squamous cell carcinoma of the head and neck. In: Harrison L, Sessions R, Hong W, editors. Head and neck cancer: a multidisciplinary approach. Philadelphia: JB Lippincott-Raven; 1999. p. 353–89.
13. Quraishi HA, Wax MK, Granke K, et al. Internal jugular vein thrombosis after functional and selective neck dissection. Arch Otolaryngol Head Neck Surg 1997;123: 969–73.
14. Foreman NK, Laitt RD, Chambers EJ, et al. Intracranial large vessel vasculopathy and anaplastic meningioma 19 years after cranial irradiation for acute lymphoblastic leukaemia. Med Pediatr Oncol 1995;24:265–8.
15. Rockman CB, Riles TS, Fisher FS, et al. The surgical management of carotid artery stenosis in patients with previous neck irradiation. Am J Surg 1996;172:191–5.
16. Chuang VP. Radiation-induced arteritis. Semin Roentgenol 1994;29:64–9.
17. Hemar P, Kennel P, Piller P, et al. Lingual necrosis after neck irradiation. Ann Otolaryngol Chir Cervicofac 1993;110:351–4 [in French].
18. Marx RE. Osteoradionecrosis: a new concept of its pathophysiology. J Oral Maxillofac Surg 1983;41:283–8.
19. Parsons F. The effect of radiation on normal tissues in the management of head and neck cancer. In: Million RR, Cassisi NJ, editors. Management of head and neck cancer: a multidisciplinary approach. 2nd edition. Philadelphia: JB Lippincott; 1994. p. 183–4.
20. Hermans R, Pameijer FA, Mancuso AA, et al. CT findings in chondroradionecrosis of the larynx. AJNR Am J Neuroradiol 1998;19:711–8.
21. Lee EJ, Calcaterra TC, Zuckerbraun L. Traumatic neuromas of the head and neck. Ear Nose Throat J 1998;77:670–4, 676.
22. Kus H, Araszkiewicz H, Wlodarska-Araszkiewicz A, et al. Multiple post-traumatic neuromas of the cervical plexus with atypical symptoms. Neurol Neurochir Pol 1983;17:597–9 [in Polish].
23. Sung JH, Mastri AR. Aberrant peripheral nerves and microneuromas in otherwise normal medullas. J Neuropathol Exp Neurol 1983;42:522–8.
24. Iida S, Shirasuna K, Kogo M, et al. Amputation neuroma following radical neck dissection–report of 3 cases. J Osaka Univ Dent Sch 1995;35:1–4.
25. de Chalain T, Nahai F. Amputation neuromas of the great auricular nerve after rhytidectomy. Ann Plast Surg 1995;35:297–9.
26. Toriumi DM, Sykes J, Wolff A. Pathologic quiz case 1. Amputation neuroma of the great auricular nerve. Arch Otolaryngol Head Neck Surg 1987;113:888–90.
27. Rauchfuss A, Caselitz J. Scar neuroma following tumor operations of the head and neck. Immunohistologic studies, differential diagnosis, therapy. HNO 1987; 35:84–7 [in German].
28. Hobsley M. Amputation neuroma of the great auricular nerve after parotidectomy. Br J Surg 1972;59:735–6.
29. Huang LF, Weissman JL, Fan C. Traumatic neuroma after neck dissection: CT characteristics in four cases. AJNR Am J Neuroradiol 2000;21:1676–80.
30. Pitman KT, Johnson JT. Skin metastases from head and neck squamous cell carcinoma: incidence and impact. Head Neck 1999;21:560–5.
31. Hermans R, Pameijer FA, Mancuso AA, et al. Laryngeal or hypopharyngeal squamous cell carcinoma: can follow-up CT after definitive radiation therapy be used to detect local failure earlier than clinical examination alone? Radiology 2000;214: 683–7.

32. Schwartz DL, Barker J Jr, Chansky K, et al. Postradiotherapy surveillance practice for head and neck squamous cell carcinoma: too much for too little? Head Neck 2003;25:990–9.

33. van den Broek GB, Rasch CR, Pameijer FA, et al. Response measurement after intraarterial chemoradiation in advanced head and neck carcinoma: magnetic resonance imaging and evaluation under general anesthesia? Cancer 2006; 106:1722–9.

34. Hudgins PA, Burson JG, Gussack GS, et al. CT and MR appearance of recurrent malignant head and neck neoplasms after resection and flap reconstruction. AJNR Am J Neuroradiol 1994;15:1689–94.

35. Hudgins PA. Flap reconstruction in the head and neck: expected appearance, complications, and recurrent disease. Eur J Radiol 2002;44:130–8.

36. Lapela M, Eigtved A, Jyrkkio S, et al. Experience in qualitative and quantitative FDG PET in follow-up of patients with suspected recurrence from head and neck cancer. Eur J Cancer 2000;36:858–67.

37. Mukherji SK, Gapany M, Phillips D, et al. Thallium-201 single-photon emission CT versus CT for the detection of recurrent squamous cell carcinoma of the head and neck. AJNR Am J Neuroradiol 1999;20:1215–20.

38. Valdes Olmos RA, Balm AJ, Hilgers FJ, et al. Thallium-201 SPECT in the diagnosis of head and neck cancer. J Nucl Med 1997;38:873–9.

39. Di Martino E, Nowak B, Hassan HA, et al. Diagnosis and staging of head and neck cancer: a comparison of modern imaging modalities (positron emission tomography, computed tomography, color-coded duplex sonography) with panendoscopic and histopathologic findings. Arch Otolaryngol Head Neck Surg 2000;126:1457–61.

40. Lell M, Baum U, Greess H, et al. Head and neck tumors: imaging recurrent tumor and post-therapeutic changes with CT and MRI. Eur J Radiol 2000;33:239–47.

41. Mukherji SK, Mancuso AA, Kotzur IM, et al. Radiologic appearance of the irradiated larynx. Part II. Primary site response. Radiology 1994;193:149–54.

42. Glazer HS, Niemeyer JH, Balfe DM, et al. Neck neoplasms: MR imaging. Part II. Posttreatment evaluation. Radiology 1986;160:349–54.

43. Tomura N, Watanabe O, Hirano Y, et al. MR imaging of recurrent head and neck tumours following flap reconstructive surgery. Clin Radiol 2002;57:109–13.

44. Loevner LA, Sonners AI, Schulman BJ, et al. Reinterpretation of cross-sectional images in patients with head and neck cancer in the setting of a multidisciplinary cancer center. AJNR Am J Neuroradiol 2002;23:1622–6.

45. Delikatny EJ, Russell P, Hunter JC, et al. Proton MR and human cervical neoplasia: ex vivo spectroscopy allows distinction of invasive carcinoma of the cervix from carcinoma in situ and other preinvasive lesions. Radiology 1993; 188:791–6.

46. Gill SS, Thomas DG, Van Bruggen N, et al. Proton MR spectroscopy of intracranial tumours: in vivo and in vitro studies. J Comput Assist Tomogr 1990;14: 497–504.

47. Negendank WG, Brown TR, Evelhoch JL, et al. Proceedings of a national cancer institute workshop: MR spectroscopy and tumor cell biology. Radiology 1992; 185:875–83.

48. Shah GV, Gandhi D, Mukherji SK. Magnetic resonance spectroscopy of head and neck neoplasms. Top Magn Reson Imaging 2004;15:87–94.

49. Vogl T, Peer F, Schedel H, et al. 31P-spectroscopy of head and neck tumors: surface coil technique. Magn Reson Imaging 1989;7:425–35.

50. Yeung DK, Fong KY, Chan QC, et al. Chemical shift imaging in the head and neck at 3T: initial results. J Magn Reson Imaging 2010;32:1248–54.

51. King AD, Yeung DK, Yu KH, et al. Monitoring of treatment response after chemo-radiotherapy for head and neck cancer using in vivo 1H MR spectroscopy. Eur Radiol 2010;20:165–72.
52. Lee TY. Functional CT: physiological models. Trends Biotechnol 2002;20:8.
53. Lee TY, Purdie TG, Stewart E. CT imaging of angiogenesis. Q J Nucl Med 2003; 47:171–87.
54. Bisdas S, Baghi M, Smolarz A, et al. Quantitative measurements of perfusion and permeability of oropharyngeal and oral cavity cancer, recurrent disease, and associated lymph nodes using first-pass contrast-enhanced computed tomography studies. Invest Radiol 2007;42:172–9.
55. Vandecaveye V, De Keyzer F, Nuyts S, et al. Detection of head and neck squamous cell carcinoma with diffusion weighted MRI after (chemo)radiotherapy: correlation between radiologic and histopathologic findings. Int J Radiat Oncol Biol Phys 2007;67:960–71.
56. Abdel Razek AA, Kandeel AY, Soliman N, et al. Role of diffusion-weighted echo-planar MR imaging in differentiation of residual or recurrent head and neck tumors and posttreatment changes. AJNR Am J Neuroradiol 2007;28:1146–52.
57. Vandecaveye V, de Keyzer F, Vander Poorten V, et al. Evaluation of the larynx for tumour recurrence by diffusion-weighted MRI after radiotherapy: initial experience in four cases. Br J Radiol 2006;79:681–7.
58. Lacerda S, Law M. Magnetic resonance perfusion and permeability imaging in brain tumors. Neuroimaging Clin N Am 2009;19:527–57.
59. Ludemann L, Warmuth C, Plotkin M, et al. Brain tumor perfusion: comparison of dynamic contrast enhanced magnetic resonance imaging using T1, T2, and T2* contrast, pulsed arterial spin labeling, and H2(15)O positron emission tomography. Eur J Radiol 2009;70:465–74.
60. Cao Y, Popovtzer A, Li D, et al. Early prediction of outcome in advanced head-and-neck cancer based on tumor blood volume alterations during therapy: a prospective study. Int J Radiat Oncol Biol Phys 2008;72:1287–90.
61. Fukui MB, Blodgett TM, Snyderman CH, et al. Combined PET-CT in the head and neck. Part 2. Diagnostic uses and pitfalls of oncologic imaging. Radiographics 2005;25:913–30.
62. Wong RJ, Lin DT, Schoder H, et al. Diagnostic and prognostic value of [(18)F]flu-orodeoxyglucose positron emission tomography for recurrent head and neck squamous cell carcinoma. J Clin Oncol 2002;20:4199–208.
63. Ong SC, Schoder H, Lee NY, et al. Clinical utility of 18F-FDG PET/CT in assessing the neck after concurrent chemoradiotherapy for locoregional advanced head and neck cancer. J Nucl Med 2008;49:532–40.
64. Al-Ibraheem A, Buck A, Krause BJ, et al. Clinical applications of FDG PET and PET/CT in head and neck cancer. J Oncol 2009;20:872–5.

Interventional Neuroradiology Applications in Otolaryngology, Head and Neck Surgery

Gaurav Jindal, MD[a],*, Joseph Gemmete, MD[b],
Dheeraj Gandhi, MD[a]

KEYWORDS

• Interventional neuroradiology • Head and neck

KEY POINTS

• Interventional Neuroradiology can play a vital role in the diagnosis and treatment of vascular and non-vascular pathology in the head and neck. Continuing advancements in and increasing awareness of this field have allowed for the assessment and treatment of epistaxis, hypervascular tumors, vascular malformations, trauma, and bleeding in the head and neck. Percutaneous image guided interventions include biopsy and sclerosis. Radiofrequency ablation and cryoablation of head and neck tumors are evolving disciplines.

• The most common dangerous vascular anastomoses in the head and neck involve communications of the internal carotid artery and/or vertebral artery with the first-order and second-order branches of the external carotid artery; these anastomoses may not be evident on an initial angiogram but may reveal themselves as changes in local blood flow occur during embolization.

• Complications resulting from the described treatments are usually minor, including groin hematoma, facial numbness or pain, mucosal necrosis, and sinusitis. Serious major complications can be associated with head and neck embolization procedures if care is not taken to identify dangerous vascular anastomoses.

INTRODUCTION

Interventional neuroradiology is a rapidly evolving field encompassing several procedures that can be valuable assets in the diagnosis, treatment, and surgical management of a variety of disorders affecting the extracranial head and neck. Continuing advancements in medical imaging and devices have allowed the interventionalist to perform procedures not possible only 1 to 2 decades ago. New embolic materials,

The authors have nothing to disclose.
[a] Department of Radiology, University of Maryland Medical Center, 22 South Greene Street, Baltimore, MD 21201, USA; [b] Department of Radiology, University of Michigan Health System, 1500 East Medical Center Drive, Ann Arbor, MI 48109, USA
* Corresponding author.
E-mail address: drjindal@gmail.com

guide catheters, microcatheters, stents, and other devices have resulted in expanding applications of this discipline in treating both intracranial and extracranial vascular lesions of the head and neck. The minimally invasive nature of the field is a driving force for embracing novel methods to treat these abnormalities. With the use of high-quality imaging and meticulous technique, the incidence of major complications can be very low.

Interventions in the head and neck can be performed via a percutaneous, endovascular, or combination approach. Procedures that typically require percutaneous access include biopsies, aspirations, sclerotherapy, and relatively newer techniques, such as radiofrequency ablation and cryoablation. An endovascular approach is used to treat vascular pathology, such as dissection, pseudoaneurysm, arteriovenous fistula, and bleeding, as well as in the presurgical treatment of hypervascular tumors of the head and neck, such as paragangliomas, juvenile nasopharyngeal angiofibroma, and other tumors. Transarterial chemotherapy administration for head and neck neoplasms is another growing application. A combination percutaneous and endovascular approach may be needed in the embolization of high-flow craniofacial vascular malformations (VMs) and hypervascular tumors. This article provides a review of the current clinical applications of a variety of percutaneous and endovascular interventional procedures of the extracranial head and neck.

GENERAL PRINCIPLES

A thorough understanding of cross-sectional and vascular anatomy with a keen awareness of collateral pathways and potential collateral pathways between the extracranial and intracranial vessels is essential for ensuring safe and successful endovascular procedures in the head and neck. Anastomotic pathways exist between the external carotid artery (ECA), internal carotid artery (ICA), vertebral artery (VA), ophthalmic artery, ascending cervical artery, deep cervical artery, and spinal arteries. The most common dangerous anastomoses involve communications of the ICA and/or VA with the first-order and second-order branches of the ECA, such as the ascending pharyngeal artery, occipital artery, middle meningeal artery, accessory meningeal artery, and internal maxillary artery. These anastomoses may not be evident on an initial angiogram but may reveal themselves as changes in local blood flow occur during embolization. Moreover, branches of the ECA serve as the primary blood supply to many of the cranial nerves; palsies of cranial nerves V, VII, IX, X, XI, and/or XII may result from inadvertent embolization of feeding branches to the vasa nervorum. The middle meningeal artery supplies the vasa nervorum of cranial nerve VII. The ascending pharyngeal artery provides supply to the vasa nervorum of cranial nerves IX, X, XI, and XII via its posteriorly directed neuromeningeal trunk. Appropriate selection of embolic agents, and, if necessary, provocative testing before embolization, may help avoid damage to the cranial nerves.

Embolic Agents

Embolic agents are classified into the categories of mechanical devices, particles, and liquids. The optimal embolic agent may be chosen depending on hemodynamic and angioarchitectural factors.

Mechanical devices

Mechanical devices include balloons, which are useful in the permanent occlusion of large vessels, such as the carotid and vertebral arteries, and are useful in transarterial embolization of large direct arteriovenous fistulas.[1–3] Detachable coils can be deployed by means of electrolysis and are primarily used for embolization of intracranial aneurysms.[4] They can also be used in the embolization of arteriovenous fistulas to safely form the initial meshwork into which pushable coils will be placed. Pushable coils tend to be more thrombogenic and less expensive than detachable coils and can be used to occlude relatively larger vessels, such as the ICA or VA, which may be desirable in certain clinical scenarios, such as trauma.[5]

Particles

Particles, such as polyvinyl alcohol particles, embospheres, or gelfoam, can be used for the embolization of hypervascular tumors and in the treatment of epistaxis, as they are able to penetrate into the small vascular interstices of these lesions while allowing for delayed recanalization of embolized tissue and, thereby, also diminishing the risks of nontarget tissue embolization.[6,7] The tendency to recanalize can be advantageous in the setting of nontarget embolization, as opposed to nontarget embolization with permanent embolic agents.[6] Choosing particulate size is dependent on multiple factors. Larger particles tend to embolize more proximally than smaller particles and, thereby, may avoid ischemic complications to nontarget tissue seen with smaller particles and with permanent liquid embolics. This is because small particles or liquid embolic agents can penetrate capillaries, such as the vasa nervorum beyond the point of effective anastomoses and, therefore, induce nerve ischemia.[8] Small particles, on the other hand, by penetrating into the tiny vascular interstices of target hypervascular lesions, can more optimally embolize target tissue.[6] If an arteriovenous shunt within an arteriovenous malformation (AVM), fistula, and/or hypervascular mass is larger than the particle diameter being used, the particles may travel through the lesion and embolize to the lungs.[8]

Liquids

Liquid embolic agents include cyanoacrylates, ethylene vinyl alcohol copolymer (EVAC), dehydrated ethanol, Ethibloc (Ethnor Laboratories, Norderstedt, Germany), and sodium tetradecyl sulfate.[9] Cyanoacrylates, such as N-butyl cyanoacrylate (n-BCA), also commonly referred to as "glue," are not entirely permanent[10] but are one of the longest lasting embolic agents and are generally referred to as "permanent" agents.[11] Glue polymerizes on contact with ionic solutions, such as saline or blood, and can be difficult to use for a nonexperienced operator. Polymerization time can be controlled by the addition of various concentrations of ethiodol. Nevertheless, delivery of glue demands extensive familiarity with the substance and with the procedure and careful control of polymerization time, velocity of injection, and microcatheter manipulation. Inherent in the use of glue is the risk of gluing the microcatheter in place in the vessel with the associated risks of thrombosis or vessel rupture.[12] To avoid gluing the microcatheter into the vessel, the operator must inject glue relatively quickly and continuously, thereby often sacrificing precise control.

Onyx

EVAC, also known by its trade name of "Onyx," is a liquid embolic agent that was approved by the Food and Drug Administration in 2005 for the use of endovascular embolization. Similar to glue, Onyx polymerizes when injected into the vasculature. It is delivered as a mixture in solution with dimethyl sulfoxide (DMSO). It is radiopaque and is manufactured in established concentrations and viscosities. The least-concentrated Onyx solution is the least viscous and is expected to have the most distal penetration.

Onyx has several advantages over glue.[13,14] Onyx carries a lower risk of gluing the catheter into the vessel because of its cohesive and yet *nonadhesive* properties. Injection of Onyx can be performed slowly for precise delivery. Injection of EVAC can be and is often stopped intermittently to check the degree of embolization. In contrast to glue, Onyx is advanced as a single column, thereby lowering the risk of involuntary venous migration. Onyx has less tendency to fragment in high-flow lesions. These characteristics of Onyx make embolization with this material more controllable and, according to many users, safer in comparison with glue.[13,14]

Onyx does have its own drawbacks. Long injection times require prolonged exposure to xray fluoroscopy. Rapid injection of DMSO or Onyx can induce vasospasm, which can hinder Onyx penetration or even trap the catheter within the vessel. DMSO is angiotoxic if not used appropriately.[14,15] Onyx cannot always be injected a long distance in a small-diameter or slow-flow vessel. Onyx injection into a large arteriovenous fistula does entail risk of unwanted venous migration, although glue and particles carry this risk as well. To overcome this limitation in high-flow lesions, partial embolization can first be performed with coils to slow the blood flow and provide a meshwork before embolization with other agents. Embolization with DMSO and Onyx can be painful, and general anesthesia is often recommended to provide patient comfort and prevent patient movement. Onyx embolization requires the use of special DMSO-compatible microcatheters. The microcatheter cannot be reused and has to be changed after each vessel embolization. Microcatheters for the use of glue also have to be changed after each vessel embolization. Embolization with particles, on the other hand, does not require the changing of microcatheters after each embolization.

ENDOVASCULAR MANAGEMENT OF EPISTAXIS

Epistaxis is a common clinical problem, with 60% of individuals in the normal population experiencing an episode of varying severity in their lifetime.[16] Epistaxis can be managed conservatively in most cases; only 6% of cases require medical or surgical attention.[17] Intractable epistaxis is relatively uncommon. The idiopathic or spontaneous form of epistaxis is the most common cause, accounting for at least 70% of cases and is often related to cigarette use, hypertension, and atherosclerotic disease.[18] Other causes of epistaxis include hereditary hemorrhagic telangiectasia (HHT), craniofacial trauma, infections, tumors, bleeding disorders, vascular abnormalities, and anticoagulation therapy.[19]

In most of these cases, findings of angiography will be normal. Although hypervascularity is commonly seen, angiographic demonstration of the point of extravasation is rare.[20] This normal initial angiographic finding may relates in part to the nasal packing material that is generally in place to tamponade bleeding.

The arterial supply to the nasal fossa involves branches from both the ECA and ICA. The terminal branch of the internal maxillary artery (IMA), the sphenopalatine artery, provides the dominant supply to the nasal cavity. The roof of the nasal cavity is supplied by the anterior ethmoidal artery (AEA) and posterior ethmoidal artery, which branch off the ophthalmic artery. The floor of the nasal cavity is supplied by the ascending palatine artery and decending palatine artery, branches of the facial artery and IMA, respectively. Minor supply is provided anteriorly by the superior labial artery, a branch of the facial artery, and posteriorly by branches from the ascending pharyngeal artery (**Fig. 1**).

Epistaxis in Anterior Septal Area (Little Area)

Most cases of epistaxis arise from the anterior septal area, also known as the Little area. This area is vascularized by the Kiesselbach plexus, which is supplied by second-order branches of the ECA, including the sphenopalatine artery, descending

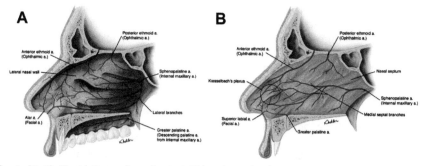

Fig. 1. (A, B). Illustrations of nasal arterial blood supply. The terminal branch of the internal maxillary artery, the sphenopalatine artery, provides the dominant arterial supply to the nasal cavity. The roof of the nasal cavity is supplied by the anterior and posterior ethmoidal arteries, which branch off the ophthalmic artery. The floor of the nasal cavity is supplied by the ascending palatine artery (not shown) and descending palatine artery, branches of the facial artery, and internal maxillary artery, respectively. Minor supply is provided anteriorly by the superior labial artery, a branch of the facial artery, and its alar branch artery.

palatine artery, and superior labial artery, as well as the anterior and posterior ethmoidal arteries[20] (see **Fig. 1**). Hemorrhage from this region can usually be managed by applying pressure to the nostrils, chemical or electrocautery, topical hemostatic or vasoconstricting agents, cryotherapy, hot water irrigation, or anterior nasal packing together with the management of underlying risk factors, such as hypertension and oral anticoagulation.[21]

Epistaxis from Posterior Nasal Cavity

In only approximately 5% of cases, the origin of the epistaxis lies more posteriorly on the nasal cavity, causing these initial measures to fail.[22] In most cases, an attempt will be made to control such posterior bleeding with the application of anterior and posterior packs. These packs should be applied with care because they can lead to nasal trauma, cartilage necrosis, vagal response, aspiration, infection, sepsis, and airway obstruction, which can lead to hypoxia, cardiac arrhythmia, myocardial infarction, and, rarely, even death.[21,23] The success rate of nasal packs in this setting has been reported to lie between 48% and 83%.[24-26] In the remaining patients, bleeding either continues despite packing or recurs after removal of the packs. Subsequent treatment can consist of either surgical ligation or endovascular embolization of the arteries supplying the posterior nasal fossa. Historically, the definitive treatment for intractable posterior epistaxis consisted of transantral surgical ligation of branches of the IMA, with or without ligation of the AEA. A failure rate of up to 24% has been described with this technique.[17] Endoscopic surgical procedures have been described more recently for direct cauterization of the active bleeding site or ligation of the sphenopalatine artery.[27]

Endovascular Embolization for Epistaxis

Endovascular embolization for epistaxis is an effective alternative to surgery and is associated with few complications.[17,28] The procedure was first presented as an alternative to surgery by Sokoloff and colleagues[29] in 1974 and consisted of particle embolization of the ipsilateral IMA. The technique was later refined by Lasjaunias and colleagues,[30] stressing the need for a standardized angiographic and therapeutic approach. It has gained increased acceptance, and several large series have been reported.[31,32]

Reported success rates range from 71% to 100%.[17,31–33] The ability to halt bleeding with embolization therapy immediately following the procedure has been reported to be between 93% and 100%.[31–37] When early rebleeds were taken into account, the success rate dropped to 77% to 95%.[32–37] Retrospective reviews that took late rebleeds into account reported a further drop in the success rate to 71% to 89%.[31–37] In general, these success rates best represent the results in idiopathic posterior epistaxis. Failure of endovascular treatment of epistaxis is often related to continued bleeding from the ethmoidal branches of the ophthalmic artery (**Fig. 3A**). Embolization of these branches is relatively contraindicated because ophthalmic artery embolization carries a risk of blindness (**Fig. 2**). The ethmoidal vessels can, however, be surgically ligated, as they perforate the medial wall of the orbit.[26] In comparison, the failure rate of surgical ligation to treat intractable epistaxis has been reported to be between 4.3% and 33.0%.[25–27] Success rates are comparable between surgical ligation and embolization.[38]

Endovascular Embolization Procedure

The endovascular embolization procedure can often be done safely using either conscious sedation or general anesthesia.

Selective angiography of the bilateral ICAs and ECAs is first performed with 4F or 5F catheters. In a minority of cases, this may reveal specific abnormalities indicating the cause and location of the hemorrhage. These include contrast extravasation, a tumor blush, a vascular malformation, a traumatic pseudoaneurysm, or another unusual ICA source of epistaxis (**Figs. 2, 3** and **4**). Furthermore, angiography enables identification of vascular anomalies, variants, or anastomoses between the ECA and ICA and/or ophthalmic artery that could increase the risk of complications, such as stroke or blindness during embolization. Embolization through the ICA, ophthalmic artery, and ascending pharyngeal artery is not considered safe. Although uncommon,

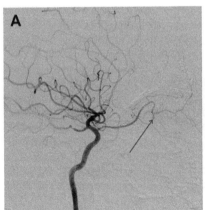
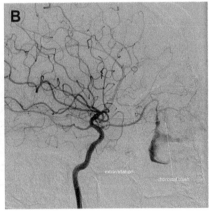

Fig. 2. Epistaxis from traumatic injury to the anterior ethmoidal artery (AEA) (*A*). With posterior nasal packs in place, the site of bleed appears to be a small pseudoaneurysm arising off an anterior ethmoidal artery (*arrow*). (*B*) After removal of nasal packs, the extravasation is more obvious (*arrow*). The choroidal blush is also demonstrated (*arrow*). Embolization of the AEA off of the ophthalmic artery carries a risk of damage to the retina, although in this case the central retinal artery arises proximal to the site of extravasation. It was deemed safer to treat this case via a surgical approach given the risk of catheter manipulation in the ophthalmic artery as well as the risk of reflux of embolic material into the central retinal artery.

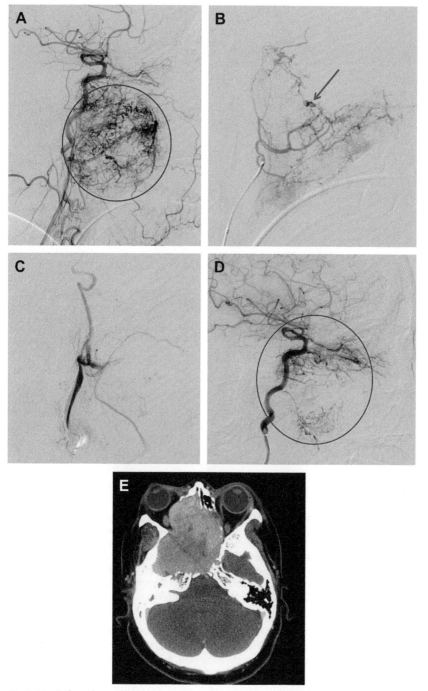

Fig. 3. Epistaxis from large facial leiomyosarcoma. (*A*) Digital subtraction angiogram (DSA) on common carotid injection reveals severe neohypervascularity over the posterior nasal fossa and nasopharynx consistent with hypervascular tumor (*circle*). (*B*) DSA on selective catheterization of the IMA reveals neohypervascularity in addition to a small pseudoaneurysm (*arrow*), which may have been the site of the patient's epistaxis. (*C*) DSA of the external carotid artery and internal carotid artery (*D*) after particle embolization demonstrates significant reduction in tumor vascularity (*circle*) and nonvisualization of the previously seen IMA pseudoaneurysm. (*E*) Axial contrast-enhanced CT demonstrates the large skull base and nasal mass lesion.

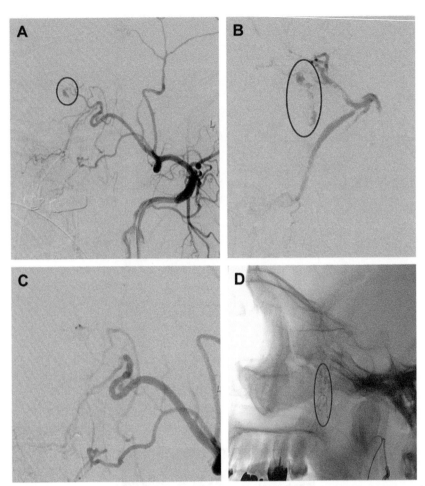

Fig. 4. Epistaxis status postembolization of internal maxillary artery pseudoaneurysm. (*A*) DSA image with nasal packing in place demonstrates small pseudoaneurysm (*circle*) arising from the distal IMA. (*B*) DSA image after removal of nasal packing demonstrates gross extravasation (*oval*) of contrast material from site of pseudoaneurysm. (*C*) After emboliza-tion with *n*-BCA, this DSA image shows that previously seen pseudoaneurysm and extrava-sation are no longer present. (*D*) Unsubtracted angiographic image after embolization demonstrates cast of *n*-BCA (*oval*) from the embolization.

embolization of the ophthalmic artery can occur if it is supplied by the ECA instead of the ICA. Therefore, one can confirm the choroidal blush from the ICA before emboli-zation. The angiographic findings may influence the embolization protocol or even lead to aborting the procedure.

In idiopathic cases of bleeding, a routine embolization protocol is used, with the goal of diminishing flow to the bleeding mucosa but allowing sufficient collateral flow to avoid mucosal necrosis. The most important vessel to embolize is the ipsilateral IMA and its branches. Because of anastomoses between the ICA and ECA described previously, embolization should be performed only with a stable microcatheter posi-tion sufficiently distal to the origins of the accessory meningeal artery and the middle meningeal artery. Placing the microcatheter distal to the middle deep temporal artery also may avoid postembolization pain and trismus. Additional embolization of the ipsilateral facial artery has been reported to increase the success rate.[34] In this case, the catheter should be placed beyond the submandibular artery to avoid embolization of the submandibular gland.[39] Some investigators will also embolize the contralateral IMA and even the contralateral facial artery, especially when these show substantial collateral supply.[35]

The microcatheter is positioned just proximal to the branches supplying the nasal mucosa, and care is taken to avoid nontargeted vessel embolization. Embolization is performed by injecting a suspension of embolic and contrast material under fluoroscopic guidance until significant flow reduction is noted in the artery and its branches. Injection of embolic material should be gentle to avoid reflux of embolic material into dangerous anastomoses. A wedged catheter position should also be avoided, as this may allow buildup of injection pressure with the subsequent opening of potential dangerous anastomoses.[35]

Embolization is generally performed using particles sized 150 to 500 μm. If smaller particles (50–150 μm) are chosen, they are typically used in small quantities because aggressive embolization with small particles is associated with a risk of necrosis of the embolized territory, owing to the greater degree of distal penetration of particles into tiny mucosal vessels; smaller particles are also more likely to enter dangerous anastomoses. Gelfoam pledgets may be placed in the vessel lumen after completing embolization with particulate agents. Permanent occlusion of vessels with mechanical devices, such as coils, is avoided in patients with epistaxis unless the bleeding is related to trauma, pseudoaneurysm, or nasal AVMs, because permanent occlusion of vessels in epistaxis will not allow the operator access for reembolization of the target territory should bleeding recur because of collateral flow and/or intrinsic regrowth of vascular pathology.

Complications with Endovascular Embolization

Complications resulting from the treatment are usually minor, including groin hematoma, facial numbness or pain, mucosal necrosis, and sinusitis. A cerebrovascular accident or blindness can occasionally occur as a complication of the treatment, although the incidence of this complication is very low.[33,40] Serious major complications can be associated with embolization if care is not taken to identify dangerous vascular anastomoses. Larger series report minor transient complications in 25% to 59% of cases, major transient complications in 0% to 1% of cases, and persistent complications in 2% or fewer cases.[31–37] With the advent of endoscopic surgery, complication rates of surgery have decreased, with only minor complications being reported.[25,27] Thus, success and complication rates are comparable between surgical ligation and embolization.

Hereditary Hemmorhagic Teleangiectasia

Recurrent bleeding is not uncommon in patients with HHT; however, embolization often decreases the severity of hemorrhage and improves the quality of life in these patients.[28] The difficulty in treating recurrent epistaxis in patients with HHT is reflected by the multitude of reported treatment options, including chemical, electrical, or ultrasonic cauterization; local or systemic hormone therapy; topical application of fibrin glue; photocoagulation; transarterial embolization; brachytherapy; septal dermoplasty; vessel ligation; bleomycin injections; and the use of nasal obturators.[41] Because none of these provide a definite cure, treatment is aimed at reducing the number and severity of epistaxis episodes. Although transarterial embolization may achieve this goal, recurrence rates requiring reembolization or surgery are generally higher in patients with HHT than in patients without HHT.[28] Therefore, permanent proximal occlusion with coils is not advised because this may preclude reembolization when distal collaterals result in recurrent bleeding episodes.[28] Embolization at a time when the patient is not actively bleeding will generally not yield long-term control.[31]

EMBOLIZATION OF VASCULAR HEAD AND NECK TUMORS

The tumors that most frequently require embolization in the head and neck include glomus tumors, angiofibromas, and meningiomas. Other tumors that may benefit from preoperative embolization include hypervascular metastases, esthesioneuroblastomas, schwannomas, rhabdomyosarcomas, plasmacytomas, chordomas, and hemangiopericytomas.

Preoperative embolization has been shown to be cost-effective and tends to shorten operative time by reducing blood loss and the period of recovery.[42,43] Moulin and colleagues[44] demonstrated a statistically significant difference in blood loss between embolized and nonembolized surgical groups of patients with high-grade tumors. The benefit is less clear for smaller, less vascular tumors.[44] Embolization is ideally performed 24 to 72 hours before surgical resection to allow maximal thrombosis of the occluded vessels and to prevent recanalization of the occluded arteries or formation of collateral arterial channels.[44]

Blood supply to tumors of the head and neck is derived primarily from branches of the ECA, which can vary greatly in size depending on local tumoral influences. Additional recruitment of vascular supply may develop from the VA, ICA, and thyrocervical and costocervical trunks.

Treatment consists of performing detailed angiography, including selective injections of the ICA and the ECA. A microcatheter is advanced into the artery supplying the tumor and angiography is performed to assess flow dynamics and to identify any potentially dangerous vascular anastomoses. The embolic agent is then injected under constant fluoroscopic monitoring, making sure to avoid both reflux of embolic material and possibly opening of previously occult potential anastomoses. Ideally, the embolic material is deposited at the arteriolar/capillary level. If there is arteriovenous shunting, particle size may need to be increased to prevent passage into the venous side. Proximal arterial occlusion alone is inadequate because it allows arterial collateralization into the tumor bed between the time of embolization and surgery and may make surgical resection more difficult.[42] If critical anastomoses are present, the anastomotic connection may first be occluded with coils followed by particulate embolization of the tumor.

Embolization of Vascular Head and Neck Tumors with Particles

Particles are most frequently used at our institution for the embolization of hypervascular head and neck tumors. Small particles, such as those in the 100-um to 300-um range, allow more distal penetration into the tumor bed and better devascularization.[45] One should always be aware of the possible risk of devascularizing the cranial nerves with small particles that may penetrate into the tiny vasa nervorum, however. Therefore, when embolizing the arterial pedicles that might also supply the cranial nerves (for example, the stylomastoid branch of the occipital artery or neuromeningeal trunk of the ascending pharyngeal artery), increasing particle size to 300 to 500 μm is generally preferred. Smaller particles may also increase the risk of tumoral hemorrhage and swelling.[46] In addition, undesired embolization of normal ECA territory tissue can cause harm to mucosa, tongue, larynx, and orbit.[16] Anastomoses to the ophthalmic and central retinal arteries may exist from the IMA, middle meningeal artery, facial artery, and superficial temporal artery. Of utmost concern during embolization of a juvenile nasopharyngeal angiofibroma, for example, is central retinal artery occlusion secondary to the presence of dangerous collaterals from the IMA into the orbit via nasal to ethmoidal and/or other potential collateral pathways.

Embolization of Vascular Head and Neck Tumors with Liquids

Liquid embolic agents are generally not used in this setting via a transarterial approach because liquid has greater potential to occlude the vasa nervorum of the cranial nerves and may also pass through tiny anastomoses into the intracranial circulation.[9,13] Moreover, the advantageous permanent quality of liquid embolics need not be used in this setting if surgical resection of the embolized tumor is planned to be within 24 to 72 hours postembolization.

Embolization of Vascular Head and Neck Tumors with Percutaneous Puncture

Direct percutaneous puncture under fluoroscopic guidance, computed tomography (CT), or sonography has also been described to embolize head and neck tumors. This method was initially reported for use in tumors in which conventional transarterial embolization was technically impossible because of the small size of the arterial feeders or in the setting of dangerous vascular anastomoses to the ICA or VA.[47] Excellent results obtained by this technique have extended its application to smaller and less complex tumors.[48] Direct and easy access to the vascular tumor bed that is not hampered by arterial tortuosity, small size of the feeders, atherosclerotic disease, or catheter-induced vasospasm is the main advantage of this direct percutaneous technique. Complete or near complete devascularization of the tumor can be obtained with decreased risk to the patient by direct tumoral injection of n-BCA or Onyx[47,48] (**Fig. 5**). Serious complications occur in fewer than 2% of patients and include dangerous nontarget migration of embolic material. These are usually related to particle reflux, poor technique, or nonvisualization of dangerous anastomoses resulting in blindness or irreversible neurologic deficits.[47–49]

EMBOLIZATION OF CERVICOFACIAL VASCULAR MALFORMATIONS
High-Flow Vascular Malformations

True high-flow AVMs of the extracranial head and neck are rare in contrast to low-flow vascular anomalies, such as venous malformations or hemangiomas. Angiographically, craniofacial high-flow VMs may consist of a nidus or direct communications between arteries and veins, although the precise distinction between these 2 types may not always be possible.[50]

Clinical presentation

The clinical presentation can be cosmetic defects, pain, bleeding, ischemic ulceration, and congestive heart failure.

Management

The management of high-flow vascular anomalies is challenging because of their unpredictable biologic behavior and a relatively high incidence of recurrence if not managed correctly.[51] Although smaller lesions can be managed by endovascular embolization alone, larger and complex lesions may require additional surgical resection. Additionally, because of the rarity of high-flow VMs in the soft tissues of the head and neck, there is a lack of consensus on the optimal method of treatment. Nevertheless, embolization forms an integral part of treatment (**Fig. 6**).

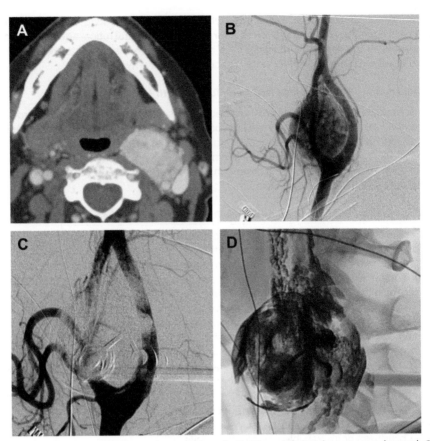

Fig. 5. Percutaneous hypervascular tumor embolization. (*A*) Axial contrast-enhanced CT demonstrates hypervascular mass at the level of the left carotid bulb consistent with a carotid body glomus tumor. (*B*) DSA image demonstrates hypervascular mass splaying the internal and external carotid arteries. (*C*) DSA image after percutaneous Onyx embolization of the mass reveals no residual hypervascularity. (*D*) Fluoroscopic image demonstrates the Onyx cast within the embolized tumor.

Embolization of cervicofacial VMs with liquids

Liquid embolic agents, such as *n*-BCA and Onyx, are generally used for high-flow AVM embolization, as these agents are more effective and permanent[50]; however, staged procedures may be necessary and distal microcatheter access may be difficult when there is excessive vascular tortuosity. Coils may be used in addition to liquid embolic agents; using coils alone for these lesions is not feasible, given that adequate penetration into the interstices of the AVM nidus is generally not possible with coils.[50] Embolization with particles is not effective because of both frequent incomplete closure and recanalization of the VM.[6]

Embolization of cervicofacial VMs with percutaneous puncture

Direct-puncture, or percutaneous, embolization can be used for direct access into the vascular nidus or the adjacent vein.[52] The nidus and/or the draining vein can be embolized with *n*-BCA or Onyx by using this approach. Flow-modification techniques are frequently required to limit the venous egress of the embolic material and to facilitate complete filling of the nidus. This can be accomplished by manual

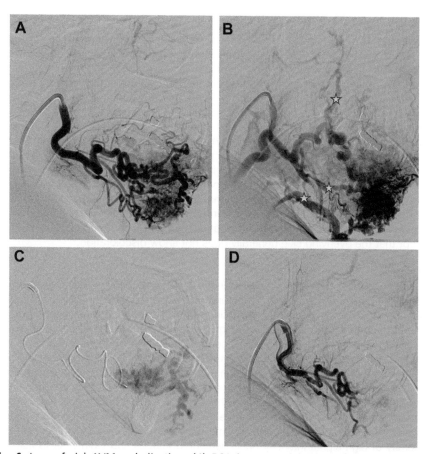

Fig. 6. Large facial AVM embolization. (*A*) DSA image on injection of the facial artery demonstrates a large soft tissue arteriovenous malformation nidus overlying the mandible. (*B*) DSA image slightly later demonstrates early-draining veins (*stars*). (*C*) DSA image after superselective injection of distal facial arterial feeder to the AVM. (*D*) After embolization with particles, a facial arterial angiogram demonstrates resolution of the facial AVM. The AVM recurred on a follow-up angiogram 1 month later and was reembolized with particles. Particle embolization allows for recanalization of the lesion but tends to preserve the adjacent soft tissues and skin from damage in the setting of a large lesion embolization such as this one. Multiple embolization procedures with particles are often required to promote thrombosis within a lesion of this size.

compression of the vein if there is a single large outflow channel; however, when an AVM has multiple venous drainage channels, a compression device for circumferential flow reduction can be more effective than manual digital compression.[52] Alternatively, a temporary balloon may be inflated in the feeding artery to decrease the rate of shunt surgery and limit the backward reflux of embolic material in the feeding vessel. Direct-puncture embolization of an AVM is often technically easier compared with transarterial embolization, reduces the procedure time, and has the advantage of reducing the risk of ischemic complications, such as skin necrosis and brain or retinal ischemia.[52] If Onyx is used for percutaneous injection, care should be taken to avoid subcutaneous extravasation, as this may result in skin discoloration.

Low-Flow VMs

Low-flow VMs of the head and neck include venous, lymphatic, and capillary congenital VMs.[53] These can involve the soft tissue structures of the face and neck and/or the maxillofacial skeleton. Venous and lymphatic malformations are often treated by percutaneous embolization.[54–56] Capillary malformations are rarely treated via endovascular or percutaneous techniques.

Clinical presentation

Symptoms can range from pain, swelling, infection, or bleeding; or the problem can be cosmetic. Functional impairment may be present, depending on the size, location, hemodynamic effects, and type of vessel involved. Large lesions may compress the aerodigestive tract and can sometimes present with compromise of the airway.[54] VMs consist of dilated venous channels that enlarge in a dependent position or with the Valsalva maneuver. The overlying skin may have a bluish-purple discoloration, and the lesions are compressible on palpation. Lymphatic malformations are similar, except that the overlying skin generally does not show discoloration.[54]

Evaluation

Evaluation is best performed with magnetic resonance (MR) imaging. Sequences should include T1-weighting with fat saturation before and after the infusion of gadolinium, inversion-recovery, or T2-weighting with fat saturation, and gradient-echo. Dynamic and/or time-resolved MR imaging with gadolinium could be obtained to study the timing and hemodynamics of contrast uptake within these lesions.[57,58]

VMs demonstrate high signal intensity with septations on T2-weighted images. Phleboliths may be evident as areas of signal-intensity void and are best seen on the gradient-echo images or on CT. Contrast administration results in a variable enhancement pattern, ranging from attenuated enhancement similar to that in adjacent veins to nonhomogeneous or delayed enhancement.[57,58] Lymphatic malformations are generally classified as macrocystic, microcystic, or mixed. On MR imaging, lesions are generally of high signal intensity on T2-weighted images and isointense to fluid on T1-weighted sequences. Unlike venous malformations, lymphatic malformations generally do not enhance.[57,58]

Management of low-flow VMs

Treatment of low-flow VMs is challenging and often multidisciplinary, with involvement of the plastic surgeon, pediatric surgeon, otolaryngologist, and interventional radiologist.[51] Therapeutic options include compression, laser photocoagulation, resection, radiofrequency ablation, and obliteration of the lesion by percutaneous injection of a sclerosant agent.[51] The most commonly used sclerosant agents are ethanol, sodium tetradecyl sulfate, and polidocanol. Lyphmatic malformations may be treated with OK-432 or doxycycline.[59] Larger lesions may be treated with multistaged sclerotherapy sessions, which are usually spaced weeks to months apart.

The procedure is typically performed in the interventional suite with conscious sedation or general anesthesia. General anesthesia is preferable when the lesion is large and may involve the airway. Percutaneous catheterization of vascular channels or cysts is generally performed under direct visualization or sonography. Contrast material is then injected under fluoroscopic guidance to assess the lesion and its venous drainage, exclude arterial cannulation, and calculate the volume of the sclerosant that can be injected before filling the draining vein. Injected contrast material is then aspirated out of the malformation and replaced with a slightly lower amount of the sclerosing agent (**Fig. 7**). Foaming the sclerosant agent can be performed by mixing

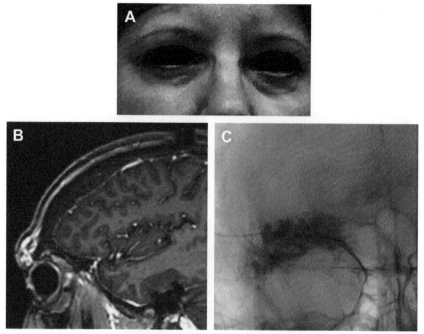

Fig. 7. Low-flow VM. (*A*) Photograph demonstrates mild superior right periorbital soft tissue swelling. (*B*) Sagittal contast-enhanced T1-weighted image demonstrates enhancing vessels above the globe consistent with vascular malformation. (*C*) Fluoroscopic image after injection of contrast material and alcohol demonstrates opacification of the venous malformation.

it with air, which may allow more prolonged displacement of the blood within the lesion and better contact of the sclerosant with the walls of the lesion.

Other Applications for Sclerosants

The mechanism of action of sclerosing agents involves producing an inflammatory reaction of the adjacent tissue as well as endothelial necrosis. Because of these properties, sclerosing agents have been used with variable success in many other cystic lesions of the head and neck, including plunging ranulas, sialoceles, benign lymphoepithelial cysts of the parotid gland, branchial cysts, and other benign cysts of the head and neck[59] (**Fig. 8**). Complications are generally minor, including fever and tender swelling for a few days. Extracystic extravasation of sclerosants should be avoided, especially in the oral cavity and oropharynx because it can cause mucosal swelling, discomfort, and swallowing difficulties. Sclerotherapy should be withheld for the acutely infected cysts, and the infection should be controlled first.

ENDOVASCULAR MANAGEMENT OF HEAD AND NECK TRAUMA AND BLEEDING

Traumatic vascular injuries in the head include arterial dissection, pseudoaneurysm, arteriovenous fistula, arterial occlusion, and bleeding. Endovascular treatments, when indicated, generally involve stenting of the dissected artery, embolization with or without stenting of a pseudoaneurysm, embolization of arteriovenous fistulae, and vessel sacrifice if deemed necessary and feasible.[60] If there is extensive damage to the vessel, reconstructive endovascular treatment may not be possible, and vessel

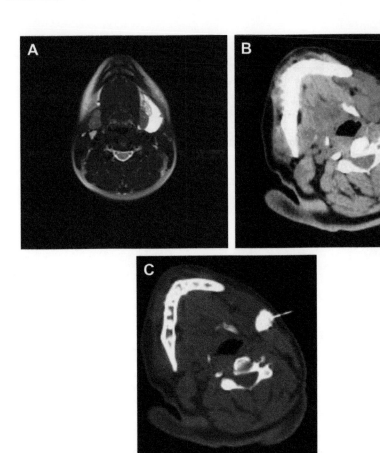

Fig. 8. Sclerosis of a cystic facial venolymphatic malformation. (*A*) T2-weighted axial MR image demonstrates a hyperintense lesion within the subcutaneous tissues of the left face surrounding the mandible and extending into the parapharyngeal and sublingual spaces. (*B*) Axial CT image during needle placement demonstrates the needle tip in the lesion with a small amount of hypodense air introduced into the lesion. (*C*) Axial CT after contrast material injection into the lesion confirms route of spread of injected material. A sclerosis was then performed using Ethanolamine.

sacrifice may be necessary. This technique is safe if contralateral supply to the brain from the ICA or VA is sufficient in the setting of an arterial occlusion. VA occlusion can often be safely performed below the level of the posterior inferior cerebellar artery.[61] A temporary balloon occlusion test can be performed before sacrificing an artery and may help in identifying patients at risk for immediate or delayed ischemic complications from arterial occlusion.[62]

Traumatic vascular injuries in the head and neck occur in the setting of both penetrating and nonpenetrating trauma and may present as a pulsatile neck mass, enlarging hematoma, transient ischemic attack, and/or stroke. Arteriovenous fistula often lack direct symptoms at presentation but can present with findings of a thrill or symptoms related to vascular steal phenomenon.[63]

CT angiography has a preponderant role in the evaluation of vascular neck trauma[64]; however, conventional angiography remains the study of choice for equivocal cases and for treatment planning. Conventional angiography better evaluates the degree of collateral circulation and can detect arteriovenous shunting given the temporal nature of image acquisition in conventional angiography.[65,66]

Dissection

Trauma accounts for a minority of cervical arterial dissections in comparison with spontaneous dissections. Nevertheless, a history of a minor precipitating event is frequently elicited in patients with a spontaneous cervical arterial dissection. Antithrombotic agents are generally considered first-line therapy for uncomplicated cervical arterial dissection.[63] The decision to use antiplatelets versus anticoagulants is based on a number of different clinical factors, including presence of stroke and its severity, severity of imaging findings, extension of dissection intracranially, and contraindications to either treatment. Prognosis tends to be favorable with conservative management; resolution of stenosis from spontaneous dissection can be seen in 90% of cases within the first 3 to 6 months.[63] Traumatic dissections have an overall worse prognosis in comparison with spontaneous dissections.[67]

Endovascular management of cervical arterial dissection is typically reserved for those cases that are refractory to medical management or that are deemed to be incurable and of significant risk without endovascular intervention. Endovascular therapy generally involves stenting of the dissected vessel, embolization of a dissecting pseudoaneurysm with or without a stent, and vessel sacrifice if deemed appropriate (**Figs. 9** and **10**). Endovascular stent reconstruction of a dissected cervical artery is considered safe and effective according to data from several retrospective case series and case reports. Pham and colleagues[68] recently reported a technical success rate of 99% to 100% with minimal complication.

Pseudoaneurysms

Carotid and vertebral arterial pseudoaneurysms are uncommon lesions that may occur as sequelae of blunt trauma, cancer/radiation necrosis, or mycotic infection. Historically, treatment of pseudoaneurysms has been primarily surgical[69]; however, because surgical intervention requires proximal and distal control of the artery, pseudoaneurysms near the skull base may be very difficult to repair and pose greater risk to the patient.[70] As a result, endovascular techniques have evolved in an effort to reduce morbidity associated with surgical techniques. More recently, endovascular techniques have become more appealing with encouraging results.

Pseudoaneurysms of the extracranial head and neck can be treated with the use of detachable coils with or without a stent as well as with the use of single or multiple overlapping bare or covered stents with good success rates and relatively low complications. There have been numerous case series describing the use of bare or covered stents with or without coils to treat traumatic cervical arterial pseudoaneurysms.[71–75] Although covered stents have been used with high rates of success, they are felt to carry a higher risk of delayed thromboembolic complications.[75]

Consensus does not exist as to the ideal anticoagulation/antiplatelet regimen for use with stent placement for cervical arterial injury. Generally, patients are placed on dual antiplatelets for 3 to 6 months following stent placement, after which they continue on lifelong daily aspirin.

Arteriovenous Fistulae

Traumatic arteriovenous fistulae in the neck can occur after either penetrating or blunt trauma. Surgical access can be difficult, and a wide exposure is often needed to obtain proximal and distal control. Access to the vessels at the level of the skull

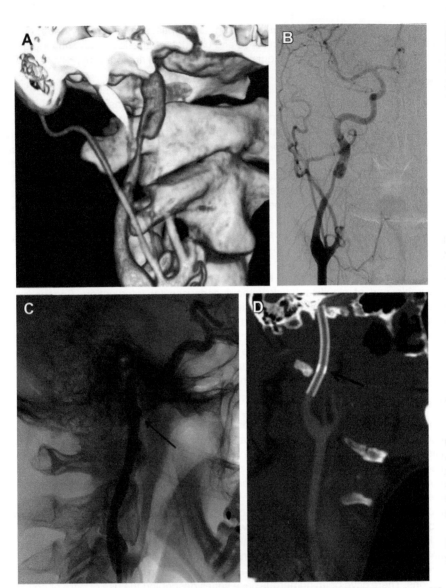

Fig. 9. Traumatic internal carotid artery dissection and dissecting pseudoaneurysm. (*A*) Three-dimensional volume-rendered contrast-enhanced reconstructed CT image and (*B*) DSA image show luminal stenosis of the midcervical ICA consistent with dissection and associated distal cervical internal carotid artery dilation consistent with a dissecting pseudoaneurysm. (*C*) Fluoroscopic image after stenting shows minimal contrast material permeating through the stent interstices into the pseudoaneurysm (*arrow*). (*D*) Follow-up CT angiogram reveals stent patency without evidence of pseudoaneurysm consistent with bare stent-related flow diversion away from the pseudoaneurysm with resultant pseudoaneurysmal thrombosis. Overlapping segments of the 2 deployed stents centrally demonstrate hyperdensity (*arrow*).

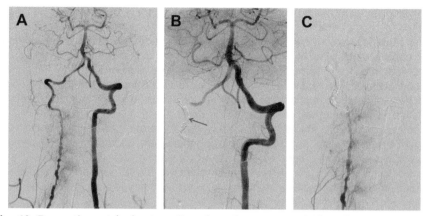

Fig. 10. Traumatic vertebral artery dissection after motor vehicle collision. (*A*) Digital subtraction angiography after selection of both vertebral arteries with separate catheters demonstrates severe irregularity of the right vertebral artery consistent with long-segment, flow-limiting dissection. (*B*) DSA image on left vertebral artery injection status post right vertebral artery embolization with coils demonstrates coils within the distal cervical right vertebral artery (*arrow*) without compromise of contrast opacification of the posterior fossa intracranial branch arteries. (*C*) DSA image on right vertebral artery injection status post right vertebral artery embolization with coils demonstrates residual dissection of the proximal right vertebral artery without distal flow from this vessel into the intracranial compartment.

base is challenging. As such, endovascular techniques have largely replaced surgical treatments for cervical arteriovenous fistulas.[76]

The ideal treatment for these lesions is exclusion of the fistula with preservation of the parent vessel. The use of covered stents for this application has been described and is the preferred method when the normal artery distal to the site of the fistula can be safely catheterized, although this is commonly not possible.[77] When parent vessel preservation is not possible, endovascular sacrifice of the parent vessel can be performed, and a variety of techniques have been used, including coil embolization, detachable balloons, and, less commonly, liquid embolics.[78] In the setting of a vertebral artery to vertebral venous plexus fistula, the possibility of steal phenomena into the lesion from the contralateral vertebral artery exists; it is, therefore, important to occlude both the proximal and distal aspects of the fistula.[78]

Bleeding and Carotid Blowout Syndrome

Traumatic arterial extravasation in the head and neck is a life-threatening condition that often requires immediate attention. Carotid blowout is a term that has commonly been applied to cases of rupture of the extracranial carotid artery or its branches. Usually, carotid blowout results from trauma or as a complication of head and neck cancer therapy, with resulting extravasation, pseudoaneurysm, or AVF. Morbidity and mortality rates associated with this complication are high and survival is usually less than 2 years.[79] Surgical ligation of the bleeding artery with or without a bypass has been the traditional form of treatment, although this can be technically demanding, depending on the location of the lesion and extent of injury. Moreover, surgical repair of carotid blowout lesions may be technically demanding because exploration and repair of a previous surgical and irradiated field can be difficult.[79,80]

Endovascular therapy is an excellent alternative to surgery in these settings and is the method of choice when feasible[81] (**Figs. 11** and **12**).

Permanent occlusion of the carotid artery is usually performed with coils or a detachable balloon. Approximately 15% to 20% of patients treated with permanent vessel occlusion may have immediate or delayed cerebral ischemia.[80–82] A temporary balloon occlusion test can be performed before sacrificing the carotid artery and may help in identifying patients at risk for immediate or delayed ischemic complications from occlusion of the carotid artery.[83]

The use of covered stents has been reported in carotid blowout syndrome with a high rate of technical success in achieving immediate hemostasis[82,84]; however, unfavorable long-term outcomes because of rebleeding, delayed thrombosis, and abscess formation from contamination of the stent with the skin or oral flora has limited the usefulness of endovascular stent reconstruction of these vessels.[85] These findings

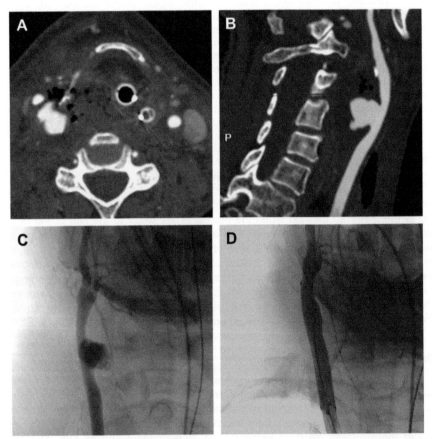

Fig. 11. Carotid blowout syndrome. Internal carotid pseudoaneurysm repair with a covered stent-graft. (*A*) Axial contrast-enhanced CT demonstrates large enhancing pseudoaneurysm arising from the medial aspect of the right ICA adjacent a necrotic mass lesion. (*B*) Coronal oblique contrast-enhanced CT image redemonstrates the pseudoaneurysm. (*C*) Angiographic image redemonstrates the pseudoaneurysm. (*D*) Angiographic image after covered stent grafting demonstrates exclusion of the pseudoaneurysm from the parent vessel with wide patency of the parent vessel.

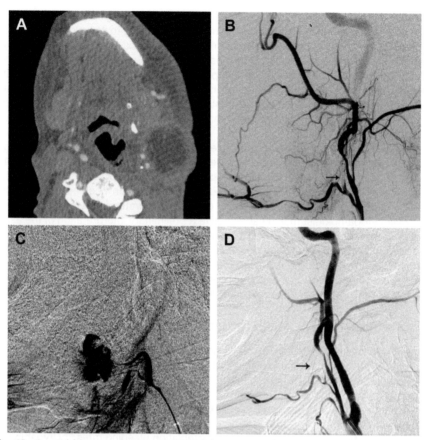

Fig. 12. Carotid blowout syndrome. (A) Axial contrast-enhanced CT demonstrates a hypo-dense metastasis from head and neck squamous cell carcinoma adjacent multiple external carotid arterial branches containing hyperdense intraluminal contrast material. (B) DSA image demonstrates proximal lingual arterial branch vessel irregularity consistent with site of bleeding (arrow). (C) DSA image after superselective injection of the injured vessel demonstrates gross extravasation of contrast material. (D) DSA image after coil emboliza-tion sacrifice of injured vessel (arrow) demonstrates no residual extravasation with patency of the lingual artery.

suggest that stent-graft placement may be beneficial for temporary rather than perma-nent management for patients with carotid blowout syndrome.[85] Appropriate candi-dates for the use of stent-grafts may include those at high risk of neurologic morbidity from carotid occlusion, patients with acute massive bleed that prevents temporary balloon test occlusion, or those with a short life expectancy.[85]

PERCUTANEOUS BIOPSY WITHIN THE HEAD AND NECK

Percutaneous biopsies of the head and neck can be performed with the use of imaging guidance. The most common techniques use CT imaging for the assessment of needle placement into the deeper spaces of the head and neck during the procedure. Ultra-sound guidance is often used to localize and help guide needle trajectory for superfi-cial lesions. Many superficial lesions that are palpable may be biopsied in the office setting without the use of imaging guidance as well. MR imaging may also be used for guidance, but experience with this technique is limited owing to its lack of widespread availability, because it is technically more difficult in comparison with "CT fluoroscopy" techniques, which are becoming more readily available, and because of the lower spatial resolution of MR imaging in comparison with CT.[86] With both high-quality imaging often obtained with the use of intravenous contrast material to delineate vascular structures and a thorough understanding of head and neck anatomy, nearly all of the spaces of the head and neck may be safely accessible for percutaneous biopsy.[86,87]

A coaxial needle technique is often useful in obtaining a stable system through which to obtain multiple samples. We generally use an introducer needle of 18 or 19 gauge to traverse the superficial and deep soft tissues and position it adjacent the lesion. We follow this with 20-gauge or 22-gauge aspiration needles, such as the Chiba, Westcott, or Franseen needles for obtaining aspirates for cytologic analysis. An onsite cytopathologist may be able to give a preliminary interpretation of the aspirates and may help determine if a core biopsy is needed. If required, a core biopsy can be obtained with a 20-gauge cutting needle. The introducer needle itself may also be used to obtain core biopsy samples (**Fig. 13**). Most head and neck biopsies we perform are done using local anesthesia and moderate sedation, whereas transoral biopsies of prevertebral or upper cervical vertebral lesions require general anesthesia.

RADIOFREQUENCY ABLATION AND CRYOABLATION OF TUMORS

Radiofrequency and cryoablation can be used as focal tumor ablation strategies and are most often used for the palliative treatment of unresectable malignancies or resectable lesions in patients who are poor surgical candidates. Radiofrequency ablation is performed using percutaneous probes to create an alternating electric current that produces frictional heat and subsequent tissue necrosis. This technique has gained wide acceptance in the treatment of solid tumors of the liver, lung, kidney, and bone with fairly low complication and postablation bleeding rates.[88] Cryoablation produces rapid freezing of tissue with resultant cell death.[89] It has been widely reported in the treatment of primary and metastatic tumors, most notably in the liver

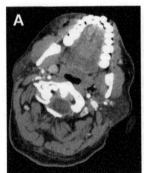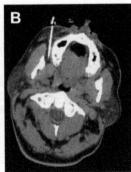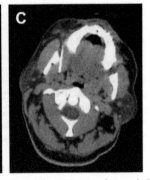

Fig. 13. CT-guided parapharyngeal space needle biopsy. (*A*) Axial contrast-enhanced CT image demonstrates a small enhancing rounded mass within the right parapharyngeal fat. (*B, C*) Spot "CT fluoro" images demonstrate the 19-gauge needle with its tip at the edge of the mass. Fine-needle aspirations were obtained through a small inner biopsy needle using a coaxial technique. A core biopsy sample was also obtained through the larger introducer needle itself. Pathology revealed pleomorphic adenoma.

and the prostate.[90] Treated tissue can be visualized with a variety of imaging modalities, including sonography, CT, and/or MR imaging during the procedure to determine treatment success.

Experience with radiofrequency ablation and cryoablation techniques in the head and neck is in its early stages. Although it is an evolving and exciting treatment option in the head and neck, consensus on appropriate indications is currently unclear. Published literature is limited to case descriptions and review articles.[91,92] Brook and colleagues[92] reported the use of radiofrequency ablation as a palliative measure in 14 patients with advanced unresectable head and neck cancers. Their technical success was reported to be 100% with 3 major complications, including stroke and carotid blowout related to the proximity of the electrodes to the carotid artery. The investigators from this series cautioned that tumors surrounding or adjacent to the carotid artery should be treated at relatively lower energy levels and that greater distances between the tumor and the electrodes may be helpful in preventing these complications.

REFERENCES

1. Gobin YP, Garcia-de-la-Fuente JA, Herbreteau D, et al. Endovascular treatment of external carotid-jugular fistulae in the parotid region. Neurosurgery 1993;33:812–6.
2. Debrun G, Lacour P, Caron JP, et al. Detachable balloon and calibrated-leak balloon techniques in the treatment of cerebral vascular lesions. J Neurosurg 1978;49:635–49.
3. Ricolfi F, Gobin YP, Aymard A, et al. Giant perimedullary arteriovenous fistulas of the spine: clinical and radiologic features and endovascular treatment. AJNR Am J Neuroradiol 1997;18:677–87.
4. Guglielmi G, Vinuela F, Dion J, et al. Electrothrombosis of saccular aneurysms via endovascular approach. II. Preliminary clinical experience. J Neurosurg 1991;75:8–14.
5. Quinones D, Duckwiler G, Gobin PY, et al. Embolization of dural cavernous fistulas via superior ophthalmic vein approach. AJNR Am J Neuroradiol 1997; 18:921–8.
6. Sorimachi T, Koike T, Takeuchi S, et al. Embolization of cerebral arteriovenous malformations achieved with polyvinyl alcohol particles: angiographic reappearance and complications. AJNR Am J Neuroradiol 1999;20:1323–8.
7. Nichols DA, Rufenacht DA, Jack CR, et al. Embolization of spinal dural arteriovenous fistula with polyvinyl alcohol particles: experience in 14 patients. AJNR Am J Neuroradiol 1992;13:933–40.
8. Repa I, Moradian GP, Dehner LP, et al. Mortalities associated with use of a commercial suspension of polyvinyl alcohol. Radiology 1989;170:395–9.
9. Dion JE. Principles and methodology. In: Vinuela F, Halbach VV, Dijon JE, editors. Interventional neuroradiology. New York: Raven; 1992. p. 1–17.
10. Rao VR, Mandalam KR, Gupta AK, et al. Dissolution of isobutyl 2-cyanoacrylate on long-term follow-up. AJNR Am J Neuroradiol 1987;10:135–41.
11. Wikholm G. Occlusion of cerebral arteriovenous malformations embolized with n-butyl cyanoacrylate is permanent. AJNR Am J Neuroradiol 1995;16:479–82.
12. Debrun GM, Aletich V, Ausman JI, et al. Embolization of the nidus of brain arteriovenous malformations with n-butyl cyanoacrylate. Neurosurgery 1997;40:112–21.
13. Thiex R, Wu I, Mulliken JB, et al. Safety and clinical efficacy of Onyx for embolization of extracranial head and neck vascular anomalies. Am J Neuroradiol 2011; 32(6):1082–6.
14. Ayad M, Eskioglu E, Mericle RA. Onyx: a unique neuroembolic agent. Expert Rev Med Devices 2006;3(6):705–15.

15. Loh Y, Duckwiler GR, Onyx Trial Investigators. A prospective, multicenter, randomized trial of the Onyx liquid embolic system and N-butyl cyanoacrylate embolization of cerebral arteriovenous malformations. Clinical article. J Neurosurg 2010;113(4):733–41.
16. Turowski B, Zanella FE. Interventional neuroradiology of the head and neck. Neuroimaging Clin N Am 2003;13:619–45.
17. Andersen PJ, Kjeldsen AD, Nepper-Rasmussen J. Selective embolization in the treatment of intractable epistaxis. Acta Otolaryngol 2005;125:293–7.
18. Pallin DJ, Chng YM, McKay MP, et al. Epidemiology of epistaxis in US emergency departments, 1992 to 2001. Ann Emerg Med 2005;46:77–81.
19. Walker TW, Macfarlane TV, McGarry GW. The epidemiology and chronobiology of epistaxis: an investigation of Scottish hospital admissions 1995–2004. Clin Otolaryngol 2007;32:361–5.
20. Koh E, Frazzini VI, Kagetsu NJ. Epistaxis: vascular anatomy, origins, and endovascular treatment. AJR Am J Roentgenol 2000;174:845–51.
21. Tan LK, Calhoun KH. Epistaxis. Med Clin North Am 1999;83:43–56.
22. Viducich RA, Blanda MP, Gerson LW. Posterior epistaxis: clinical features and acute complications. Ann Emerg Med 1995;25:592–6.
23. Monte ED, Belmont MJ, Wax MK. Management paradigms for posterior epistaxis: a comparison of costs and complications. Otolaryngol Head Neck Surg 1999; 121:103–6.
24. Pollice PA, Yoder MG. Epistaxis: a retrospective review of hospitalized patients. Otolaryngol Head Neck Surg 1997;117:49–53.
25. Klotz DA, Winkle MR, Richmon J, et al. Surgical management of posterior epistaxis: a changing paradigm. Laryngoscope 2002;112:1577–82.
26. Schaitkin B, Strauss M, Houck JR. Epistaxis: medical versus surgical therapy— a comparison of efficacy, complications, and economic considerations. Laryngoscope 1987;97:1392–6.
27. Holzmann D, Kaufmann T, Pedrini P, et al. Posterior epistaxis: endonasal exposure and occlusion of the branches of the sphenopalatine artery. Eur Arch Otorhinolaryngol 2003;260:425–8.
28. Layton KF, Kallmes DF, Gray LA, et al. Endovascular treatment of epistaxis in patients with hereditary hemorrhagic telangiectasia. AJNR Am J Neuroradiol 2007;28:885–8.
29. Sokoloff J, Wickbom I, McDonald D, et al. Therapeutic percutaneous embolization in intractable epistaxis. Radiology 1974;111:285–7.
30. Lasjaunias P, Marsot-Dupuch K, Doyon D. The radio-anatomical basis of arterial embolisation for epistaxis. J Neuroradiol 1979;6:45–53.
31. Elden L, Montanera W, Terbrugge K, et al. Angiographic embolization for the treatment of epistaxis: a review of 108 cases. Otolaryngol Head Neck Surg 1994;111:44–50.
32. Tseng EY, Narducci CA, Willing SJ, et al. Angiographic embolization for epistaxis: a review of 114 cases. Laryngoscope 1998;108:615–9.
33. Strutz J, Schumacher M. Uncontrollable epistaxis, angiographic localization and embolization. Arch Otolaryngol Head Neck Surg 1990;116:697–9.
34. Vitek J. Idiopathic intractable epistaxis: endovascular therapy. Radiology 1991; 181:113–6.
35. Fukutsuji K, Nishiike S, Aihara T, et al. Superselective angiographic embolization for intractable epistaxis. Acta Otolaryngol 2008;128:556–60.
36. Duncan IC, Fourie PA, le Grange CE, et al. Endovascular treatment of intractable epistaxis: results of a 4-year local audit. S Afr Med J 2004;94:373–8.

37. Sadri M, Midwinter K, Ahmed A, et al. Assessment of safety and efficacy of arterial embolisation in the management of intractable epistaxis. Eur Arch Otorhinolaryngol 2006;263:560–6.
38. Cullen MM, Tami TA. Comparison of internal maxillary artery ligation versus embolization for refractory posterior epistaxis. Otolaryngol Head Neck Surg 1998;118: 636–42.
39. Duncan IC, Spiro FI, van Staden D. Acute ischemic sialadenitis following facial artery embolization. Cardiovasc Intervent Radiol 2004;27:300–2.
40. Christensen NP, Smith DS, Barnwell SL, et al. Arterial embolization in the management of posterior epistaxis. Otolaryngol Head Neck Surg 2005;133:748–53.
41. Guttmacher AE, Marchuk DA, White RI Jr. Hereditary hemorrhagic telangiectasia. N Engl J Med 1995;333:918–24.
42. Dean BL, Flom RA, Wallace RC, et al. Efficacy of endovascular treatment of meningiomas: evaluation with matched samples. AJNR Am J Neuroradiol 1994; 15:1675–80.
43. Macpherson P. The value of pre-operative embolization of meningiomas estimated subjectively and objectively. Neuroradiology 1991;33:334–7.
44. Moulin G, Chagnaud C, Gras R, et al. Juvenile nasopharyngeal angiofibroma: comparison of blood loss during removal in embolized group versus nonembolized group. Cardiovasc Intervent Radiol 1995;18(3):158–61.
45. Wakhloo AK, Juengling FD, Delthoven VV. Extended preoperative polyvinyl alcohol microembolization of intracranial meningiomas: assessment of two embolization techniques. AJNR Am J Neuroradiol 1993;14:571–82.
46. Kallmes DF, Evans AJ, Kaptain GJ, et al. Hemorrhagic complications in embolization of a meningioma: case report and review of the literature. Neuroradiology 1997;39:877–80.
47. Quadros RS, Gallas S, Delcourt C, et al. Preoperative embolization of a cervico-dorsal paraganglioma by direct percutaneous injection of Onyx and endovascular delivery of particles. AJNR Am J Neuroradiol 2006;27:1907–9.
48. Abud DG, Mounayer C, Benndorf G, et al. Intratumoral injection of cyanoacrylate glue in head and neck paragangliomas. AJNR Am J Neuroradiol 2004;25:1457–62.
49. Casasco A, Houdart E, Biondi A, et al. Major complications of percutaneous embolization of skull-base tumors. AJNR Am J Neuroradiol 1992;20(1):179–81.
50. Arat A, Cil BE, Vargel I, et al. Embolization of high-flow craniofacial vascular malformations with Onyx. AJNR Am J Neuroradiol 2007;28:1409–14.
51. Erdmann MW, Jackson JE, Davies DM, et al. Multidisciplinary approach to the management of head and neck arteriovenous malformations. Ann R Coll Surg Engl 1995;77:53–9.
52. Ryu CW, Whang SM, Suh DC, et al. Percutaneous direct puncture glue embolization of high-flow craniofacial arteriovenous lesions: a new circular ring compression device with a beveled edge. AJNR Am J Neuroradiol 2007;28:528–30.
53. Mulliken JB, Glowacki J. Hemangiomas and vascular malformations in infants and children: a classification based on endothelial characteristics. Plast Reconstr Surg 1982;69:412–20.
54. Turkbey B, Peynircioğlu B, Arat A, et al. Percutaneous management of peripheral vascular malformations: a single center experience. Diagn Interv Radiol 2011; 17(4):363–7.
55. Love Z, Hsu DP. Low-flow vascular malformations of the head and neck: clinicopathology and image guided therapy. J Neurointerv Surg 2011.
56. Renton JP, Smith RJ. Current treatment paradigms in the management of lymphatic malformations. Laryngoscope 2011;121(1):56–9.

57. Legiehn GM, Heran MK. Venous malformations: classification, development, diagnosis, and interventional radiologic management. Radiol Clin North Am 2008;46(3):545–97.
58. Legiehn GM, Heran MK. A step-by-step practical approach to imaging diagnosis and interventional radiologic therapy in vascular malformations. Semin Intervent Radiol 2010;27(2):209–31.
59. Kim KH, Sung MN, Rho JL, et al. Sclerotherapy for congenital lesions in the head and neck. Otolaryngol Head Neck Surg 2004;131:307–16.
60. Ohta H, Natarajan SK, Hauck EF, et al. Endovascular stent therapy for extracranial and intracranial carotid artery dissection: single-center experience. J Neurosurg 2011;115(1):91–100.
61. Sadato A, Maeda S, Hayakawa M, et al. Endovascular treatment of vertebral artery dissection using stents and coils: its pitfall and technical considerations. Minim Invasive Neurosurg 2010;53(5–6):243–9.
62. Van Rooij WJ, Sluzewski M, Slob MJ, et al. Predictive value of angiographic testing for tolerance to therapeutic occlusion of the carotid artery. Am J Neurorad 2000;21(7):1280–92.
63. Schievink WI. Spontaneous dissection of the carotid and vertebral arteries. N Engl J Med 2001;344(12):898–906.
64. Schneidereit NP, Simons R, Nicolau S, et al. Utility of screening for blunt vascular neck injuries with computed tomographic angiography. J Trauma 2006;60:209–16.
65. Goodwin RB, Beery PR, Dorbish RJ, et al. Computed tomographic angiography versus conventional angiography for the diagnosis of blunt cerebrovascular injury in trauma patients. J Trauma 2009;67(5):1046–50.
66. O'Brien PJ, Cox MW. A modern approach to cervical vascular trauma. Perspect Vasc Surg Endovasc Ther 2011;23(2):90–7.
67. Biffl W, Moore E, Offner P, et al. Blunt carotid injuries: implications of a new grading scale. J Trauma 1999;45:845–66.
68. Pham MH, Rahme RJ, Arnaout O, et al. Endovascular stenting of extracranial carotid and vertebral artery dissections: a systematic review of the literature. Neurosurgery 2011;68(4):856–66.
69. Pearce WH, Whitehill TA. Carotid and vertebral arterial injuries. Surg Clin North Am 1988;68:705–23.
70. Müller B, Luther B, Hort W, et al. Surgical treatment of 50 carotid dissections: indications and results. J Vasc Surg 2000;31:980–8.
71. Coldwell DM, Novak Z, Ryu RK, et al. Treatment of posttraumatic internal carotid arterial pseudoaneurysms with endovascular stents. J Trauma 2000;48:470–2.
72. Maras D, Lioupis C, Magoufis G, et al. Covered stent-graft treatment of internal carotid artery pseudoaneurysms: a review. Cardiovasc Intervent Radiol 2006; 29:958–68.
73. Duane TM, Parker F, Stokes GK, et al. Endovascular carotid stenting after trauma. J Trauma 2002;52:149–53.
74. Wang W, Li MH, Li YD, et al. Treatment of traumatic internal carotid artery pseudoaneurysms with the Willis covered stent: a prospective study. J Trauma 2011; 70(4):816–22.
75. Yi AC, Palmer E, Luh GY, et al. Endovascular treatment of carotid and vertebral pseudoaneurysms with covered stents. AJNR Am J Neuroradiol 2008;29(5): 983–7.
76. Herrera DA, Vargas SA, Dublin AB. Endovascular treatment of penetrating traumatic injuries of the extracranial carotid artery. J Vasc Interv Radiol 2011;22(1): 28–33.

77. Redekop G, Marotta T, Weill A. Treatment of traumatic aneurysms and arteriovenous fistulas of the skull base by using endovascular stents. J Neurosurg 2001; 95(3):412–9.

78. Herrera DA, Vargas SA, Dublin AB. Endovascular treatment of traumatic injuries of the vertebral artery. AJNR Am J Neuroradiol 2008;29(8):1585–9.

79. Chaloupka JC, Roth TC, Putman CM, et al. Recurrent carotid blowout syndrome: diagnosis and therapeutic challenges in a newly recognized subgroup of patients. AJNR Am J Neuroradiol 1999;30:1069–77.

80. Chaloupka JC, Putman CM, Citardi MJ, et al. Endovascular therapy of the carotid blowout syndrome in head and neck surgical patients: diagnostic and managerial considerations. AJNR Am J Neuroradiol 1996;17:843–52.

81. Mcdonald S, Gan J, Mckay AJ, et al. Endovascular treatment of acute carotid blowout syndrome. J Vasc Interv Radiol 2000;11:1184–8.

82. Lesley WS, Chaloupka JC, Weigele JB, et al. Preliminary experience with endovascular reconstruction for the management of carotid blowout syndrome. AJNR Am J Neuroradiol 2003;24:975–81.

83. Mathis JM, Barr JD, Jungreis CA, et al. Temporary balloon test occlusion of the internal carotid artery: experience in 500 cases. AJNR Am J Neuroradiol 1995; 16:749–54.

84. Chang FC, Lirng JF, Luo CB, et al. Carotid blowout syndrome in patients with head-and-neck cancers: reconstructive management by self-expandable stent-grafts. AJNR Am J Neuroradiol 2007;28:181–8.

85. Pyun HW, Lee DH, Yoo HM, et al. Placement of covered stents for carotid blowout in patients with head and neck cancer: follow-up results after rescue treatments. AJNR Am J Neuroradiol 2007;28:1594–8.

86. Gupta S, Henningsen JA, Wallace MJ, et al. Percutaneous biopsy of head and neck lesions with CT guidance: various approaches and relevant anatomic and technical considerations. Radiographics 2007;272:371–90.

87. Sherman PM, Yousem DM, Loevner LA. CT-guided aspirations in the head and neck: assessment of the first 216 cases. AJNR Am J Neuroradiol 2004;25: 1603–7.

88. van Vledder MG, van Aalten SM, Terkivatan T, et al. Safety and efficacy of radiofrequency ablation for hepatocellular adenoma. J Vasc Interv Radiol 2011;22(6): 787–93.

89. Erinjeri JP, Clark TW. Cryoablation: mechanism of action and devices. J Vasc Interv Radiol 2010;21(Suppl 8):S187–91.

90. Webb H, Lubner MG, Hinshaw JL. Thermal ablation. Semin Roentgenol 2011; 46(2):133–41.

91. Wyse G, Hong H, Murphy K. Percutaneous thermal ablation in the head and neck: current role and future applications. Neuroimaging Clin N Am 2009;19(2):161–8.

92. Brook A, Gold MM, Miller TS. CT-guided radiofrequency ablation in the palliative treatment of recurrent advanced head and neck malignancies. J Vasc Interv Radiol 2008;19:725–35 [Epub 2008 Mar 17].

Index

Note: Page numbers of article titles are in **boldface** type.

A

Abscess, in retropharyngeal space, 1302, 1304
Acinic cell carcinoma, of parotid gland, 1265
Adenoid cystic carcinoma, of larynx, 1348, 1349
    of parotid gland, 1264–1265
Adenoma, pleomorphic, 1261–1263, 1319–1320
Air collection, in prevertebral space, 1298, 1299
Amyloidosis, of larynx, 1354–1355
Arteriovenous fistulae, endovascular management of, 1439–1441

B

Branchial cleft cysts, of retropharyngeal space, 1302
    of submandibular and sublingual spaces, 1315

C

Carcinoma ex pleomorphic adenoma, 1262
Carotid artery dissection, 1276, 1277, 1278
Carotid blowout syndrome, endovascular management of, 1441–1443
Carotid pseudoaneurysms, endovascular management of, 1439
Carotid space, benign tumors of, 1278–1287, 1288, 1289, 1290
    imaging of, **1273–1292**
    infectious processes of, 1276–1277
    malignant tumors of, 1287–1291
    meningiomas of, 1286–1287, 1290
    neurofibromas of, 1285–1286, 1288, 1289
    paragangliomas of, 1279–1284
    pseudotumor of, 1274
    schwannomas of, 1284–1285, 1286, 1287
    vascular lesions of, 1275–1276
Cellulitis/abscess, of submandibular space, 1315, 1316
Cervical arterial dissection, endovascular management of, 1439, 1440, 1441
Cervical lymph nodes, classification of, 1365–1368
    contrast-enhanced CT of, 1374–1375, 1376, 1377
    diffusion-weighted MRI of, 1375–1376
    diseases of, invasion of adjacent structures, 1374, 1375
    drainage of, patterns of, 1368–1371
    evaluation and diagnosis of, **1363–1383**
    pathologic, imaging characteristics of, 1371–1373
    positron emission tomography and [^{18}F]fluorodeoxyglucose of, 1377–1378
    ultrasound of, 1375

Otolaryngol Clin N Am 45 (2012) 1451–1458
http://dx.doi.org/10.1016/S0030-6665(12)00152-1
0030-6665/12/$ – see front matter © 2012 Elsevier Inc. All rights reserved.

oto.theclinics.com

United States Postal Service

Statement of Ownership, Management, and Circulation
(All Periodicals Publications Except Requestor Publications)

1. Publication Title	2. Publication Number								3. Filing Date
Otolaryngologic Clinics of North America	4	6	6	-	5	5	5	0	9/14/12

4. Issue Frequency	5. Number of Issues Published Annually	6. Annual Subscription Price
Feb, Apr, Jun, Aug, Oct, Dec	6	$335.00

7. Complete Mailing Address of Known Office of Publication (Not printer) (Street, city, county, state, and ZIP+4®)

Elsevier Inc.
360 Park Avenue South
New York, NY 10010-1710

Contact Person
Stephen R. Bushing
Telephone (Include area code)
215-239-3688

8. Complete Mailing Address of Headquarters or General Business Office of Publisher (Not printer)

Elsevier Inc., 360 Park Avenue South, New York, NY 10010-1710

9. Full Names and Complete Mailing Addresses of Publisher, Editor, and Managing Editor (Do not leave blank)

Publisher (Name and complete mailing address)

Kim Murphy, Elsevier, Inc., 1600 John F. Kennedy Blvd. Suite 1800, Philadelphia, PA 19103-2899

Editor (Name and complete mailing address)

Joanne Husovski, Elsevier, Inc., 1600 John F. Kennedy Blvd. Suite 1800, Philadelphia, PA 19103-2899

Managing Editor (Name and complete mailing address)

Barbara Cohen – Kligerman, Elsevier, Inc., 1600 John F. Kennedy Blvd. Suite 1800, Philadelphia, PA 19103-2899

10. Owner (Do not leave blank. If the publication is owned by a corporation, give the name and address of the corporation immediately followed by the names and addresses of all stockholders owning or holding 1 percent or more of the total amount of stock. If not owned by a corporation, give the names and addresses of the individual owners. If owned by a partnership or other unincorporated firm, give its name and address as well as those of each individual owner. If the publication is published by a nonprofit organization, give its name and address.)

Full Name	Complete Mailing Address
Wholly owned subsidiary of	1600 John F. Kennedy Blvd., Ste. 1800
Reed/Elsevier, US holdings	Philadelphia, PA 19103-2899

11. Known Bondholders, Mortgagees, and Other Security Holders Owning or Holding 1 Percent or More of Total Amount of Bonds, Mortgages, or Other Securities. If none, check box ☐ None

Full Name	Complete Mailing Address
N/A	

12. Tax Status (For completion by nonprofit organizations authorized to mail at nonprofit rates) (Check one)
The purpose, function, and nonprofit status of this organization and the exempt status for federal income tax purposes:
☐ Has Not Changed During Preceding 12 Months
☐ Has Changed During Preceding 12 Months (Publisher must submit explanation of change with this statement)

PS Form 3526, September 2007 (Page 1 of 3 (Instructions Page 3)) PSN 7530-01-000-9931 PRIVACY NOTICE: See our Privacy policy in www.usps.com

13. Publication Title	14. Issue Date for Circulation Data Below
Otolaryngologic Clinics of North America	August 2012

15. Extent and Nature of Circulation		Average No. Copies Each Issue During Preceding 12 Months	No. Copies of Single Issue Published Nearest to Filing Date
a. Total Number of Copies (Net press run)		1501	1239
b. Paid Circulation (By Mail and Outside the Mail)	(1) Mailed Outside-County Paid Subscriptions Stated on PS Form 3541. (Include paid distribution above nominal rate, advertiser's proof copies, and exchange copies)	642	583
	(2) Mailed In-County Paid Subscriptions Stated on PS Form 3541 (Include paid distribution above nominal rate, advertiser's proof copies, and exchange copies)		
	(3) Paid Distribution Outside the Mails Including Sales Through Dealers and Carriers, Street Vendors, Counter Sales, and Other Paid Distribution Outside USPS®	404	411
	(4) Paid Distribution by Other Classes Mailed Through the USPS (e.g. First-Class Mail®)		
c. Total Paid Distribution (Sum of 15b (1), (2), (3), and (4))	▶	1046	994
d. Free or Nominal Rate Distribution (By Mail and Outside the Mail)	(1) Free or Nominal Rate Outside-County Copies Included on PS Form 3541	110	87
	(2) Free or Nominal Rate In-County Copies Included on PS Form 3541		
	(3) Free or Nominal Rate Copies Mailed at Other Classes Through the USPS (e.g. First-Class Mail)		
	(4) Free or Nominal Rate Distribution Outside the Mail (Carriers or other means)		
e. Total Free or Nominal Rate Distribution (Sum of 15d (1), (2), (3) and (4))	▶	110	87
f. Total Distribution (Sum of 15c and 15e)	▶	1156	1081
g. Copies not Distributed (See instructions to publishers #4 (page #3))	▶	345	158
h. Total (Sum of 15f and g)	▶	1501	1239
i. Percent Paid (15c divided by 15f times 100)		90.48%	91.95%

16. Publication of Statement of Ownership
☐ If the publication is a general publication, publication of this statement is required. Will be printed in the December 2012 issue of this publication. ☐ Publication not required

17. Signature and Title of Editor, Publisher, Business Manager, or Owner

Stephen R. Bushing — Inventory/Distribution Coordinator

Date September 14, 2012

I certify that all information furnished on this form is true and complete. I understand that anyone who furnishes false or misleading information on this form or who omits material or information requested on the form may be subject to criminal sanctions (including fines and imprisonment) and/or civil sanctions (including civil penalties).

PS Form 3526, September 2007 (Page 2 of 3)

Moving?

Make sure your subscription moves with you!

To notify us of your new address, find your **Clinics Account Number** (located on your mailing label above your name), and contact customer service at:

Email: journalscustomerservice-usa@elsevier.com

800-654-2452 (subscribers in the U.S. & Canada)
314-447-8871 (subscribers outside of the U.S. & Canada)

Fax number: 314-447-8029

Elsevier Health Sciences Division
Subscription Customer Service
3251 Riverport Lane
Maryland Heights, MO 63043

*To ensure uninterrupted delivery of your subscription,
please notify us at least 4 weeks in advance of move.

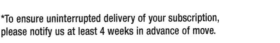

Printed and bound by CPI Group (UK) Ltd, Croydon, CR0 4YY

03/10/2024

01040440-0007